Modern Management of Cancer of the Rectum

Springer
London
Berlin
Heidelberg
New York
Barcelona
Hong Kong
Milan
Paris
Singapore
Tokyo

Riccardo A. Audisio, James G. Geraghty and
Walter E. Longo (Eds)

Modern Management of Cancer of the Rectum

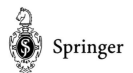 Springer

Riccardo A. Audisio, MD
University of Liverpool
Department of Surgery, Whiston Hospital, Prescot,
Merseyside L35 5DR, UK

James G. Geraghty, MD, PhD, MCh, FRCS (Irel)
Professorial Department of Surgery, Nottingham City Hospital,
Hucknall Road, Nottingham NG5 1PB, UK

Walter E. Longo, MD, FACS, FASCRS
Saint Louis University Health Sciences Center, Department of Surgery,
Section of Colon and Rectal Surgery, 3635 Vista @ Grand Blvd.,
PO Box 15250, Saint Louis, MO63110-0250, USA

British Library Cataloguing in Publication Data
Modern management of cancer of the rectum
  1. Rectum – Cancer – Treatment
  I. Audisio, Riccardo A. II. Geraghty, James G. III. Longo, Walter
  616.9'9435'06
  ISBN 1852332875

Library of Congress Cataloging-in-Publication Data
Modern management of cancer of the rectum/Ricardo Audisio, James Geraghty, and
Walter Longo (eds.).
    p.; cm.
  Includes bibliographical references and index.
  ISBN 1–85233–287–5 (alk. paper)
  1. Rectum – Cancer. I. Audisio, Riccardo A. II. Geraghty, J.G. (James G.), 1955–
III. Longo, Walter E.
  [DNLM: 1. Rectal Neoplasms – therapy. 2. Rectal Neoplasms – diagnosis. 3. Rectal
Neoplasms – surgery. WI 610 M689 2001]
  RC280.R37 M63 2001
  616.99'435 – dc21

                                                    00-053782

ISBN 1-85233-287-5 Springer-Verlag London Berlin Heidelberg
a member of BertelsmannSpringer Science+Business Media GmbH
http://www.springer.co.uk

Typeset by EXPO Holdings, Malaysia
Printed and bound at The Cromwell Press, Trowbridge, Wiltshire, UK
28/3830-543210 Printed on acid-free paper SPIN 10682016

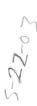

To Frank W. Longo, M.D.

a 31-year survivor of rectal cancer

Foreword

The management of rectal cancer has changed very considerably over the last twenty years. New imaging techniques have improved pre-operative assessment which have facilitated treatment planning that should lead to a reduction in local recurrence. Radiotherapy used in appropriate cases has been shown to reduce local treatment failure which is also potentially reducible by modern surgery based upon anatomical and pathological principles of locoregional spread.

Modern Management of Cancer of the Rectum covers the entire field of the disease from the history of its development to aetiology, pathology, imaging, treatment, quality of life and palliative care. Radiotherapy is considered in two excellent chapters devoted to pre and post-operative treatment respectively. There are separate chapters on aspects of surgical technique dealing with restorative and non-restorative major procedures, laparoscopic resection and minimal access surgery. The role of chemotherapy is described with a clear review of the present position. The important question of follow up is considered in detail and there are chapters on the management of treatment failure both local and distant.

Each chapter is written by acknowledged experts of world standing reputation. The referencing is excellent supplying a bibliography including classical publications leading on to an invaluable list of modern citations. The book is well laid out with excellent tables and illustrations. As a statement of the present position regarding all aspects of rectal cancer, this is an excellent book which will be an invaluable source of information, opinion and references to all practitioners involved in management of the disease. It shows the importance of multidisciplinary care from screening to treatment of the primary disease and the management of failure.

R.J. Nicholls
MA, MB, M.Chair, FRCS(Eng), FRCS(Glasg)
Consultant Surgeon, St Mark's Hospital, London
Professor of Colorectal Surgery, Imperial College of Science,
Technology and Medicine, London

Contents

List of Contributors

R.A. Audisio
University of Liverpool
Department of General Surgery
Whiston Hospital
Prescot
Merseyside L35 5DR
UK

R.W. Beart Jr
USC Dept of Surgery
1510 San Pablo St 514
Los Angeles
CA 90033-4612
USA

K.F. Birbeck
Institute of Pathology
Leeds General Infirmary
Great George Street
Leeds LS1 3EX
UK

A. Cairns
Institute of Pathology
Leeds General Infirmary
Great George Street
Leeds LS1 3EX
UK

H.J. Cho
Division of Colorectal Surgery
Department of Surgery
The Mount Sinai Medical Center
Box 1259
5 East 98th Street, 11th Floor
New York
NY 10029-6574
USA

D. Cunningham
The Royal Marsden NHS Trust
Downs Road
Sutton
Surrey SM2 5PT
UK

W.E. Enker
Beth Israel Medical Center
Division of Colorectal Surgery
Department of Surgery
350 East 17th Street, 16th Floor
New York
NY 10003
USA

F. Fazio
Department of Nuclear Mecicine
IRCCS S Raffaele
University Hospital
Milan
Italy

V.W. Fazio
Department of Colorectal Surgery
The Cleveland Clinic Foundation
9500 Euclid Avenue
Desk A-111
Ohio
OH 44195
USA

C. Ferrero
Department of Radiology
Multimedica-Hospital
300 via Milanese
20099 SSG Milan
Italy

A. Filiberti
Department of Pathological Behaviour
Omegna City Hospital
Omegna
Italy

J.G. Geraghty
Professorial Department of Surgery
Nottingham City Hospital
Hucknall Road
Nottingham NG5 1PB
UK

L. Gianolli
Department of Nuclear Mecicine
IRCCS S Raffaele
University Hospital
Milan
Italy

S.M. Goldberg
Division of Colon and Rectal Surgery
University of Minnesota
Minneapolis
MN 55455
USA

C. Greco
Department of Radiative Oncology
European Institute of Oncology
435 Via Ripamonti
20141 Milan
Italy

E.M. Grossmann
Saint Louis University Health Sciences
    Center
Department of Surgery
Section of Colon and Rectal Surgery
3635 Vista @ Grand Blvd
PO Box 15250
Saint Louis
MO 63110-0250
USA

J.G. Guillem
Memorial Sloan-Kettering Cancer Center
1275 York Avenue
Room C986
New York
NY10021
USA

F.E. Johnson
Saint Louis University Health Sciences
    Center
Department of Surgery
3635 Vista @ Grand Blvd
PO Box 15250
Saint Louis
MO 63110-0250
USA

N.J. Kafka
Beth Israel Medical Center
Division of Colorectal Surgery
Department of Surgery
350 East 17th Street, 16th Floor
New York
NY 10003
USA

C.H. Köhne
Universität Rostock
Ernst-Heydemann-Str. 6
18055 Rostock
Germany

C. Landoni
Department of Nuclear Mecicine
IRCCS S Raffaele
University Hospital
Milan
Italy

W.E. Longo
Saint Louis University Health Sciences
    Center
Department of Surgery
Section of Colon and Rectal Surgery
3635 Vista @ Grand Blvd
PO Box 15250
Saint Louis
MO 63110-0250
USA

F. López-Kostner
Department of Digestive Surgery
Catholic University School of Medicine
Marcoleta 367
Santiago
Chile

A. Del Maschio
Department of Radiology
IRCCS S Raffaele
University Hospital
Milan
Italy

J.W. Milsom
Division of Colorectal Surgery
Department of Surgery
The Mount Sinai Medical Center
Box 1259
5 East 98th Street
11th Floor
New York
NY 10029-6574
USA

B.D. Minsky
Department of Radiation Oncology
Memorial Sloan-Kettering Cancer Center
1275 York Avenue
New York
NY 10021
USA

D.E. Nadig
Saint Louis University Health Sciences
    Center
Department of Surgery
3635 Vista @ Grand Blvd
PO Box 15250
Saint Louis
MO 63110-0250

H. Nelson
Division of Colon and Rectal Surgery
Mayo Clinic
200 First Street SW
Rochester
MN 55905
USA

R.J. Nicholls
St. Marks' Hospital
Northwick Park
Watford Road
Harrow HA1 3UJ
UK

P. Quirke
Department of Histopathology
Algernon Firth Building
University of Leeds
Leeds LS2 9JT
UK

C.A. Paterson
Division of Colon and Rectal Surgery
Mayo Clinic and Mayo Foundation
200 First St SW
Rochester
MN 55905
USA

J. Puig-La Calle Jr
Department of Surgery
Memorial Sloan–Kettering Cancer Center
New York
NY 10021
USA

P.L. Roberts
Department of Colon and Rectal Surgery
Lahey Clinic Medical Center
Burlington
MA 01805
USA

D. Rosenfeld
USC Dept of Surgery
1510 San Pablo St 514
Los Angeles
CA 90033-4612
USA

A. Sbanotto
Medical Oncology Division
European Institute of Oncology
435 via Ripamonti
20144 Milan
Italy

D.J. Schoetz Jr
Department of Colon and Rectal Surgery
Lahey Clinic Medical Center
Burlington
MA 01805
USA

A.A. Shelton
Division of Colon and Rectal Surgery
University of Minnesota
Minneapolis
Minnesota
MN 55455
USA

S. Sironi
Department of Radiology
Multimedica-Hospital
300 via Milanese
20099 SSG
Milan
Italy

K.A. Sumpter
The Royal Marsden NHS Trust
Downs Road
Sutton
Surrey SM2 5PT
UK

K.S. Virgo
Saint Louis University Health Sciences
    Center
Department of Surgery
3635 Vista @ Grand Blvd
PO Box 15250
Saint Louis
MO 63110-0250
USA

A. Zbar
FRACS Kaplan Medical Center
Rehovot 76100
Israel

Introduction

The management of rectal cancer has changed dramatically since decompressive procedures of the colon were initially performed. Although excisional procedures date back to the 1800s, when various transanal and subsequently abdominal procedures were carried out, it was not until 1908 that Ernest Miles presented his results of abdominoperineal resection, establishing a therapeutic standard on the base of his personal investigations. His practical suggestions were rapidly popularized and little changed until the 1960s, when the understanding of the psychological burden of satisfactory sphincteric continence was appreciated, adding important details involving quality of life issues to clinical outcomes. Several years have passed since restorative procedures were introduced in maintaining bowel continuity and anal function. In the meanwhile, new technical tools have become part of the surgeon's armamentarium; stapling guns and new suture devices have allowed the performance of lower anastomoses while still respecting oncological criteria.

Surgical oncology has been expanding rapidly, at the same time achieving a proper role in the treatment of rectal cancer while maintaining the dignity of the patient. The rapid and dramatic evolution of our knowledge of cancer development, prevention, growth, diffusion, host interaction, patterns of recurrence and many other issues have directed the surgeons who care for patients with rectal cancer to interact proactively with medical oncologists, pathologists and radiation therapists. New personnel have been entering into the daily scenario: basic scientists and geneticists, epidemiologists and economists, oncology nurses and therapists with oncological expertise.

It is under this light that we felt the need to collect and review critically the many recent advancements in the management of rectal cancer. This includes the areas of clinical and pathological staging, screening and chemoprevention, diagnostic imaging, preoperative neoadjuvant therapy, surgery, postoperative adjuvant therapy, follow-up and the management of surgical strategies, including both restorative and non-restorative abdomino-pelvic procedures employing total mesorectal excision, laparoscopic surgery and minimal access local surgery. The purpose of this book is not to provide guidelines or gold standards that may become obsolete as a consequence of the continuing evolution of knowledge. We have attempted to discuss and interpret results and experiences, so that the scientific evidence is put together logically for the clinician who is caring for rectal cancer patients. We hope that this textbook will allow the general practitioner and the surgical trainee to appreciate the complexity of the newly available data, while the surgical specialist will enjoy a broad approach to this increasingly prevalent disease.

Riccardo A. Audisio, M.D.
James G. Geraghty, M.D., Ph.D., M.Ch., F.R.C.S. (Ireland)
Walter E. Longo, M.D., F.A.C.S., F.A.S.C.R.S.

1. Evolution of the Surgical Management of Rectal Cancer

A.A. Shelton and S.M. Goldberg

A bubo is a tumour developing within the anus in the rectum – of great hardness but little aching. I will first say that the ulceration of it is nothing other than a concealed canker, that may not in the beginning be recognized by inspection, for it is completely hidden within the anus, and it is therefore called bubo for just as bubo, i.e. an owl, is a beast dwelling in hiding places, so this sickness lurks within the anus in the beginning, but after the passage of time it ulcerates and emerges eroding the anus. And often it erodes and consumes the whole circumference of it, so that faeculent excrements pass out continually until death, so that it may never be cured with human treatment, unless it pleases God to help, who made man out of nothing with his ineffable power. It is recognized as follows: the doctor should put his finger into the anus of this patient and if he finds within the anus something as hard as a stone, sometimes just on one side, sometimes on both, so that it hinders the patient from passing excrement, then this is certainly a bubo. The signs of its ulceration are these: the patient cannot keep himself from the privy because of the aching and sharp pains, and this occurs twice or thrice in an hour, and pus exudes out of it as if it were mixed with stinking and water blood ... be careful not to manage these cases except by the administration of enemas, as is said before which considerably alleviates these above mentioned patients as I have experienced, and always give warning to them or to their friends of death as well as of incurability. Such a warning to them or to their friends will do honour to the profession of the doctor, avarice will be shunned in this way and you should abstain from false promises.

John of Arderne c. 1376

Introduction

Although John of Arderne recognized rectal cancer, its signs and symptoms, and natural history, no form of excisional surgery was performed for nearly

another 400 years. The surgical treatment of rectal cancer has evolved significantly over the last 250 years, paralleling the evolution of the art and science of surgery in general. The first procedures were local excisions and were nearly always palliative in nature. Improvements in anesthesia and antisepsis allowed the development of radical extirpative procedures done with curative intent. The present time again finds local therapy as an integral technique in the armamentarium of the surgeon treating patients with rectal cancer.

Perineal Approach

Although Morgagni reportedly proposed the removal of the rectum for carcinoma in the early eighteenth century, and Faget attempted a posterior proctectomy in 1739, Jacques Lisfancz was probably the first surgeon to excise the rectum successfully in 1826 [1,2]. The earliest operations were essentially an amputation of the anus and lower rectum, resulting in an incontinent perineal anus.

In 1880 William Harrison Cripps of St Bartholomew's Hospital described patients deemed suitable for operation:

To sum up briefly the general outline of cases suitable for operation, I should say that the disease must be within four inches of the anus, and in women must not have extended on the anterior wall further than three inches, and the rectum must be fairly movable on the neighboring parts, and there must be no sign of hepatic infection. Each case will, however, have to be decided upon its own merits, after due consideration has been given to the surrounding circumstances [3].

The operation described is as follows:

The patient, being prepared for the operation by a purgative and warm-water enema, is placed fully

1

under the influence of an anaesthetic and arranged in the lithotomy position … The left forefinger being passed into the rectum feels for the tip of the coccyx, the curved bistoury [knife], held in the right hand, is passed into the bowel, the point being guarded by the finger nail, the handle of the knife is then raised, and, with a little jerk, the point is made to protrude through the skin on a level with the tip of the coccyx and exactly in the mid-line. The whole of the intervening tissue between this point and the margin of the anus is cut through … The left hand of the operator is now placed on the right side of the buttock, so as to draw the anus outwards and stretch the tissues at the line of junction of the mucous membrane with the skin. The portion of the rectum or anus through which the lateral incision is to be made must depend upon the distance from the anus of the lower margin of the disease, and if possible, should be at least half an inch from the growth. The point being selected, the knife is made to cut deeply by using firm pressure, a crescentic incision extending from the margin of the first cut round the anus to a point in the middle of the anterior margin … The forefinger thrust into this incision will readily separate the bowel from the surrounding tissue, except at the insertion of the levator ani, which should be divided with scissors … the opposite side is treated in a similar manner … the lateral and posterior portion of the bowel being freed from their attachments, the next, and most delicate step in the operation is the separation of the bowel from its anterior connections … when the dissection has been carried to a sufficient distance beyond the disease … the bowel is slowly cut through and removed [3].

After establishing hemostasis, the operation was essentially over, and all that remained was perioperative care:

I employ no dressings of any kind, nor do I put any plug or lint into the wound. Any attempt to draw down the cut end of the bowel and stitch it to the anal margin is perfectly useless; the stitches are sure to give way, and before they do so prevent a free discharge from the wound … the patient when put to bed, should lie on his back, his head and shoulders well raised, while the knees are bent and supported by pillows underneath … in this position there is free drainage from the wound … the patient should be left quiet till the morning following the operation, when the wound should be gently, but very thoroughly syringed … the patient usually convalesces rapidly, and can leave his bed in two or three weeks [3].

Cripps then goes on to describe the condition of the rectum after complete healing:

The cut ends of the bowel quickly form attachments to the sides of the cavity that remain as the result of the operation, and seem during the process of cicatrization to be drawn considerably downwards … the lining of the canal for the remainder of the distance is

composed of a tissue similar to the ordinary scar tissue found on cutaneous surfaces, but of a softer consistency … this tissue has sometimes a great tendency to contract thus narrowing considerably the outlet [3].

Nearly 100 years after the operation had initially been described, John Percy Lockhart-Mummery, of St Mark's Hospital, reported his revision of the operation. The operation was done in two stages. A permanent colostomy was done either 1 week prior to resection or at the time of proctectomy. The patient was placed in a prone position and a perineal proctectomy was performed, removing the entire rectum and the lower portion of the sigmoid colon. The proximal portion of the sigmoid colon was closed and left in place as a blind spur. Lockhart-Mummery reported on 200 patients operated on in this manner, with a mortality of 8.5% [4].

Transanal Excision

Richard Von Volkmann, somewhat less well known than his student Kraske, also reported on perineal excision of rectal cancer. However, he also noted certain tumors that were amenable to transanal excision. He described three different approaches that may be utilized, depending on the location and the extent of the tumor. One of these was:

A well-circumscribed tumor, the removal of which requires excision of a small portion of the rectum and permits the wound in the rectum to be closed primarily by suture … care must be taken to create a wound in such a manner that the anastomosis itself is located in a transverse direction, so that the entrance to the rectum should not be narrowed [5].

Transsacral Resection

In 1876 Theodore Kocher resected the rectum and performed a primary anastomosis after removal of the coccyx and a portion of the sacrum. This technique has become associated with Paul Kraske, who introduced the technique in Germany in 1885. Kraske recognized that certain cancers of the rectum were situated too low down for removal at laparotomy when using the available techniques and too high for removal from the perineal approach. The death of two patients with high rectal cancers after attempted transperineal excision led Kraske to revisit the technique of sacral resection previously reported by Kocher. Kraske first experimented on cadavers. He found that, by detaching the gluteal muscles, dividing the sacrospinous and sacrotuberous ligaments, and resecting the coccyx and a portion of the left wing of the sacrum, the proximal rectum could be mobilized quite easily. In 1886 Kraske reported two patients operated on using this method. Both survived the operation and, at follow-up at 3 months, had good sphincter control. However, both patients did have small draining perineal fistulas. Neither had any disturbance related to the resection of the sacral ligaments or sacral bone [6].

Abdominosacral Resection

With the sacral approach alone, it was often difficult to anastomose the colon to the anorectal stump. In 1912, William Mayo described a two-stage abdominosacral resection, in which the colon was pulled through a rectal stump from which the mucosa had been removed [7]. Charles Pannett, of London, reported using the abdominosacral resection and creation of an end-to-end anastomosis [8]. In more recent years, Arthur Localio has popularized this approach, avoiding the need to reposition the patient by placing the patient in the right lateral position with the hips flexed [9].

Abdominoperineal Resection

The abdominoperineal resection is associated with the name of Sir Ernest Miles, who discussed the operation in 1908 [10]. However, the first reported combined operation using both an abdominal and a perineal approach was performed by Vincenz Czerny in Germany in 1884 [1]. Charles Mayo reported his technique of abdominoperineal resection in 1904 and then again in 1906, emphasizing the importance of resecting the lymphatics as high up as the sacral promontory [11,12].

However, it was Sir Ernest Miles who provided the most convincing evidence for the use of the abdominoperineal approach. Prior to 1906 Miles had relied solely on the perineal methods of excision of the rectum, but was dissatisfied with the results and noted that "recurrence of the disease was a rule to which there were few exceptions". He found that recurrences in the field of operation were relatively uncommon, but that post-mortem examinations showed recurrence in the pelvic peritoneum, the pelvic mesocolon, and the lymph nodes situated over the bifurcation of the left common iliac artery. Miles considered that these structures represented the "zone of upward spread" of rectal cancer, and that their removal was essential to the prevention of recurrence. Miles noted in his 1908 paper:

The study of the spread of cancer from the rectum has led me to formulate certain essentials in the technique of the operation which must be strictly adhered to if satisfactory results are to be obtained – namely: 1) that an abdominal anus is a necessity; 2) that the whole of the pelvic colon, with the exception of the part from which the colostomy is made, must be removed because its blood supply is contained in the zone of upward spread; 3) that the whole of the pelvic mesocolon below the point where it crosses the common iliac artery, together with a strip of peritoneum at least an inch wide on either side of it, must be cleared away; 4) that the group of lymph nodes situated over the bifurcation of the common iliac artery are in all instances to be removed; and lastly 5) that the perineal portion of the operation should be carried out as widely as possible so that the lateral and downward zones of spread may be effectively extirpated [10].

If there was obstruction by the tumor, Miles would create a colostomy at least 2 weeks before the resection. If not placed previously, the operation would begin by the creation of a loop colostomy with division of the bowel 2 inches below it. Miles thought that and end colostomy was more prone to prolapse. The inferior mesenteric artery was then divided and the bowel mobilized until it could be pushed into the pelvis and the peritoneum covered over it. The patient was then place in the right lateral position and the operation completed from the perineal approach [10].

In 1908 Miles presented his first 12 patients operated on using this approach. There were five deaths for an operative mortality of 42%. It was only after the better 5-year survival statistics were known that the procedure became widely accepted [13].

Throughout the years many modifications were made to the Miles abdominoperineal resection. In 1915 Daniel Fiske Jones proposed a two-stage operation, performing the perineal phase 5–7 days after the abdominal phase. Jones considered that this would decrease sepsis and he reported an 18% mortality in 16 patients [14]. The need for repositioning the patient was eliminated in 1937 when Sir Hugh Devine introduced adjustable leg rests so that the operation could be performed in the lithotomy position. In 1938 Lloyd-Davies introduced the synchronous combined abdominoperineal procedure, with one surgeon performing the abdominal operation and another surgeon the perineal operation [15,16].

Abdominoanal Approach

H. Widenham Maunsell of New Zealand described in 1892 a method for anastomosing the sigmoid colon to the anus. The anal sphincters were divided in the posterior mid-line. After abdominal mobilization of the colon and rectum, the rectosigmoid was invaginated out of the enlarged anus, the tumor was resected, and the two ends of the bowel anastomosed [17].

Robert Weir of Columbia University modified this technique in 1901. Weir was dissatisfied with Kraske's approach for high-lying tumors of the rectum. He noted:

> I ventured to practice such an extirpation after the plan of Maunsell … but it did not work with me in my trial of it, the hitch being that the tumor would not pass through the divided anus … I therefore changed the plan of the procedure in this way: My fingers had freely detached the divided peritoneum so that the bowel and the entire contents of the sacral curve were liberated behind nearly to the tip of the coccyx and in front to the edge of the prostate; this gave me room to tie around the bowel some three inches from the anus, a couple of iodoform tapes, about an inch apart. The intestine was here cut through and, being free was readily raised out of the abdominal wound and held aside by an assistant. The lower end of the rectum was then seized by the forceps in the hands of another assistant, who drew it down and out of the anus in an inverted condition. Untying the tape that closed the everted bowel, its lumen was opened so that a longer forceps could be carried through it into the pelvis when the end of the upper bowel was brought down within its clasp and by it the latter was drawn through the lower bowel out into the world. A couple of needles passed through the invaginated ends of the bowel – near their margins – allowed easy union by sutures of their edges and replacement of the same followed [18].

Weir initially reported on three patients operated on in this manner. Two survived and were alive at 18 months and 9 months without evidence of recurrence. One patient died "not from peritonitis, but from persistent diarrhea without temperature elevation". The two surviving patients both developed stenosis of the anastomosis requiring periodic dilatation [18].

In 1961 Turnbull and Cuthbertson, at the Cleveland Clinic, described a two-stage abdomino-anal pullthrough procedure [19]. Turnbull had been using this technique since 1952 for both mid-rectal cancers and Hischprung's disease. After resection of the rectum, the colon was pulled through the everted rectal stump. The rectum was then sutured to the seromuscular layer of the colon with 2 inches of colon left protruding and wrapped in gauze. In the second stage, 10 days later, the bowel was excised just above the dentate line and an end to end anastomosis performed. This two-stage procedure was

thought to decrease the incidence of anastomotic leaks and pelvic sepsis.

In 1972 Sir Alan Parks introduced a technique of transanal anastomosis. From an abdominal approach the rectum was clamped distal to the tumor and traction applied. The rectum was divided at the level of the pelvic floor. An anal mucosectomy was then carried out, starting at the dentate line. A self-retaining anoscope was then used to anastomose the colon to the dentate line after it had been drawn through the muscular cuff. This technique avoids possible neuromuscular injury from eversion of the anal canal.

Anterior Resection

In 1833 Rebard, a French surgeon, reported a resection of a portion of the sigmoid colon followed by an end to end anastomosis. For this he was severely criticized by his colleagues [1]. William J. Mayo was reported to be the first surgeon to perform an anterior resection in the USA early in the twentieth century. His technique involved a two-layer anastomosis performed over a rectal tube, which was left in place for approximately 6 days [2].

In 1921 Henri Hartmann described an operation for high rectal lesions, an anterior resection without end anastomosis. After resection of the involved segment and its mesentery, the rectum was inverted and left in place. This procedure was associated with less blood loss and mortality than the abdominoperineal resection [2].

In 1948 Claude Dixon, of the Mayo Clinic, reported on his experience with anterior resection performed without a rectal tube. The operation was carried out routinely with a covering colostomy, either as a three-stage procedure, when the colostomy was created before resection, or as a two-stage procedure, when the colostomy was created at the time of resection. A hand-sewn anastomosis, using one row of sutures posteriorly and two rows anteriorly, was performed after resection with at least a 3–4 cm distal margin. Dixon reported his results on 523 patient in 1948. Anastomotic leaks occurred in 12 patients (2.3%) but Dixon noted that "with the proximal temporary colonic stoma, there is little febrile reaction and there is merely a delay of an extra week or two for the fistula to close before proceeding with closure of the stoma". Mortality fell from 8.5% during the period 1930–1935 to 2.6% for 1941–1947, after the introduction of sulfa antibiotics. Five-year survival for all patients was 67.7% [20].

In 1975 Fain described his experience with a Soviet-designed circular stapling apparatus employing metallic staples for low colorectal anastomosis [21]. Time-consuming cleaning and reloading of the Soviet stapling machine led to the development of the American end to end anastomosis stapling instrument, together with its preloaded, presterilized and disposable staple cartridges. This instrument became available in 1978 and has had a dramatic impact on the management of rectal cancer. It has reduced the need for the use of a permanent colostomy.

The Present

… always give warning to them or to their friends of death as well as of incurability. Such a warning to them or to their friends will do honour to the profession of the doctor, avarice will be shunned in this way and you should abstain from false promises.

John of Arderne c. 1376

Thankfully, much has been learned about the biology, natural history and optimal treatment of rectal cancer in the nearly 700 years since John of Arderne made this statement regarding cancer of the rectum. Physicians managing this condition have a number of perioperative and operative techniques at their disposal for the better treatment of these patients.

Improvements in anesthetic technique, perioperative care and the availability of antibiotics have had a significant impact on operative morbidity and mortality. Major refinements have been made in operative technique, but many of the operations currently used in the management of rectal cancer are very similar to those utilized by the surgeons who originally described them. The use of preoperative endorectal ultrasound and computed tomographic scanning now allows therapy to be individualized to the patient. Transanal excision is frequently used today for the treatment of early rectal cancer. Radical abdominal surgery remains the mainstay of treatment for advanced disease. The importance of "negative margins", especially a negative radial margin, is being increasingly recognized. Heald and others have emphasized the importance of complete excision of the mesorectum in surgical management. He has reported an enviable 4% local recurrence rate by using this technique. The use of the circular stapler allows many patients with cancer of the distal rectum to retain intestinal continuity and avoid a permanent colostomy. Adjuvant chemotherapy and radiation therapy play an integral role in the modern management of advanced rectal cancer.

References

1. Rankin FW. How surgery of the colon and rectum developed. Surg Gynecol Obstet 1937;64:705–10.
2. Breen RE, Garnjobst W. Surgical procedures for carcinoma of the rectum: a historical review. Dis Colon Rectum 1983;26:680–5.
3. Cripps WH. Cancer of the rectum: its pathology, diagnosis and treatment. London: J and A Churchill, 1880:133–64.
4. Lochart-Mummery JP. Two hundred cases of cancer of the rectum treated by perineal excision. Br J Surg 1926;14:110–24.
5. Von Volkmann R. Concerning rectal cancer and the removal of the rectum. Chirurgie 29–53:1113–27.
6. Kraske P. Zur extirpatio hochsitzender mastdarmkrebse. Arch Klin Chir (Berlin) 1886;33:563–73.
7. Mayo WJ. The radical operation for the relief of cancer of the rectum and rectosigmoid. Ann Surg 1912;56:240–55.
8. Pannett CA. Resection of the rectum with restoration of continuity. Lancet 1935;ii:423–5.
9. Localio SA, Stahl WM. Simultaneous abdominotranssacral resection and anastomosis for midrectal cancer. Am J Surg 1969;117:282–9.
10. Miles WE. A method of performing abdominoperineal excision for carcinoma of the rectum and the terminal portion of the pelvic colon. Lancet 1908;ii:1812–3.
11. Mayo CH. Cancer of the large bowel. Med Sentinel 1904;12:466–73.
12. Mayo CH. Cancer of the sigmoid and rectum. Surg Gynecol Obstet 1906;3:236–41.
13. Miles WE. Technique of the radical operation for cancer of the rectum. Br J Surg 1914;2:292–305.
14. Jones DF. A two-staged combined abdominoperineal operation for carcinoma of the rectum. JAMA 1915;65:757–64.
15. Devine H. Excison of the rectum. Br J Surg 1937;25:351–81.
16. Lloyd-Davies OV. Lithotomy-Trendelenberg position for resection of the rectum and the lower pelvic colon. Lancet 1939;ii:74–6.
17. Maunsell HW. A new method of excising the two upper portions of the upper rectum and lower segment of the sigmoid flexure of the colon. Lancet 1892;ii:473–6.
18. Weir RF. An improved method of treating high seated cancers of the rectum. JAMA 1901;37:801–3.
19. Turnbull RB, Cuthbertson A. Abdominorectal pull-through resection for cancer and for Hirschprung's disease. Cleveland Clin Q 1961;28:109–15.
20. Dixon CF. Anterior resection for malignant lesions of the upper part of the rectum and lower part of the sigmoid. Ann Surg 1948;128:425–42.
21. Fain SN, Patin CS, Marganstern L. Arch Surg 1975.

2. Pathology and Staging

K.F. Birbeck, A. Cairns and P. Quirke

Introduction

According to latest figures there are approximately 8500 new diagnoses of rectal cancer in England and Wales each year (Office for National Statistics, 1999, personal communication) and about 4000 deaths from the disease [1]. This compares to predictions made for the USA, which estimated that a total of about 36 000 new diagnoses of rectal cancer would be made during 1998, with approximately 8800 deaths from the disease [2]. At diagnosis one-fifth of these patients already have distant metastases, which automatically confers on them a much poorer prognosis. Nowadays we make this comment almost casually, but it should be borne in mind that, while generally being a good indicator of prognosis, disease stage is not an infallible predictor. Indeed, after stage has been taken into account, survival can be very variable between surgeons and institutions, with some patients who would be expected to do well succumbing to the disease at a relatively early stage and vice-versa.

One of the major factors influencing survival in rectal cancer is local recurrence. Increased local recurrence results in lower survival. Hence it is vital that in our management of rectal cancer we constantly strive to find ways of reducing local recurrence rates. The pathologist and the surgeon form a vital partnership in this respect, particularly in the light of the many recent changes in the management of rectal cancer. Later in this chapter we will discuss how the surgeon and pathologist can work together to reduce local recurrence rates and improve outcomes.

Resection Specimen

A resection undertaken for the treatment of rectal cancer may range from being a straightforward local excision through to a complete rectal resection with total mesorectal excision and possibly resection of other attached organs. Here we intend to limit our discussion to major resection specimens only. The histological features that we discuss later obviously relate for the most part as much to locally resected tumours as those contained within larger specimens.

Total Mesorectal Excision

Traditionally in many institutions, standard rectal cancer surgery has consisted of removal of the rectum by techniques involving a combination of blunt digital dissection and traction. This method has great potential for leaving substantial amounts of mesorectal tissue behind in the pelvis and has often been responsible for the production of resection specimens in which large areas of muscularis propria have been left bare and exposed at the outer surface. In such cases there is a significant risk of leaving mesorectal tumour deposits behind (discontinuous islands of tumour or lymph nodes containing metastases can be present in the mesorectum away from the macroscopic primary tumour) or creating a circumferential resection margin (CRM) that is involved by tumour. This problem has been resolved by Heald and colleagues who described the technique of total mesorectal excision (TME) in 1982 [3].

The mesorectum, which is derived from the dorsal mesentery from which the primitive gut tube is suspended, is the integral visceral mesentery that surrounds the rectum. A layer of visceral fascia encloses both the rectum and mesorectum within a package that thus forms a separate compartment within the pelvis. With TME the surgeon is aiming

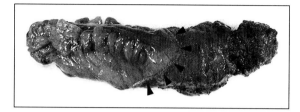

Fig. 2.1. An abdominoperineal resection specimen viewed from the anterior aspect. Towards the distal end of the specimen (to the right side of the picture) the specimen has acquired a narrow "waist" where there is reduced perirectal tissue. This is the point at which the levator muscles insert into the rectal wall and where such tapering inwards of the mesorectal tissues is unavoidable. Proximal to this, however, and below the peritoneal re ection (arrowed), this is a good total mesorectal excision.

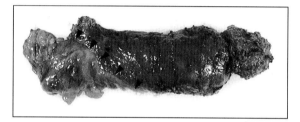

Fig. 2.2. The posterior aspect of the specimen seen in Fig. 1. The arrowheads indicate the site of the peritoneal reflection which, on this view, is seen running obliquely upwards and around the back of the specimen. Note the smooth surface of the mesorectum with its glistening, intact covering of mesorectal fascia.

to define and completely remove this entire rectal/mesorectal package, using sharp retroperitoneal dissection to separate the apposed visceral and parietal fascial layers. Ideally such a resection specimen should have a regular and smooth mesorectal surface with an intact mesorectal fascia. A good TME showing these features is an indicator of good quality surgery, which in turn has an influence on local recurrence rates (Figs 2.1 and 2.2).

The anterior peritoneal reflection represents the point at which the rectum exits the peritoneal cavity and becomes entirely retroperitoneal. Below this level there is a mesorectal, or circumferential, resection margin all around the rectum. Above it the CRM is in fact only partially present, at the back of the upper rectum (Figs 2.1 and 2.2). Tumours may lie above or below, or straddle the reflection. This relationship is important because tumours below it have a higher rate of local recurrence. Generally speaking, as tumour distance from the anus increases, local recurrence rate decreases [4].

As more data emerge, the advantages of total mesorectal excision are now becoming evident, and with more and more surgeons adopting the technique, particularly in Europe, it is gradually gaining acceptance as the new standard in rectal cancer surgery.

Histological Features of Rectal Cancer and Their Prognostic Significance

There have been many pathological factors reported to be of prognostic significance in colorectal cancer. Most prognostic factors are not independent or are subject to a degree of interobserver variation, making direct comparison of different cases meaningless. The most important prognostic factors remain those recognized in Cuthbert Dukes' original staging system: the extent of local spread and lymph node involvement, together with completeness of excision.

Histological Type

The vast majority (over 90%) of colorectal cancers are adenocarcinomas, characterized histologically by the presence of well-formed glandular structures. They are composed of a variety of cell types including columnar and goblet cells, with occasional endocrine cells and paneth cells. Mucinous and signet ring carcinoma are both variants of adenocarcinoma and account for some 10% of all colorectal cancers. Mucinous carcinomas, by definition, contain large lakes of extracellular mucin, which make up at least 50% of the tumour [5]. They occur most commonly in the rectum, present at a more advanced stage than ordinary adenocarcinomas [6], and are more frequently associated with adenomas elsewhere in the large bowel [7]. Signet ring carcinoma grows diffusely through the bowel wall and tends to occur in younger individuals. In contrast to mucinous carcinoma, the mucin is mostly intracellular, displacing the nucleus and giving the cell the characteristic signet ring appearance. Signet ring carcinomas spread via peritoneal dissemination and common sites of metastases include lymph nodes and the ovary, rather than the liver. The possibility of a metastasis from a gastric primary must always be considered before making a diagnosis of primary signet ring carcinoma of the colon or rectum.

The subdivision of rectal cancers into ordinary adenocarcinomas, mucinous carcinomas and signet ring carcinomas appears to confer no independent predictive value [8].

Other types of tumour do occur in the rectum but they are rare. Squamous differentiation can occur in colorectal tumours, most notably caecal tumours, but this is usually associated with a glandular component (adenosquamous carcinoma) [9]. Pure squamous carcinomas are rare and have been described in association with long-standing idiopathic inflammatory bowel disease [10]. The possibility of upward extension from an anal primary must always be considered when presented with a squamous carcinoma located in the low rectum.

Small cell carcinoma is similar to its pulmonary counterpart, both in its histological appearance and its behaviour. It is usually seen in the right side of the colon.

Carcinoid tumours of the rectum can occur, usually as non-ulcerating plaques or polyps, and are infrequently associated with the carcinoid syndrome [11,12]. They tend to be small (less than 1 cm in diameter) and are usually located on the anterior or lateral wall of the rectum. Several cases of primary malignant melanoma of the rectum have been reported [13,14].

Tumour Differentiation

The most important parameter in grading colorectal cancers is tubular configuration [15]. An absence of tubules defines a tumour as poorly differentiated. There are, however, problems in grading, including a degree of interobserver variation and the presence of varying differentiation within the same tumour. The predominant grade is thought to be the most important [16]. Small foci of poor differentiation in an otherwise well-differentiated tumour are not considered to be significant.

It is important to recognize poorly differentiated tumours because of their worse prognosis. Tumours should be graded as either poorly differentiated or other (well- or moderately differentiated).

Invasive Growth Pattern and Peritumoral Lymphocytic Infiltration

The quality of the advancing tumour margin and the lymphocytic infiltrate associated with it have been shown to be powerful prognostic indicators in rectal cancer [17]. The majority of rectal cancers show a well- or moderately well-circumscribed (so-called "expanding") margin. Demonstration of an infiltrative margin, however, is frequently associated with perineural and lymphatic invasion and confers a significantly worse prognosis [15]. An infiltrative margin also predicts an increased risk of local recurrence [18].

Tumours with a well-formed peritumoral lymphocytic infiltrate are associated with a 5-year survival of >90% [19].

Completeness of Excision

Completeness of excision depends upon two factors: the extent of tumour spread beyond the confines of the wall of the rectum and the technique of the surgeon (as discussed later). The surgeon is, in fact, one of the most important variables in the prediction of local recurrence [20].

Serosal Involvement

Serosal involvement (defined as the presence of tumoral ulceration of the serosa or tumour cells on the peritoneal surface) is an independent prognostic factor in rectal cancer, conferring a poorer prognosis if present [21,22]. Serosal involvement is applicable only to tumours that originate or extend above the peritoneal reflection. They should not be confused with circumferential margin involvement.

Lymph Node Metastases

Lymph node involvement is an important prognostic variable and there is a strong correlation between the number of lymph node metastases and survival [15]. The presence of tumour within the apical lymph node (the lymph node closest to the main vascular tie) indicates an increased likelihood of residual tumour and is associated with a poor prognosis.

The role of special techniques in the detection of lymph node metastases remains controversial and they are not used routinely by most laboratories. Fat clearance has been recommended by a small number of authors [23] but is seen by others as time-consuming, expensive and of little benefit [24]. Likewise, the benefits of detecting micrometastases using immunohistochemical or molecular techniques remain uncertain, with some evidence that immunohistochemically detected micrometastases have no bearing on prognosis [25].

Extramural Vascular Invasion

Extramural venous invasion (tumour within vessels located outside the muscular wall of the rectum, within the fat) has been reported by some to be an adverse predictive factor [26], although in multivariate analysis it has been suggested to have no independent prognostic value [17]. Nevertheless, it is usually reported because it may have future predictive value with respect to adjuvant therapy or the risk of developing liver metastases.

Surgical Resection Margins and Local Recurrence

Local Recurrence

Local recurrence is defined as regrowth of tumour in or around the tumour bed after previous removal of all visible tumour. It includes regrowth within the suture or staple line of an anastomosis, the adjacent mesorectum or adjacent lymph nodes. If a patient with rectal cancer develops local recurrence the prognosis is poor, with a 90% chance of death as a result.

In a recently reported Medical Research Council (MRC) trial in the UK, comparing surgery alone and surgery with postoperative radiotherapy in patients with mobile Dukes' stage B and C rectal cancers, 33% of the patients treated by surgery alone had developed local recurrence by 5 years [27]. The trial population for this series ($n = 469$) was drawn from a total of 46 hospitals in the UK and the Republic of Ireland. Local recurrence to this extent is not an uncommon finding within the literature but, in contrast, Heald and colleagues have recently reported results from a single-surgeon series involving 519 patients (all operated on by Mr Heald himself) with a local recurrence rate of only 6% at 5 years [28]. The reason for this markedly more favourable outcome, which defies even differences in casemix between these two studies and the fact that a small proportion of the more recent cases in the latter study received preoperative radiotherapy ($n = 49$), appears to lie in Mr Heald's employment of meticulous surgical technique, of which TME forms a part. This wide variation in outcomes should perhaps come as little surprise in the light of results from the German Prospective Multicentre Study of the Study Group Colorectal Carcinoma, conducted between 1984 and 1992, which showed that the frequency of local recurrence was determined not only by tumour-related factors but also by department and individual surgeon [20].

Results such as these add weight to the view that high local recurrence rates in rectal cancer often occur as a result of inadequate surgery. With this in mind numerous authors have suggested that the key to reducing rates of local recurrence significantly is first and foremost to achieve complete tumour excision. In relation to this there are two surgical resection margins to consider: longitudinal and circumferential.

The Longitudinal Resection Margin

The longitudinal resection margin, which assumes most importance in this context, is virtually always the distal resection margin. Several studies have shown that rectal cancers may extend further distally than their surface appearance leads one to believe. This spread may occur either within the wall of the rectum (distal intramural spread) or within the mesorectal tissues (distal mesorectal spread) [29–32]. Scott et al. [32] reported distal mesorectal spread extending further than intramural spread, with tumour deposits being present as far as 3 cm distal to the primary tumour. In this study, concomitant CRM involvement was also seen in two of the four cases showing distal mesorectal spread, but in only two of the other 16, suggesting a least a partial relationship between distal spread and CRM involvement. Indeed, both are now recognised as markers of advanced local disease. When a tumour is highly infiltrative, shows extensive extramural vascular or lymphatic invasion or extensive mesorectal spread, or is of an aggressive histological type, even allowing a distance of 3 cm between it and the distal resection margin may not be sufficient. Preoperative biopsy and imaging of a tumour can guide the surgeon with regard to how far beyond it the distal limit of resection should be.

Circumferential Resection Margin

Careful assessment of the CRM of a rectal cancer specimen allows prediction of local recurrence. CRM status is an independent prognostic variable in rectal cancer, with involvement of this margin by tumour predicting a 12-fold increased risk of local recurrence and a threefold increased risk of death [18]. Tumours at or within 1 mm of the CRM (measured histologically using the microscope Vernier scale) should be regarded as being incompletely excised (Fig. 2.3). Involvement need not necessarily be the result of direct or discontinuous spread of the primary tumour, but may be because of tumour within a lymph node or vessel approaching to within 1 mm of the margin [18,33]. At present it is not known whether any one mode of CRM involvement is of greater significance than the others.

In one study Adam et al. [18] reported that 25% of patients thought to have had curative surgery at the time of operation were found to have tumour involvement of the CRM on subsequent histological examination. They also found that, after a median follow-up of 5 years, 78% of patients with an involved circumferential margin had developed

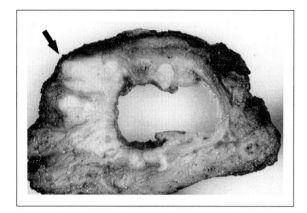

Fig. 2.3. A transverse slice from an abdominoperineal resection specimen at a site of significant extramural tumour spread. Tumour is seen invading the mesorectal fat on the left side of the picture. In the arrowed area it is seen extending to within 1 mm of the circumferential resection margin, which had been painted with black ink prior to slicing.

local recurrence compared with only 10% of those who were considered to have had a clear margin histologically. Other authors have also demonstrated significant increases in local recurrence for patients with CRM involvement by tumour [34,35]. It is results such as these that have led to the treatment strategy, now adopted by a significant number of surgeons, of administering postoperative radiotherapy to patients with an involved circumferential margin.

The Staging of Rectal Cancer

There are four ways in which rectal cancer may spread:

1. By direct invasive growth through the wall of the rectum
2. Via lymphatics
3. Via blood vessels
4. By seeding across the peritoneal cavity

The various staging systems currently in use tend to assess degree of spread by these routes to a greater or lesser extent, resulting ultimately in the assigning of a specific stage. Accurate staging is important for the following reasons:

1. *It influences subsequent treatment strategy.* Both the extent of surgery undertaken and the decisions made with respect to offering adjuvant

therapy are influenced by staging. To quote an example, current guidelines in the UK suggest that a tumour that has been locally excised in its entirety (i.e. all surgical margins are more than 1 mm from the tumour) and staged as pT1 using the TNM system may, in general, be regarded as having been adequately treated. In contrast, for locally excised tumours staged as pT2 it is suggested (at least until further data from radiotherapy trials are available) that further radical surgery should be performed [36]. (Of course there are always exceptions to rules and the presence of certain histological features when associated with the pT1 tumour described above, such as vascular invasion, extensive submucosal invasion or poor differentiation, would demand that further surgery be carried out.) The influence of stage on the decision to offer adjuvant therapy is illustrated by the fact that virtually all patients with Dukes' C rectal cancer now go on to receive adjuvant chemotherapy, whereas patients with a Dukes' A or B cancer do not.

2. *It allows a prognosis to be given.* Prognosis is of paramount importance to the patient with rectal cancer. Survival for the subdivisions of the various staging systems is now well documented, so the clinicopathological stage can be used to provide the patient with details of the extent to which they can expect to recover after surgery.

3. *It facilitates the drawing of comparisons between patients involved in cancer registry studies and clinical trials.* Accurate staging allows outcomes between different surgeons to be compared by cancer registries, and permits the grouping together for analysis purposes of patients involved in trials. The inclusion of staging data allows more meaningful comparisons to be made when considering the results of trials that are similar in design but which have been conducted separately.

Staging Systems Currently In Existence

The longest established of all the rectal cancer staging systems is the Dukes' system. Cuthbert Dukes first published this in 1932, later producing modified forms of his original system in conjunction with others [37–39]. In 1954 Astler and Coller published a similar ABC-type of staging system [40], as a modification of that proposed by Kirklin and colleagues in 1949 [41]. This is a system still based on depth of penetration of the bowel wall and lymph node involvement, but which specifies more subdivisions of direct spread and lymph node involvement by way of its B2 and C2 stages. The TNM staging system is an internationally recognised system that is now in widespread usage [42]. This classification again takes into consideration direct tumour spread and nodal involvement, but in more detail than the other systems, independently classifying tumour status, nodal status and the presence of metastases. Additionally, the TNM system now also encompasses the very important R0, R1, R2 residual tumour classification. The Australian Clinico-pathological Staging System (ACPSS), developed in the 1980s, uses similar pathological parameters to the previously described systems in conjunction with clinical information to give nine staging categories from A1 to D2 (the "A" category has three subdivisions, while the others have two) [43,44]. The system proposed by Jass et al. in 1987 is not strictly a staging system, but rather a prognostic classification system [17]. Within this the pathologist is required to assess amongst other things the nature of the advancing tumour margin, deciding whether it is of an expanding or infiltrating type and whether there is a conspicuous lymphocytic infiltrate around it or not. To date, this system remains untested by other groups in large prospective series and has not been widely adopted by pathologists. Its usefulness may be limited by interobserver variability, particularly in relation to assessment of the lymphocytic infiltrate.

In deciding which staging system(s) to employ it is important to remember that many large European and North American colorectal cancer trials have utilised the TNM system. This in itself provides a strong argument (although not the only one) for why routine hospital practice should embrace its use. By adopting the same staging system, the integration into clinical practice of new and better therapies can be carried out with precise groups of patients in mind, thus maximising any potential benefits that a new mode of treatment may offer. Dukes' staging probably represents the main rival to the TNM system, being both a simple system and one that is currently in widespread use throughout the UK and in many other countries of the world. This, together with the fact that it too is a staging system that has been used in the context of many major clinical trials, adds strength to the argument in favour of its continued usage alongside the TNM system, although, as we will outline later, in comparison to the TNM system it does have a number of shortcomings. The Astler and Coller system does not provide any further benefit if TNM has been adopted and TNM encompasses the ACPSS. Therefore, for the remainder of this section we intend to concentrate the remainder of our discussion around the Dukes' and TNM systems.

Dukes' Staging

Dukes' staging is a simple, reproducible and widely recognised staging system (Table 2.1). This is not to say, however, that it is either an ideal or a flawless system. One of its weaknesses is that the category that carries with it a confident prediction of cure (i.e. stage A) encompasses only about 16% of rectal cancers. At the opposite end of the spectrum a similar problem exists, with less than 10% of tumours falling into the C2 category, this being the stage that most strongly predicts cancer-related death. In its pure form Dukes' staging does not take into account clinical information that may lead to considerable differences in reported survival for each stage. The concept of the so-called Dukes' D category, denoting the presence of distant metastases, was introduced by Turnbull in 1967 [45] and has gone some way towards integrating clinical data into the system, but not all pathologists and clinicians accept this as being the answer, with many preferring to use a combination of Dukes' and other systems designed specifically to take clinical data into consideration. One point of vital importance in the use of Dukes' staging is that the various stages should not be confused with stages of the similar ABC systems published by other authors because this can potentially result in patients being given an incorrect prognosis [46].

TNM Staging System

This system, which has been developed over the past 40 years or so by the International Union Against Cancer (UICC) in Switzerland, is strongly favoured by clinicians in countries such as the USA and Germany. Until recently, however, it has been unpopular amongst many pathologists, especially in the UK. During the mid to late 1990s it gradually gained universal acceptance, probably as a result of its use within large-scale clinical trials involving pathological assessment of specimens, and the ever

Table 2.1. Dukes' staging of colorectal cancer

Stage	Description
A	Growth of primary tumour does not penetrate beyond muscularis propria; no nodal metastases
B	Growth of primary tumour extends beyond muscularis propria; no nodal metastases
C1	Lymph node metastases present but apical node(s) free of tumour
C2	Metastases within apical lymph node(s)

increasing pressures to provide a quality pathology service that integrates well into an overall patient management strategy. There are three basic component arms to the system, which between them take into consideration the extent of spread of the primary tumour (the T stage), the absence or presence and extent of regional lymph node metastases (the N stage), and the absence or presence of distant metastases (the M stage) [42]. When the T, N or M stage is prefixed by a "p" this indicates that the stage has been assigned using evidence obtained by pathological examination of a specimen. When there is no such prefix the stage should be taken as being based on clinical evidence only. The use of a further prefix letter "y" (not an abbreviation, of purely symbolic value only) indicates that the stage has been assigned during or following preoperative treatment (for example ypT3). TNM staging may be applied to most malignant tumours regardless of body site or system. Table 2.2 outlines how it is applied to colorectal cancer.

The issue of serosal involvement has been discussed previously [21,22]. Its presence has implications in that affected individuals are now increasingly being offered peritoneal chemotherapy. The

Table 2.2. TNM staging of colorectal cancer

Stage	Description
T stage	
TX	Primary tumour cannot be assessed
T0	No evidence of primary tumour
Tis	Carcinoma in situ: intraepithelial or invasion of lamina propria
T1	Tumour invades submucosa
T2	Tumour invades muscularis propria
T3	Tumour invades through muscularis propria into subserosa or into non-peritonealised pericolic or perirectal tissues
T4	Tumour directly invades other organs or structures and/or perforates visceral peritoneum
N stage	
NX	Regional lymph nodes cannot be assessed
N0	No regional lymph node metastases
N1	Metastasis in 1 to 3 regional lymph nodes
N2	Metastasis in 4 or more regional lymph nodes
M stage	
MX	Distant metastasis cannot be assessed
M0	No distant metastasis
M1	Distant metastasis
Residual tumour status	
RX	Presence of residual tumour cannot be assessed
R0	No residual tumour
R1	Microscopic residual tumour
R2	Macroscopic residual tumour

terms "serosal involvement" and "circumferential resection margin involvement" are not synonymous and indeed are quite unrelated features, the latter being strictly related to the retroperitoneal margin of excision. Perforated tumours are always regarded as pT4 in the TNM system.

The accuracy of the N stage assigned to a case of rectal cancer relies on the pathologist responsible making a thorough search for lymph nodes in the resection specimen. As the average number of lymph nodes recovered decreases, the likelihood of staging a case incorrectly as pN0 (i.e. no lymph node metastases present) increases. In the same scenario, the probability of staging a case correctly as pN2 decreases. With these risks in mind, the UICC now recommends that, in the assessment of rectal cancer, at least 12 separate nodes should be recovered and examined histologically before a stage of pN0 is assigned [42]. They now also recommend that extramural tumour nodules measuring 3 mm or more in diameter should be regarded as lymph node metastases, irrespective of whether or not they are accompanied by identifiable lymph node tissue [47]. After recent revisions of the system the previously used pN3 staging category no longer exists.

Although clinical and radiological evidence is sufficient to stage a tumour clinically as M1, its pathological counterpart (stage pM1) should be applied only to cases where there is histological proof of distant metastases. In tumours other than these the appropriate pathological M stage is pMX (distant metastases unknown) [48].

The Residual Tumour Classification

After recent revisions, the R0, R1, R2 classification of residual tumour status now forms part of the TNM staging system [49,50]. Under this classification, resection specimens are assigned to an R category by way of the following criteria:

R0: All tumour removed

R1: Microscopic deposits of tumour left behind (in practice this is the R category assigned to cases where, on microscopy, there is circumferential or longitudinal resection margin involvement by tumour)

R2: Macroscopic tumour left behind

The use of this classification in addition to the traditional T, N and M parameters allows the identification of non-curative resections without distant metastases. Without this extra information such cases could, in theory, go unchecked and lead to marked and potentially confusing differences in survival between studies for a particular stage of disease. The main issue that requires clarification in respect of assigning an R category relates to how microscopic involvement of a surgical resection margin should be defined. In the strict definition of the TNM guidelines, involvement is defined as tumour actually at the margin, whereas other authors have found good evidence to suggest that the presence of tumour within 1 mm of a margin is an acceptable measure of involvement [18,33]. This is an area that requires further study.

Dukes' Staging Versus TNM

Generally speaking, the TNM system has a number of important advantages over the system devised by Dukes. These are:

1. It can be applied to local excision specimens that do not contain lymph nodes and still maintain a useful degree of prognostic value. In contrast, much of the prognostic value of the Dukes' system is lost when lymph nodes cannot be assessed.

2. It provides a prognostically more useful description of extent of invasion. The T stage of a locally excised tumour, for example, can in itself provide sufficient grounds for deferring or proceeding with further surgery. In contrast Dukes' staging in isolation does not provide surgeons with enough information to allow them safely to pursue a conservative treatment strategy, for, although this may be safe for some stage A tumours, there is no way of telling exactly to which stage A tumours this applies.

3. It takes into consideration peritoneal involvement by tumour. As already discussed, the presence of peritoneal involvement confers a poorer prognosis, but within the Dukes' system there is no provision for this group of patients.

4. The residual tumour classification incorporated in the TNM system allows the identification of another group of patients who will have a poorer prognosis because they have undergone a non-curative resection. Again, no provision is made for these cases within the Dukes' system.

5. It takes into consideration the invasion of other organs by tumour. This is a further group of poor prognosis patients not separately catered for by the Dukes' system.

6. The distribution of tumours between the better prognosis N1 and the worse prognosis N2 stages of the TNM system is more even than the distribution between the C1 and C2 Dukes' stages. Consequently, the group of patients with extensive lymph node involvement who are likely to do badly after surgery is defined more accurately by the TNM system.

In spite of all the advantages TNM appears to have over Dukes' staging, the existing widespread usage, relative simplicity and ease of application of the latter system carries a great deal of weight. It is for these reasons that the Dukes' system remains universally popular. Indeed, recent guidelines issued by the Royal College of Pathologists in the UK back the continued use of Dukes' staging alongside TNM staging in colorectal cancer [48]. That said, however, particularly in the light of a continuing escalation of its use on a global scale, it is not unfeasible that a move towards the use of TNM staging alone may occur within the next 10 years.

Role of Pathology in Assessing the Quality of Rectal Cancer Surgery

The great variation in rectal cancer specimens between surgeons is reflected in differences in patient survival, with good quality surgery being associated with better survival. Arbman et al. showed that improving the quality of surgery (primarily in their series by adopting the technique of total mesorectal excision) could result in a 20% improvement in 4-year survival [51]. The pathologist receiving rectal cancer resection specimens is in an ideal position to audit the quality of surgery and it is vital, therefore, that surgeons and pathologists involved with these patients should develop good working relationships that promote constructive feedback from pathologist to surgeon on quality issues.

The quality of surgery may be assessed in three ways by the pathologist:

1. By a macroscopic visual inspection of the resection specimen
2. By recording the frequency of abdominoperineal excisions
3. By recording the frequency of perforation

With experience, the quality of surgery can be assessed by the receiving pathologist simply by paying attention to certain visual features of the resection specimen. A macroscopic photograph of the posterior and anterior aspects of the freshly received specimen can enhance the value of this assessment by providing a permanent visual record of all resections scrutinised in this way. This type of quality assessment can be made more objective by the use of particular criteria to place cases into one of a number of quality categories. The criteria and

Table 2.3. Criteria used to assess the quality of rectal surgery within the Medical Research Council CLASICC trial

Quality assessment	Criteria
Poor	Muscularis propria can be seen in any area of the posterior mesorectum
Moderate	No muscularis propria visible but irregular surface of back of mesorectum with only a moderate amount of fat May be "coning" distally
Good	Bulky mesorectum with a smooth surface covered by mesorectal fascia No "coning"

categories being utilised by the MRC CLASICC trial currently under way in the UK, comparing laparoscopic-assisted and conventional open surgery in colorectal cancer, provide as good a categorisation

system as any. In this system the quality of surgery is assessed as outlined in Table 2.3.

In our experience, on macroscopic examination the three commonest problems we see are that the mesorectum has been incised in one or two areas (but with the majority of the remaining mesorectal surface remaining intact), or that the mesorectal plane has been lost, resulting in the creation of an entirely new plane, which approaches closer to the tumour (or even passes through it), or that there is a tapering inwards of the mesorectal tissues towards the distal resection margin (so-called "coning"). In the case of abdominoperineal excisions, a degree of coning at the level where the levator muscles insert into the rectal wall is inevitable (Fig. 2.4). However, when the distal resection margin is above this level, care should be taken to transect across both the rectum and mesorectum at an angle of 90°. It is easy to see how the occurrence of any of these problems leads to an increased risk of incomplete tumour resection.

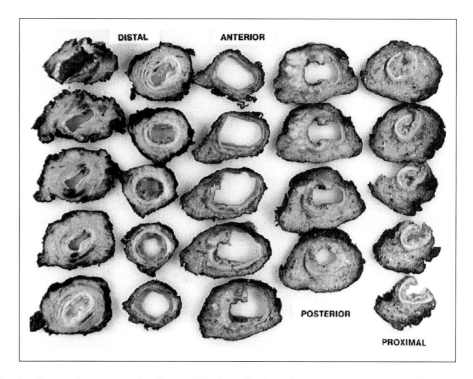

Fig. 2.4. A series of consecutive transverse slices from an abdominoperineal resection specimen, progressing from the most proximal slice in the bottom right-hand corner of the picture, upwards, through each successive column, to the most distal slice in the top left-hand corner. The top two slices in the centre column and the bottom two slices in the column immediately to its left are sequential slices through the site at which the levator muscles insert into the rectal wall, and at which there is a much thinner circumference of perirectal tissue. It is easy to appreciate how, when tumour involves this area (not seen in this instance), the risk of incomplete resection becomes high. Circumferential resection margin involvement by tumour higher up in the mesorectum is seen in this particular case. (The slice shown in Fig. 3 can be seen once again at the top of the second column from the right.)

The repeated observation of problems such as these in relation to individual surgeons may begin to raise questions regarding the quality of surgical performance; indeed, high rates of CRM involvement by tumour do often indicate poor surgical technique. In an era where neo-adjuvant therapy is being used to a greater extent, it may also raise the question of how appropriate the selection of patients for preoperative radiotherapy has been.

Even in the most skilled hands, some cases of CRM involvement by tumour are unavoidable (Fig. 2.4), particularly with some anterior tumours or when there is advanced disease. (Anteriorly, below the peritoneal reflection, it is usually possible on average for even highly proficient operators to remove mesorectal tissue only to a depth of 0.5–1.0 cm, the consequence being that low anterior wall tumours carry with them an increased risk of CRM involvement.) Because of these factors, measurement of the distance of tumour spread beyond the outer limit of the muscularis propria provides a useful indicator concerning whether or not involvement has occurred largely as a result of the adverse nature of the tumour, or simply because of poor surgery.

Abdominoperineal excision rates vary significantly between surgeons. Recording their frequency is the second way in which the pathologist can assess the quality of surgery. Sphincter-saving surgery for low rectal cancer is now a routine procedure for colorectal specialists. Tumours that may have necessitated abdominoperineal excision of the rectum 20 years ago can today be dealt with by ultralow anterior resection with subsequent restoration of colo-anal continuity. The ability of a surgeon now to avoid abdominoperineal resection in patients in whom it would once not have been possible, can be used as an indicator of quality of surgical performance. High rates of abdominoperineal resection must be justified, with the implication being that, if they cannot be, then it is an indication that performance needs to be improved. By recording the distance of tumours from the pectinate line the pathologist can provide evidence that may or may not allow the surgeon to justify why he or she has carried out a high number of abdominoperineal resections.

Currently, in many institutions the abdominoperineal excision rate still remains above 40%, whereas in centres specialising in colorectal surgery it can be as low as 15%. This is the standard to which all surgeons performing rectal cancer surgery should aspire in order for their performance to be seen as being of a high quality. In our own institution, taking into consideration all surgeons, the abdominoperineal resection rate fell from 59% in 1986 to 17% in 1997, with an even lower rate now applying to those surgeons specialising in colorectal surgery (K.F. Birbeck, et al., unpublished observations).

Perforation through a tumour (whether spontaneous or iatrogenic) is associated with a higher incidence of local recurrence and a poorer prognosis [52–55]. Although it is often associated with advanced stage or tumour fixity, the adverse effects of perforation on disease-free survival have been shown by Wiggers et al. to be independent of these factors [56]. Reported rates of inadvertent perforation during rectal cancer surgery vary from being above 25% to well under 10% [55,57–58]. In analysing this rate in relation to individual surgeons as a measure of quality of surgery, the pathologist can play an important role by contributing an assessment of both the extent of local tumour invasion and the microscopic appearances at the site of perforation. Higher rates of perforation may be explained, to a certain extent, if there is associated extensive local spread and/or reports of tumour fixity. On the other hand, in scenarios where the microscopic evidence suggests only a limited degree of local spread or provides definite evidence of damage to the rectal wall that cannot be explained, the quality of surgery must then brought into question.

In our own institution, auditing the quality of surgery by using a combination of the methods outlined above has resulted in a significant reduction in rates of CRM involvement by tumour (K.F. Birbeck, et al., unpublished observations), which is an important immediate outcome measure in this context.

Quality of Preoperative Imaging and Pathology Reporting, and the Use of Reporting Proformas

It is important that, when we are considering the quality of management of the patient with rectal cancer, it is not just the quality of the surgeon's performance that comes under scrutiny. Both the conclusions drawn from preoperative staging and the pathologist's observations influence the precise nature of the treatment a patient receives. As such, both of these areas should be scrutinised to the same extent as the work of the surgeon.

The quality of pathology reporting in colorectal cancer has been reported to be highly variable [59,60]. It has been shown to be particularly poor in terms of specifying the number of lymph nodes recovered, the number containing metastases, and reporting the presence of tumour at the CRM

Joint National Guidelines Minimum Data Set
Colorectal Cancer Histopathology Report

Patient Name:.. Date of Birth:..

Hospital:.. Hospital No:..

Histology No: .... Surgeon: ....

Gross Description

Site of Tumour...

Maximum tumour diameter ....

Distance of tumour to nearer margin (cut end) ....

	Yes	No
Presence of tumour perforation (pT4)	☐	☐

For rectal tumours

Tumour is: Above ☐   At ☐   Below ☐
the peritoneal reflection

Distance from dentate line ....

Histology
Type

	Yes	No
Adenocarcinoma	☐	☐

(to include mucinous and signet ring adenocarcinomas)

If No, Other..

Differentiation by predominant area

Poor ☐   Other ☐

Local Invasion

Submucosa (pT1)	☐
Muscularis propria (pT2)	☐
Beyond muscularis propria (pT3)	☐
Tumour cells have breached the peritoneal surface or invaded adjacent organs (pT4)	☐

Margins

Tumour involvement	N/A	Yes	No
doughnut	☐	☐	☐
margin (cut end)	☐	☐	☐
circumferential margin	☐	☐	☐

Histological measurement

from tumour to circumferential margin .... mm

Metastatic Spread

No of lymph nodes examined...................................

No of positive lymph nodes...................................
(pN1 1-3 nodes, pN2 4+ nodes involved)

	Yes	No
Apical node positive (Dukes C2)	☐	☐
Extramural vascular invasion	☐	☐

Background Abnormalities

	Yes	No
Adenoma(s)	☐	☐
Synchronous carcinoma(s)	☐	☐

Complete a separate form for each cancer

	Yes	No
Ulcerative colitis	☐	☐
Crohn's	☐	☐
Familial adenomatous polyposis	☐	☐

Other Comments...
....

Pathological Staging

	Yes	No
Complete resection at all margins	☐	☐

TNM

T ☐   N ☐   M ☐

Dukes

Dukes A	☐	(Growth limited to wall, nodes negative)
Dukes B	☐	(Growth beyond M. propria, nodes negative)
Dukes C1	☐	(Nodes positive and apical node negative)
Dukes C2	☐	(Apical node positive)

	Yes	No
Histologically confirmed liver metastases	☐	☐

Signature ....

Date......................... SNOMED code......./.................

Approved by the Royal Colleges of Pathologists and Surgeons (England),
Associations of Coloproctology and Clinical Pathologists,
the Pathology Section of the British Society of Gastroenterology, SIGN/SCTN and CROPS

Fig. 2.5. Minimum dataset proforma for the reporting of colorectal cancer.

for rectal cancer specimens. The inclusion or omission of details such as these provides some indication of the quality of the pathologist's performance in assessing the specimen. Recently, Bull et al. [60] audited the performance of pathologists in one National Health Service region of the UK. Their findings were that only 11.3% of colonic cancer and 4.0% of rectal cancer reports met the desirable minimum standards decided upon at the outset of the study. On reducing these standards to a bare minimum for an adequate report, 22% of the colonic and 53.4% of the rectal reports still failed to include all the required data.

In the light of findings such as these the Royal College of Pathologists in the UK has recently published details of a recommended minimum dataset for colorectal cancer histopathology reports, part of which advocates the use of reporting proformas [48]. These are also recommended by the United Kingdom Co-ordinating Committee on Cancer Research (UKCCCR) [61]. Fig. 2.5 shows a proforma that been found to be both useful and useable in a UK district general hospital setting. Clearly the use of such a document by the pathologist reporting a colorectal cancer case provides the easiest way to ensure the inclusion of all the desirable elements in what is a relatively complex report.

Of course, the ideal report on a major rectal cancer resection specimen can be generated only by the pathologist, be it by using a proforma or otherwise, after a thorough dissection of the specimen by an appropriate technique. The UKCCCR handbook for the clinicopathological assessment and staging of colorectal cancer [61] provides a description of such a technique, which is a modification of those previously published by Quirke and colleagues [62–64].

Conclusions

The major factors influencing outcome after rectal cancer surgery include a number of histological features of the tumour, stage of the disease and the quality of surgery. Although the pathologist clearly takes a central role in assessing factors relating to the first two areas, he or she also has an important part to play in assessing the latter. Audit of the performance of surgeons, pathologists and radiologists plays an essential part in the development of rectal cancer management strategy. Constructive criticism should be accepted by all groups as this will ultimately serve to benefit patients. The type of performance improvement that reduces rates of local tumour recurrence and hence increases survival

should be sought constantly. To this end, particular attention must be paid to obtaining a complete resection of tumour at all resection margins. The first step towards achieving this requires that preoperative imaging should concentrate on assessing the chances of complete tumour removal at operation, by identifying how close a tumour lies to irresectable organs and the mesorectal fascial plane. The results of such imaging should then be reported in conjunction with recommendations for preoperative adjuvant radiotherapy in those instances where patients are at risk of incomplete excision. The CRM should receive close attention, from both the surgeon at the time of surgery, and, subsequently, from the pathologist at the time of specimen dissection and histological assessment.

In deciding which of the many staging systems currently in existence should be used to stage a tumour, a combination of both the Dukes' and TNM systems is regarded by many as the most appropriate approach at the present time, providing both a simple and widely recognised system together with one that gives the most clinically useful information.

In conclusion, there is now strong evidence that improving the quality of preoperative assessment and surgery, together with accurate pathological assessment and staging, can confer survival benefits on patients with rectal cancer that at least equal those afforded by the adjuvant therapies currently on offer. It is therefore essential that all those involved in the management of patients suffering from rectal cancer should direct their efforts first and foremost towards providing a quality service, which will ultimately result in markedly better outcomes for this patient group.

References

1. Office for National Statistics. Mortality statistics; cause. Review of the Registrar General on deaths by cause, sex, and age, in England and Wales, 1997 (Series DH2). London: The Stationary Office, 1998:10.
2. Landis SH, Murray T, Bolden S, et al. Cancer statistics, 1998. CA Cancer J Clin 1998;48:6–29.
3. Heald RJ, Husband EM, Ryall RD. The mesorectum in rectal cancer surgery – the clue to pelvic recurrence? Br J Surg 1982;69:613–16.
4. Norstein J, Langmark F. Results of rectal cancer treatment: a national experience. In: Soreide O, Norstein J, editors. Rectal cancer surgery: optimisation, standardisation, documentation. Berlin: Springer-Verlag, 1997:17–28.
5. Connelly JH, Robey-Cafferty SS, Cleary KR. Mucinous carcinomas of the colon and rectum. An analysis of 62 stage B and C lesions. Arch Pathol Lab Med 1991;115:1022–25.
6. Younes M, Katikaneni PR, Lechago J. The value of preoperative mucosal biopsy in the diagnosis of colorectal mucinous adenocarcinoma. Cancer 1993;72:3588–92.

7. Sunblad AS, Paz RA. Mucinous carcinomas of the colon and rectum and their relation to polyps. Cancer 1982;50:2504–509.
8. Sasaki O, Atkin WS, Jass JR. Mucinous carcinoma of the rectum. Histopathology 1987;11:259–72.
9. Chevinsky AH, Berelowitz M, Hoover HC Jr. Adenosquamous carcinoma of the colon presenting with hypercalcemia. Cancer 1987;60:1111–16.
10. Kulayat MN, Doerr R, Butler B, et al. Squamous cell carcinoma complicating idiopathic inflammatory bowel disease. J Surg Oncol 1995;59:48–55.
11. Soga J. Carcinoids of the rectum: an evaluation of 1271 reported cases. Surg Today 1997;27:112–19.
12. Caldarola VT, Jackman RJ, Moertel CG, et al. Carcinoid tumours of the rectum. Am J Surg 1964;107:844–49.
13. Kuroda T, Kusana J, Iijima K, et al. Primary malignant melanoma of the rectum. J Gastroenterol 1996;31:437–40.
14. Werdin C, Limas C, Knodell RG. Primary malignant melanoma of the rectum. Evidence of origination from rectal mucosal melanocytes. Cancer 1988;61:1364–70.
15. Jass JR, Atkin WS, Cuzick J, et al. The grading of rectal cancer: historical perspectives and a multivariate analysis of 447 cases. Histopathology 1986;10:437–59.
16. Halvorsen TB, Seim E. Degree of differentiation in colorectal adenocarcinomas: a multivariate analysis of the influence on survival. J Clin Pathol 1988;41:532–37.
17. Jass JR, Love SB, Northover JM. A new prognostic classification of rectal cancer. Lancet 1987;i:1303–306.
18. Adam IJ, Mohamdee MO, Martin IG, et al. Role of circumferential resection margin involvement in the local recurrence of rectal cancer. Lancet 1994;344:707–11.
19. Jass JR. Lymphocytic infiltration and survival in rectal cancer. J Clin Pathol 1986;39:585.
20. Hohenberger W. The effect of specialization or organization of rectal cancer surgery. In: Soreide O, Norstein J, editors. Rectal cancer surgery: optimization, standardization, documentation. Berlin: Springer-Verlag, 1997:353–63.
21. Shepherd NA, Baxter KJ, Love SB. Influence of local peritoneal involvement on pelvic recurrence and prognosis in rectal cancer. J Clin Pathol 1995;48:849–55.
22. Shepherd NA, Baxter KJ, Love SB. The prognostic importance of peritoneal involvement in colonic cancer: a prospective evaluation. Gastroenterology 1997;112:1096–102.
23. Haboubi NY, Abdalla SA, Amini S, et al. The novel combination of fat clearance and immunohistochemistry improves prediction of the outcome of patients with colorectal carcinomas: a preliminary study. Int J Colorect Dis 1998;13:99–102.
24. Jass JR, Miller K, Northover JM. Fat clearance method versus manual dissection of lymph nodes in specimens of rectal cancer. Int J Colorect Dis 1986;1:155–56.
25. Keffers MD, O'Dowd GM, Mulchacy H, et al. The prognostic significance of immunohistochemically detected micrometastases in colorectal carcinoma. J Pathol 1994;172:183.
26. Talbot IC, Ritchie S, Leighton MH, et al. Invasion of veins by carcinoma of the rectum: method of dissection, histological features and significance. Histopathology 1981;5:141–63.
27. Medical Research Council Rectal Cancer Working Party. Randomised trial of surgery alone versus surgery followed by radiotherapy for mobile cancer of the rectum. Lancet 1996;348:1610–14.
28. Heald RJ, Moran BJ, Ryall RD, et al. Rectal cancer: the Basingstoke experience of total mesorectal excision, 1978–1997. Arch Surg 1998;133:894–99.
29. Williams NS, Dixon MF, Johnston D. Reappraisal of the 5 centimetre rule of distal excision for carcinoma of the rectum: a study of distal intramural spread and of patients' survival. Br J Surg 1983;70:150–54.
30. Sidoni A, Bufalari A, Alberti PF. Distal intramural spread in colorectal cancer: a reappraisal of the extent of distal clearance in fifty cases. Tumori 1991;77:514–17.
31. Shirouzu K, Isomoto H, Kakegawa T. Distal spread of rectal cancer and optimal distal margin of resection for sphincter-preserving surgery. Cancer 1995;76:388–92.
32. Scott N, Jackson P, Al-Jaberi T, et al. Total mesorectal excision and local recurrence: a study of tumour spread in the mesorectum distal to rectal cancer. Br J Surg 1995;82:1031–33.
33. Quirke P, Durdey P, Dixon MF, et al. Local recurrence of rectal adenocarcinoma due to inadequate surgical resection: histopathological study of lateral tumour spread and surgical excision. Lancet 1986;ii:996–99.
34. Ng IO, Luk IS, Yuen ST, et al. Surgical lateral clearance in resected rectal carcinomas. A multivariate analysis of clinicopathologic features. Cancer 1993;71:1972–76.
35. de Haas-Kock DF, Baeten CG, Jager JJ, et al. Prognostic significance of radial margins of clearance in rectal cancer. Br J Surg 1996;83:781–85.
36. Banerjee AK, Jehle EC, Shorthouse AJ, et al. Local excision of rectal tumours. Br J Surg 1995;82:1165–73.
37. Dukes CE. The classification of cancer of the rectum. J Pathol Bacteriol 1932;35:323–32.
38. Gabriel WB, Dukes CE, Bussey HJR. Lymphatic spread in cancer of the rectum. Br J Surg 1935;23:395–413.
39. Dukes CE, Bussey HJR. The spread of rectal cancer and its effect on prognosis. Br J Cancer 1958;12:309–20.
40. Astler VB, Coller FA. The prognostic significance of direct extension of carcinoma of the colon and rectum. Ann Surg 1954;139:846–52.
41. Kirklin JW, Dockerty MB, Waugh JM. The role of the peritoneal reflection in the prognosis of carcinoma of the rectum and sigmoid colon. Surg Gynecol Obstet 1949;88:326–31.
42. Sobin LH, Wittekind C, editors. TNM classification of malignant tumours. 5th ed. New York: Wiley-Liss, 1997.
43. Davis NC, Newland RC. Terminology and classification of colorectal adenocarcinoma: the Australian clinico-pathological staging system. Aust N Z J Surg 1983;53:211–21.
44. Newland RC, Chapuis PH, Smyth EJ. The prognostic value of substaging colorectal carcinoma. A prospective study of 1117 cases with standardised pathology. Cancer 1987;60:852–57.
45. Turnbull RB, Kyle K, Watson FR, et al. Cancer of the colon: the influence of the no touch isolation technique on survival rates. Ann Surg 1967;166:420–27.
46. Kyriakos M. The President's cancer, the Dukes' classification, and confusion. Arch Pathol Lab Med 1985;109:1063–66.
47. Hermanek P, Henson DE, Hunter RVP, et al., editors. TNM supplement 1993. A commentary on uniform use. Berlin: Springer-Verlag, 1993.
48. Royal College of Pathologists. Minimum dataset for colorectal cancer histopathology reports. London: RCP, 1998.
49. Hermanek P, Sobin LH, editors. TNM classification of malignant tumours. 4th ed., 2nd rev. Berlin: Springer-Verlag, 1992.
50. Hermanek P, Wittekind C. The pathologist and the residual tumour (R) classification. Pathol Res Pract 1994;190:115–23.
51. Arbman G, Nilsson E, Hallbröök O, et al. Local recurrence following total mesorectal excision for rectal cancer. Br J Surg 1996;83:375–79.
52. Patel SC, Tovee EB, Langer B. Twenty-five years' experience with radical surgical treatment of carcinoma of the extraperitoneal rectum. Surgery 1977;82:460–65.

53. Phillips RKS, Hittinger R, Blesovsky L, et al. Local recurrence following "curative" surgery for large bowel cancer: I. The overall picture. Br J Surg 1984;71:12–16.

54. Phillips RKS, Hittinger R, Blesovsky L, et al. Local recurrence following "curative" surgery for large bowel cancer: II. The rectum and rectosigmoid. Br J Surg 1984;71:17–20.

55. Zirngibl H, Husemann B, Hermanek P. Intraoperative spillage of tumour cells in surgery for rectal cancer. Dis Colon Rectum 1990;33:610–14.

56. Wiggers T, Arends JW, Volovics A. Regression analysis of prognostic factors in colorectal cancer after curative resections. Dis Colon Rectum 1988;31:33–41.

57. Ranbarger KR, Johnston WD, Chang JC. Prognostic significance of surgical perforation of the rectum during abdominoperineal resection for rectal carcinoma. Am J Surg 1982;143:186–88.

58. Porter GA, O'Keefe GE, Yakimets WW. Inadvertent perforation of the rectum during abdominoperineal resection. Am J Surg 1996;172:324–27.

59. Blenkinsopp WK, Stewart-Brown S, Blesovsky L, et al. Histopathology reporting in large bowel cancer. J Clin Pathol 1981;34:598–613.

60. Bull AD, Biffin AHB, Mella J, et al. Colorectal cancer pathology reporting: a regional audit. J Clin Pathol 1997;50:138–42.

61. United Kingdom Coordinating Committee on Cancer Research Colorectal Cancer Subcommittee. Handbook for the clinico-pathological assessment and staging of colorectal cancer. 2nd ed. London: UKCCCR, 1997.

62. Quirke P, Dixon MF. The prediction of local recurrence in rectal adenocarcinoma by histopathological examination. Int J Colorectal Dis 1988;3:127–31.

63. Quirke P, Scott N. The pathologist's role in the assessment of local recurrence in rectal carcinoma. Surg Oncol Clin North Am 1992;1:1–17.

64. Quirke P. Limitations of existing systems of staging for rectal cancer: the forgotten margin. In: Soreide O, Norstein J, editors. Rectal cancer surgery: optimisation, standardisation, documentation. Berlin: Springer-Verlag, 1997:63–81.

3. Genetics, Screening and Chemoprevention

J. Puig-La Calle Jr. and J.G. Guillem

Introduction

Tremendous advances in basic and clinical research, including the identification of oncogenes, tumor suppressor genes and mismatch repair (MMR) genes related to dominantly inherited syndromes such as familial adenomatous polyposis (FAP) and hereditary nonpolyposis colorectal cancer (HNPCC), have greatly improved our understanding of both sporadic and familial colorectal tumorigenesis.

This chapter reviews several of these advances and how they may impact on the early detection of preneoplastic lesions as well as the prophylactic and chemopreventive management of at-risk individuals for colorectal cancer (CRC).

Genetics

Genetic predisposition is believed to be one of the most significant risk factors for the development of CRC (Fig. 3.1) because a history of CRC in at least

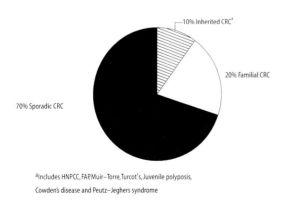

—10% Inherited CRC[a]

20% Familial CRC

70% Sporadic CRC

[a]Includes HNPCC, FAP, Muir–Torre, Turcot's, Juvenile polyposis, Cowden's disease and Peutz–Jeghers syndrome

Fig. 3.1. Distribution of CRC cases according to inheritance (modified from Guillem et al. [14]).

one first degree relative (FDR: parents, siblings and children) can be elicited in approximately 20% of young (<40 years) CRC patients [1]. It is estimated that the risk of developing CRC is twice as high in individuals with an affected FDR when compared with the general population. Furthermore, the risk is even greater when the FDR with CRC is young [2] and if more than one relative is affected.

CRC is thought to arise from the accumulation of genetic alterations that result in a growth advantage rendering an otherwise normal cell neoplastic in what is known as the adenoma-to-carcinoma sequence [3] (Fig. 3.2). These alterations can be inherited (germline) or acquired (somatic) as a result of a random de novo event or exposure to environmental factors such as diet [4]. According to Knudson's two-hit hypothesis, for a cancer to develop, both alleles of a recessive gene need to be mutated [5]. This helps to explain the difference between inherited and sporadic CRC [6]. Patients with inherited CRC (less than 10% of all CRC cases) are born with a germline mutation in one allele and undergo a somatic mutation in the other allele (Table 3.1). However, patients with sporadic CRC (approximately 70% of all cases) require two somatic mutations, one in each allele. Familial clustering of CRC that does not fit into one of the dominantly inherited syndromes such as FAP or HNPCC occurs in 20% of all CRC cases [7] and in over 35% of those with early age of onset CRC [8]. Although familial clustering of CRC may happen by chance alone, environmental influences, weakly penetrant mutations or currently unknown germline mutations may be involved.

Most genes involved in carcinogenesis codify for the synthesis of key cell cycle regulatory proteins. A mutation in any of these genes, therefore, results in either the absence of protein or the production of a truncated non-functional protein. This leads to cell

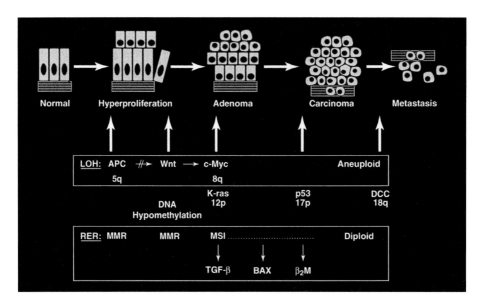

Fig. 3.2. Genetic pathways to CRC (modified from Guillem et al. [14]). LOH, loss of heterozygosity; APC, adenomatous polyposis coli gene; RER, replication error; MMR, mismatch repair; MSI, microsatellite instability; TGF-β, transforming growth factor beta-1; β_2m, beta-2-microglobulin.

Table 3.1. Genetic basis of known inherited CRC syndromes (modified from Guillem et al. [14])

Syndrome	Germline mutation
Familial adenomatous polyposis	APC gene
Hereditary non-polyposis colorectal cancer	MMR genes
Muir–Torre syndrome	MMR genes
Brain tumor–polyposis syndrome (Turcot's)	MMR genes (BTP-1) APC gene (BTP-2)
Juvenile polyposis syndrome	PTEN gene
Cowden's disease	PTEN gene
Peutz–Jeghers syndrome	STK11 gene

cycle deregulation with loss of both growth and differentiation control. The accumulation of successive mutations in other cancer-related genes enhances cell proliferation and dedifferentiation, resulting initially in cancer development and subsequently in conferring metastatic potential.

Genes responsible for CRC development include: (1) tumor suppressor genes; (2) MMR genes; and (3) oncogenes. When mutated, tumor suppressor and MMR genes undergo inactivation leading to loss or impairment of the corresponding protein function. In contradistinction, mutated oncogenes are activated, resulting in an abnormal gain or excess of a particular protein function. Most recently, the I1307K mutation in the tumor sup-

pressor gene for adenomatous polyposis coli (APC) has been shown to lead to an unstable genome, which is frequently noted in familial CRC in Ashkenazi Jews [9].

Tumor Suppressor Genes

This class of genes inhibits abnormal cell growth by slowing the cell cycle to allow for DNA repair and promote autocontrolled cell death (apoptosis) when repair is no longer possible. They are recessive genes, meaning that both alleles must be lost or mutated for the gene to be inactive and produce its phenotypic expression. Tumor suppressor genes that play a role in CRC include, among others, the APC, DCC, p53 and MCC genes.

APC

The APC gene, responsible for FAP, is located on the long arm of chromosome 5 (5q) [10]. The APC gene comprises 15 exons and codes for a 310 kDa protein recently found to play a major role in the important developmental and growth regulatory pathway called *Wnt* [11] (Fig. 3.2).

The *Wnt* pathway involves a cascade of proteins whose endpoint is to activate the transcription of a number of essential genes for normal cell growth and development. One of the most relevant proteins in the *Wnt* pathway is beta-catenin, which appears to be implicated in cell-to-cell adhesion through its interaction with E-cadherin. In the *Wnt* pathway, beta-catenin combines with several other proteins, one of which is Lef/Tcf (named Tcf-4 in the gut), a transcription factor that regulates gene expression. The normal (wild type) APC protein keeps the *Wnt* pathway in check by binding beta-catenin in a multi-protein complex along with GSK-3 beta, a kinase, which in turn degrades beta-catenin by phosphory-lating the APC protein within the complex.

In colorectal mucosa cells, damage to the APC gene, and thus the APC protein complex, results in increased levels of free beta-catenin, which accumu-late in the nucleus and induce gene overexpression and cell proliferation through Tcf-4. In addition, the cytoplasmic accumulation of beta-catenin enhances cell-to-cell adhesion and limits cell migration via its interaction with E-cadherin. As a result, the balance of cellular turnover from the lower proliferative compartment of the crypt to the upper villi is greatly impaired, leading to an accumulation of hyperproliferating cells, which would constitute a polyp [12].

A recent study has identified c-*Myc*, an oncogene mapped to the long arm of chromosome 8 (8q) and previously known to be overexpressed in CRC, as one of the genes most highly activated by beta-catenin through the *Wnt* pathway in APC mutated CRC cell lines [13]. The fact that overexpression of c-*Myc* can be rapidly repressed upon restoration of the wild type APC protein supports the paradigm that inactivation of a tumor suppressor gene can promote the activation of an oncogene.

FAP, which accounts for less than 1% of all CRC cases, is transmitted in an autosomal dominant fashion and is characterized by many hundreds of adenomatous polyps throughout the colon and rectum at an early age (average 16 years) and an estimated 100% risk of CRC by the age of 39 if untreated [14]. Extracolonic manifestations of FAP include upper gastrointestinal polyps (gastric hamartomas and duodenal adenomas), soft tissue tumors such as desmoids, osteomas or odontomas (Gardner's syndrome), medulloblastoma-like brain tumors (Turcot's syndrome) and congenital hyper-trophy of the retinal pigment epithelium (CHRPE).

These varied clinical presentations are largely dependent on the exact location of the mutation within the APC gene [14], such that mutations prox-imal to codon 1249 or distal to codon 1465 lead to sparse polyposis (less than 1000 polyps), whereas mutations between codons 1250 and 1330 lead to profuse polyposis (more than 5000). Furthermore, mutations in exons 3, 4 and at the 5′ end of the gene are associated with an attenuated form of polyposis (few polyps at a later age), whereas mutations at codons 1309 and 1328 cause a particularly aggres-sive form of the disease with a higher incidence of rectal cancer. Finally, CHRPE has been found only in patients with mutations located between exons 9 and 15.

APC gene mutations in FAP involve single base-pair mutations or single or double base-pair dele-tions or additions. These mutations create a stop codon within the aminoacidic sequence of the APC protein, resulting in a truncated, shorter than normal, protein. Truncation of the APC protein, which is readily detectable by the in vitro truncated protein (IVTP) test, is very helpful in identifying individuals with APC gene mutations [14]. The IVTP test can identify a mutation in 87% of FAP individ-uals. However, once the mutation has been identified in one affected member of an FAP kindred, the accuracy of the test for that specific mutation increases to nearly 100% for the other family members. Other methods of identifying APC gene mutations include linkage analysis, which requires prior testing of two affected family members in order to obtain adequate DNA markers for the kindred, and mutational testing, which is the direct detection of the mutation by restriction enzymes. Linkage analysis is more accurate than IVPT testing, but is restricted to known FAP families and, there-fore, cannot be used on individuals with colonic adenomatous polyposis without a family history of FAP.

When mutated, the APC gene has a very high phenotypic penetrance: over 90% of mutation carriers will ultimately develop FAP. The APC gene is also altered in over 70% of sporadic adenomas and CRC, thereby underscoring its importance in the early steps of CRC development. APC gene inactivation triggers the loss of heterozygosity (LOH) pathway of colorectal tumorigenesis (Fig. 3.2), believed to be responsible for upwards of 80% of all CRC cases.

p53

The p53 gene is located on the short arm of chromo-some 17 (17p) [17]. It functions as a gatekeeper by slowing the cell cycle to allow for DNA repair after damage by ultraviolet light, radiation or chemother-apeutic agents [6]. If DNA repair is not feasible, p53 drives the cell to autocontrolled destruction (apoptosis). In contrast to the APC gene, inactiva-tion of p53, found in 70% of CRC cases and as many as half of all carcinomas in humans, occurs late in the tumorigenic sequence. Therefore, p53 gene mutation is likely to be the limiting factor for the malignant transformation of precancerous cells in the LOH pathway. Although p53 overexpression may not be an independent prognostic marker in early (Stage I) CRC [16], p53 mutational analysis appears to have definite prognostic value in advanced (Stages III [17] and IV [18]) CRC. Most studies show significantly lower survival rates for patients with p53-negative tumors compared with those with non-mutated (wild type) p53.

DCC

The deleted in colorectal cancer (DCC) gene is located on the long arm of chromosome 18 (18q) [19] and codifies for a transmembrane protein involved in cell-to-cell adhesion. Because of this adhesion impairment, it has been hypothesized that inactivation of the DCC gene, and thus the absence of DCC protein, may enhance the metastatic potential of a CRC. Clinically, DCC protein expression may also have prognostic significance because patients with DCC-positive Stage II and III CRC were found to have a statistically significant improved overall survival when compared with those with DCC-negative cancers [20]. However, more recent studies question this prognostic significance.

MMR Genes

The recently discovered MMR genes correct base-pair errors that occur during DNA replication [21,22]. As with tumor suppressor genes, both alleles have to be lost or mutated for the MMR gene to be inactive. Phenotypic expression of an MMR gene mutation in tumor cells, namely microsatellite instability (MSI) [23], is currently detectable in the laboratory and is widely used for diagnostic purposes as a screening tool prior to genetic testing. Microsatellites are sequences of DNA base repeats scattered throughout the genome. Some are located near significant protein-encoding genes such as transforming growth factor beta-1 type II receptor, insulin-like growth factor type II receptor, BAX and beta-2-microglobulin [14]. Therefore, with MMR gene inactivation, microsatellite replication errors accumulate (instability) leading to defective protein products (Fig. 3.2). A protein truncation test, in principle similar to that used for APC gene mutation testing, is used for detecting MMR gene mutations in patients whose tumors have MSI. Linkage analysis and direct mutational analysis, although currently not widely clinically available, are other methods for detecting an MMR gene mutation.

Thus far, six MMR genes have been fully identified. Of these, four are HNPCC-related: hMSH2, hMLH1, PMS1 and PMS2, located on 2p, 3p, 2q and 7p, respectively. Germline mutations in hMSH2 and hMLH1 are, however, the two most commonly noted in HNPCC, which accounts for 1–5% of all CRC cases [14]. HNPCC is an autosomal dominantly inherited syndrome characterized by familial aggregation of early age of onset CRC and other associated malignancies such as gynecological, urological or upper gastrointestinal carcinomas, as well as an excess of right-sided, synchronous and metachronous CRC [24]. The estimated penetrance of MMR gene mutations is high, with approximately 80% of MMR gene mutation carriers ultimately developing CRC and 40% developing endometrial cancer. MMR gene mutations comprise the replication error (RER) pathway of colorectal tumorigenesis (Fig. 3.2), characterized by a predominance of diploid right-sided CRC.

As in FAP, genotype–phenotype correlations have also been determined for HNPCC. A recent study demonstrated that kindreds with hMLH1 mutations had a higher incidence of rectal cancer and fewer extracolonic manifestations when compared with those with hMSH2 mutations [25].

Oncogenes

In contradistinction to tumor suppressor and MMR genes, which require loss or mutation of both alleles for inactivation, oncogenes behave in a dominant fashion, such that a mutation in one of the two alleles is sufficient to produce activation and phenotypic expression. Besides c-*Myc* (see APC section), oncogenes implicated in CRC include *ras, neu,* and *myb.* However, relative to *ras,* the prevalence of *neu* and *myb* somatic mutations in CRC is extremely low.

ras

Of the three well-studied *ras* genes, H-*ras*, K-*ras* and N-*ras*, only K-*ras* and N-*ras* have been found to be mutated in colorectal tumors. The K-*ras* gene, which lies on the short arm of chromosome 12 (12p), encodes for p-21 *ras*, a guanosine triphosphatase protein involved in the transduction of growth and differentiation signals [6]. Therefore, when mutated and activated, K-*ras* produces overgrowth and dysplasia. About 50% of CRCs and a similar proportion of adenomas larger than 1 cm harbor *ras* mutations compared with only 9% of adenomas of less than 1 cm, suggesting that, in a proportion of CRCs, *ras* activation is an early promoter rather than an initiator of tumorigenesis [26]. Although the evidence is not as clear as with p53, K-*ras* mutations also appear to have deleterious prognostic significance in CRC patients [17].

Besides tumor suppressor genes, MMR genes and oncogenes, other genetic alterations such as DNA hypomethylation appear to be involved in colorectal tumorigenesis. It has been hypothesized that hypomethylation, one of the earliest changes identified in colonic polyps, may either facilitate overexpression of certain cell growth-related genes or interfere with cell division processes such as normal chromosome pairing [27].

Screening

The high prevalence of rectal cancer, second only to colon cancer among all estimated digestive tract malignancies in the USA, strongly underscores the need for screening. Moreover, because approximately 25% of these new rectal cancer patients will present with advanced fatal disease, early detection programs are likely to save lives as well as be cost-effective.

Since 1992, the American Cancer Society (ACS) has recommended the fecal occult blood test (FOBT) and flexible sigmoidoscopy for the early detection of CRC in asymptomatic individuals aged 50 years and over [28]. However, the importance of a properly performed digital rectal examination cannot be overemphasized because more than 50%

Table 3.2. American cancer society guidelines for CRC screening

| Risk | Classic methods | | TCE | |
	FOBT	Sigmoidoscopy	DCBE	Colonoscopy
Average: Asymptomatic 50 years of age No risk factors	FOBT yearly plus 5-year interval sigmoidoscopy beginning at age 50 years		5–10 years (alternative)	10-year interval (alternative)
Moderate: Personal history of adenomas	Small (<1 cm) single adenoma: as per average risk (after normal TCE at 3 years after initial polyp removal)		Large (>1 cm) or multiple adenomas of any size: 3 years after initial polypectomy, 5 years thereafter if normal	
Personal history of curative-intent resection of CRC	–	–	Not favored	1 year after CRC resection; if normal, in 3 years, and every 5 years thereafter
History of CRC or adenomas in FDR younger than 60 years, or in two or more FDR of any age	–	–	Every 5 years beginning at age 40 years or 10 years before youngest case in the family	
History of CRC in other relatives (not included above)	As per average risk (may consider beginning before age 50)			–
High: FAP family: genetic counseling to consider APC testing at puberty	APC negative[a]: as per average risk	APC positive, indeterminate or no testing: every 1–2 years lifetime (if polyposis consider surgery)		–
HNPCC family: genetic counseling to consider MMR testing at 21 years	MMR negative[a]: as per average risk	–	–	MMR positive, indeterminate or no testing: every 2 years until age 40, then yearly
Inflammatory bowel disease		–	–	Every 1–2 years after 8 years of pancolitis or 12–15 years of left-sided colitis

[a] In a family with a well-documented mutation.
TCE: total colon evaluation; FOBT: fecal occult blood test; DCBE: double contrast barium enema; CRC: colorectal cancer; FDR: first-degree relative; FAP: familial adenomatous polyposis; APC: adenomatous polyposis coli gene; HNPCC: hereditary non-polyposis colorectal cancer; MMR: mismatch repair genes.

of rectal cancers are within the reach of an experienced finger.

Two methods of total colon examination (TCE), colonoscopy and double contrast barium enema (DCBE), were incorporated into the new ACS screening guidelines [29].

In these guidelines (Table 3.2), individuals are stratified according to the following risk for CRC development: (1) average risk (70–80% of all CRC cases), including those who are asymptomatic, 50 years of age or older, without any other risk factor; (2) moderate risk (15–20% of all CRC cases), those with a family history of CRC in one or more FDR, or a personal history of colonic adenomas or CRC; and (3) high risk (5–10% of all CRC cases), those with a family history of FAP or HNPCC, or a personal history of inflammatory bowel disease.

Average Risk

For average risk individuals, three population-based randomized trials have shown a significant reduction in CRC-related mortality by screening with FOBT [30–32]. Although the Danish [31] and British [30] trials compared 2-year interval screening with controls, the Minnesota Colon Cancer Control Study [32] compared 1–2-year interval screening with controls and demonstrated a significant decrease in CRC mortality for the annually screened group compared with both the biennially screened and control groups. This supports the current recommendation of a yearly FOBT. It is expected that the efficacy of FOBT screening will improve with the use of newer and more sensitive tests such as Hemoccult II Sensa and HemeSelect [33] (SmithKline Diagnostics, San Jose, CA). Should the FOBT be positive on any sample, TCE by colonoscopy is currently recommended, although a DCBE with flexible sigmoidoscopy may be an alternative.

The rationale for screening sigmoidoscopy for average risk individuals comes from two case-control studies that revealed a reduced mortality from cancer of the distal colon and rectum in the screened group compared with controls [34,35]. Although one of the studies demonstrated that a 10-year interval screening might be safe [35], the current recommendation is flexible sigmoidoscopy every 5 years. Colonoscopy should be offered to those individuals found to have small (<1 cm) adenomas or large (>1 cm) polyps. Colonoscopic polypectomy has been shown to lower the incidence of CRC; it is therefore recommended that all adenomatous polyps identified should be removed [36].

Alternatives to FOBT and sigmoidoscopy include: DCBE every 5–10 years or a colonoscopy every 10 years. However, in contradistinction to FOBT and sigmoidoscopy, TCE strategies are not yet substantiated by any study showing a reduction in CRC mortality. DCBE is a safer procedure than sigmoidoscopy or colonoscopy, but has a major drawback because of its inability to remove polyps or biopsy questionable lesions. Moreover, DCBE will also miss more small polyps and produce more false positives than colonoscopy.

Moderate Risk

Those who are at moderate risk for CRC include individuals with family members affected with CRC or adenomatous polyps or a personal history of CRC or adenomatous polyps.

Individuals with close relatives affected by CRC or adenomatous polyps should begin screening at the age of 40 years or 10 years before the youngest case in the family, whichever is the earlier. As the risk of developing CRC is greater with increasing numbers of young and closely affected family members, meticulous screening in kindreds with one or more affected FDR or an index CRC case in a patient younger than 55 years of age (60 for adenomatous polyps) should be strongly enforced.

The recommendation for individuals with a previously resected CRC is to undergo TCE within 1 year of resection if complete evaluation of the colon was not performed preoperatively. If this is normal, subsequent TCE should be offered 3 years later, and every 5 years thereafter. If the rest of the colon was appropriately examined before surgery, a TCE should be done 3 years after resection and, if normal, every 5 years thereafter. Because of its higher sensitivity and ability to procure biopsy specimens, colonoscopy rather than DCBE (even with the addition of flexible sigmoidoscopy) is favored in this subset of patients.

People with previously excised adenomatous polyps are recommended to undergo a TCE 3 years after the initial polypectomy. If the initial adenoma was small (<1 cm) and single and the follow-up TCE is normal, the patient is subsequently screened as per average risk recommendations. If the initial adenoma was large (>1 cm) or there were multiple adenomas of any size, and the first follow-up TCE is normal, it should be repeated every 5 years thereafter. For this subset of patients, DCBE (with or without a flexible sigmoidoscopy) appears to be a good alternative to colonoscopy.

Increased Risk

Members of an FAP kindred should be tested for APC gene mutation status at puberty. Genetic counseling should be offered prior to genetic testing in order to discuss testing-related issues, including alternatives for long-term surveillance and prophylactic surgical management. A positive test result mandates lifetime annual sigmoidoscopy until the development of disease. If colonic polyposis is present, a prophylactic colectomy is indicated, with regular screening for upper gastrointestinal polyps. The most appropriate time for colectomy should be discussed and decided together with the patient and family. However, unless there is bleeding, large (>1 cm) adenomas or atypia, the period between high school and college is favored. Because FAP usually involves the entire colorectum, there is a risk of developing rectal cancer in the rectal mucosa of those who have undergone total abdominal colectomy and ileorectal anastomosis. In these patients, frequent bi-annual endoscopic follow-up of the rectal remnant should be offered. It is important to emphasize the need to survey the ileo-anal pouch and anastomosis of FAP patients because recent reports clearly document the development of both polyps [37] and malignant neoplasms [38] in these two sites.

A negative test result rules out FAP in a non-affected individual only if an affected family member has a well-documented mutation. In these circumstances, family members who test negative have been reassured about their normal status and spared further screening until age 50, at which point screening as per average risk (Table 3.2) has been recommended.

Individuals with an indeterminate test result as well as members of an FAP kindred in whom genetic testing is not feasible should be offered annual sigmoidoscopy. It is estimated that the risk of developing the disease decreases to 50% by age 20 and 8% by age 30.

Members of an HNPCC family should be offered genetic counseling and consider genetic testing for MMR gene mutations. However, in upwards of 65% of HNPCC kindreds a mutation cannot be detected. In 1991, the Amsterdam criteria were established [39]. These criteria, commonly referred to as the rule of 3, 2, 1, require: at least *three* relatives with histologically proven CRC in at least *two* generations, one of them an FDR of the other two; at least *one* CRC diagnosed before the age of 50; and FAP excluded.

Recently, the recognition of MSI as phenotypic expression of MMR gene mutations has led to the development of the Bethesda guidelines for testing colorectal tumors for MSI. The following list is modified from Rodriguez-Bigas et al. [40] and applies to individuals with:

A colorectal tumor in families that meet the Amsterdam criteria

Two HNPCC-related cancers, including synchronous and metachronous colorectal cancers or associated extracolonic cancers

Colorectal cancer and a first-degree relative with colorectal cancer and/or HNPCC-related extracolonic cancer and/or a colorectal adenoma; one of the cancers diagnosed at age <45 years, and the adenoma diagnosed at age <40 years

Colorectal cancer or endometrial cancer diagnosed at age <45 years

Right-sided colorectal cancer with an undifferentiated pattern (solid/cribiform) on histopathology diagnosed at age <45years

Signet ring cell-type (>50% signet ring cells) colorectal cancer diagnosed at age <45 years

Adenomas diagnosed at age <40 years

These guidelines should enable the identification of HNPCC families that do not fulfill the Amsterdam criteria. In addition to testing for MSI in CRC patients whose families meet the Amsterdam criteria, these guidelines also suggest testing CRC patients with a strong family history of CRC, patients with early age of onset CRC or adenomatous polyps or HNPCC-associated extracolonic cancers, as well as CRC patients with the classic clinicopathological features of HNPCC. If the tumor displays MSI, the patient is considered to be a candidate for MMR mutation testing.

Individuals with a positive MMR gene mutation test, an indeterminate test result or a family history of HNPCC in a non-tested individual should have a TCE every 1–2 years, starting between the ages of 20 and 30 years, and then every year after 40 years of age. Because of the predominance of right-sided tumors in HNPCC, colonoscopy is the procedure of choice. However, a DCBE together with flexible sigmoidoscopy is a good alternative. The apparently accelerated adenoma-to-carcinoma sequence noted in patients with HNPCC relative to those with sporadic CRC is the basis for the recommended shorter surveillance intervals. A negative test result rules out the disease only if a well-documented mutation has been previously identified in the family. In the absence of such a mutation, a negative test result has to be interpreted with great caution.

Although a total abdominal colectomy is recommended for HNPCC patients presenting with colon cancer, a prophylactic colectomy in healthy MMR gene mutation carriers with a normal colon remains controversial because current estimates anticipate that perhaps 20% of these individuals will never develop CRC. Furthermore, because there is an estimated 1% per year risk of developing rectal cancer in HNPCC patients after a total abdominal colectomy with ileorectal anastomosis, a total abdominal proctocolectomy in carefully selected HNPCC patients with early stage rectal cancer appears appropriate [41].

Although the optimal method has not been determined, annual screening for endometrial cancer beginning at age 25–35 years is recommended for MMR gene mutation carriers. Routine prophylactic hysterectomy and bilateral salpingo-oophorectomy for all healthy MMR gene mutation carriers also remains controversial. Screening for other HNPCC-related extracolonic cancers such as ovarian or genitourinary is recommended, especially when there is a family history of the cancer.

It is recommended that patients with inflammatory bowel disease should undergo screening colonoscopy on a regular basis to rule out CRC. Dysplasia is the marker of CRC risk and the most important factor for considering colectomy. Colonoscopies with random biopsies are recommended every 1–2 years beginning after 8 years of disease in patients with pancolitis or after 15 years in patients with segmental disease limited to the left colon.

Chemoprevention

Chemoprevention is the use of specific natural or synthetic chemical agents to prevent, inhibit or reverse tumorigenic progression to invasive cancer. It is not intended to treat invasive carcinomas and, therefore, should be clearly distinguished from chemotherapy. The main goals of chemoprevention are to block the original initiation of the carcinogenic process, to arrest or reverse further progression of premalignant cells into becoming invasive or metastatic.

Agents investigated for chemopreventive activity in CRC include: (1) non-steroidal anti-inflammatory drugs (NSAIDs) such as aspirin, ibuprofen, piroxicam, sulindac or the new selective cyclo-oxygenase (COX)-2 inhibitors such as celecoxib; (2) calcium; (3) antioxidant vitamins; (4) curcumin; (5) perillyl alcohol; (6) oltipraz; and (7) selenium. Although most chemopreventive agents have been studied in CRC animal models, many trials in humans are currently under way that focus on FAP patients, those with prior resections of early stage CRC, those with a history of adenomatous colonic polyps, and healthy individuals.

NSAIDs

Studies in rodents exposed to chemical carcinogens have shown that NSAIDs inhibit the development of colorectal tumors by blocking prostaglandin (a group of essential mediators of many physiological functions) synthesis through the inhibition of COX [42], which is also important because COX itself has been demonstrated to stimulate angiogenesis induced by colorectal cancer cells [43].

Sulindac

Although several epidemiological studies have shown that aspirin can decrease the risk of CRC, sulindac is probably the most extensively studied NSAID in relation to CRC chemoprevention. It inhibits COX activity through its metabolite sulindac sulfate. A key study in humans demonstrated sulindac's efficacy, at doses ranging from 150 to 400 mg daily, for eliminating colorectal polyps in FAP and patients with Gardner's syndrome [44]. Although the polyps re-grew when the drug was discontinued, they disappeared again after its reinstitution, suggesting the need for lifelong therapy. No effect was observed in gastric or small bowel polyps.

More recently, a randomized, double-blind trial of sulindac 300 mg daily for 9 months versus placebo in 22 FAP patients has demonstrated a 56% decrease in the baseline number of colorectal polyps and a 65% decrease in the baseline size of the polyps for those patients who received this agent [45]. However, complete resolution of polyposis was not observed in any patient. As in previous studies, 3 months after discontinuation of the drug, both the number and size of polyps in sulindac-treated patients increased.

In contrast to the previous studies, which did not report any side effects, a recent trial of sulindac 300 mg daily (subsequently reduced to 100 mg) in six Japanese FAP patients identified five with drug-related complications [46]. These ranged from severe nausea and vomiting to multiple ulcers of the small bowel and stomach, prompting premature stoppage of therapy in four patients. The investigators concluded that response to sulindac might be race specific.

Nevertheless, according to a German study conducted on 28 FAP patients who had undergone total abdominal colectomy and ileorectal anastomosis, the dose of sulindac (suppositories) can be progressively decreased from 300 mg daily to a mean of 67 mg daily after 3 years of treatment in the majority of responding patients. This maintains excellent control of the rectal polyposis with very mild side effects [47]. This study also demonstrated a permanent antiproliferative effect of low-dose sulindac on rectal mucosa, as well as its influence on tumor suppressor genes and apoptosis markers, further stressing the importance of gene interaction and apoptosis mediation in NSAID-related chemoprevention.

Selective COX-2 inhibitors

The COX enzyme family is currently believed to be comprised of two isoenzymes: cyclo-oxygenase 1 (COX-1) and cyclo-oxygenase 2 (COX-2) [48]. COX-1, which is involved in several physiologic functions, was characterized in 1976 as constitutively expressed and responsible for the secondary effects of COX inhibition, such as gastrointestinal bleeding.

The discovery in 1991 of COX-2, the inducible isoenzyme of COX and the one with anti-inflammatory activity, generated much excitement for a variety of reasons. First, COX-2 mRNA and protein are overexpressed in upwards of 80% of CRC and almost 50% of gastrointestinal adenomas, in contradistinction to COX-1, which remains unchanged in CRC and adenomas when compared with normal mucosa [49]. It is interesting to note that COX-2 overexpression is significantly more common in CRC arising through the loss of the heterozygosity pathway when compared with CRC arising through the replication error–MSI pathway [50]. Concordantly, clinicopathological features significantly associated with low COX-2 staining include those typical of MMR-deficient CRC, such as right-sided predisposition, tumor infiltrating lymphocytosis, and solid/cribiform or signet ring histological patterns. In essence, these biological differences suggest that patients with FAP will benefit more than those with HNPCC from selective COX-2 chemoprevention.

In addition, recent experiments with mice carrying a mutant APC gene resulting in a truncated, non-functional APC protein, demonstrated high levels of COX-2 in even the smallest gastrointestinal polyps, whereas the levels of COX-1 in the same polyps were similar to those in normal mucosa [49]. Moreover, when APC-deficient mice were rendered COX-2 deficient via knockout mechanisms, they developed significantly less and smaller polyps than APC-deficient mice with normal COX-2, suggesting that COX-2 plays an important role in polyp growth.

Furthermore, selective inhibition of COX-2 does not appear to induce as many side effects as other NSAIDs. Although all NSAIDs inhibit the activity of both COX-1 and COX-2, groups can be distinguished based on a COX-1 to COX-2 inhibition ratio. Selective COX-1 inhibitors include aspirin and indomethacin. Equipotent inhibitors include sulindac, diclofenac and naproxen, while selective COX-2 inhibitors include experimental drugs such as BF 389 or MF tricyclic, or the commercially available celecoxib [48]. Because of their specificity and lack of gastrointestinal side effects, these selective COX-2 inhibitors appear to be the future of NSAID-based chemoprevention, particularly in FAP patients.

Finally, a recent study has shown that the tumor suppressive effect of the COX-inhibiting NSAIDs is not likely to be related to a reduction of prostaglandin synthesis but rather to an elevation of the prostaglandin precursor and COX substrate arachidonic acid [51]. Arachidonic acid is a potent stimulator of the conversion of sphingomyelin to ceramide, which happens to be a powerful inducer of apoptosis. Therefore, ceramide could possibly prevent the malignant transformation of adenomatous colonic crypt cells by driving them to apoptosis. It appears that lipids such as arachidonic acid and ceramide play key roles in preventing colorectal tumorigenesis. It is anticipated that their manipulation may, in fact, turn out to be one of the most promising future directions in CRC chemoprevention.

Calcium

Although calcium is certainly involved in basic steps such as differentiation, proliferation and signaling, its potential chemopreventive activity in CRC arises from its ability to bind enteral bile acids and fatty acids to form insoluble calcium soaps, thus eliminating their carcinogenic effect on the colonic epithelium. This is supported by several rodent studies that have shown a decrease in bile acid- and fatty acid-induced colon crypt cell hyperproliferation after calcium supplementation [52].

Unfortunately, randomized studies in humans have not been successful thus far. One of them [53], conducted in the USA on 21 patients with histologically documented sporadic colonic adenomas, showed, after 8 weeks of treatment, no difference in rectal epithelial cell proliferation between the group taking a calcium supplement and the group that received a calcium-free placebo. Furthermore, a more recent British study on 79 patients with adenoma who were randomized to receive calcium or placebo for 2 years reported comparable results regarding rectal mucosal proliferation [54]. Moreover, this study also demonstrated that the occurrence of de novo colonic adenomas was similar in both groups after 2 years. The authors concluded that calcium supplementation did not show any antineoplastic effect [55].

In summary, the antiproliferative effect of physiological amounts of calcium noted in vitro does not appear to occur in vivo. Furthermore, the cells show no response to calcium after their dedifferentiation to adenoma or carcinoma [52]. Nevertheless, to define its role better, a number of trials studying the effect of calcium, alone or in combination with other chemopreventive agents such as vitamin D or

NSAIDs, on adenomas and CRC are currently in progress.

Antioxidant Vitamins

Although several epidemiological studies suggest that the antioxidant vitamins found abundantly in fruits and vegetables reduce CRC risk, the results from several clinical trials remain, thus far, inconclusive.

An Italian study demonstrated that dietary supplements with vitamins A, C and E taken for 6 months significantly decreased cell proliferative abnormalities in the upper 40% of rectal mucosa crypts when compared with placebo [56]. However, this study failed to show any significant variation in overall rectal mucosa labeling index. Moreover, the beneficial effect disappeared 6 months after the cessation of treatment, when differences in proliferative parameters were not significant.

In addition, a clinical trial conducted in the USA by the Polyp Prevention Study Group in patients previously diagnosed with colorectal adenomas demonstrated no reduction in the relative risk of developing new adenomas after beta-carotene (a vitamin A precursor) and vitamins C and E supplementation for 4 years [57]. The investigators suggest that components other than antioxidant vitamins, such as fiber or folate, may better explain the CRC protective effect of fruits and vegetables.

Curcumin

Curcumin, a component of the turmeric plant (*Curcuma longa* Linn), has been used for centuries as a natural remedy for a wide variety of diseases. It is also a commonly used spice and food additive, constituting the main yellow pigment in curry and mustard, and has been shown in several animal tumor models to have chemopreventive properties against stomach, small intestine and colorectal cancer.

In a recent study, curcumin decreased equally the proliferative rate of cell lines, with and without prostaglandin synthetic ability [58], suggesting an effect independent from the COX pathway. This reduction in proliferation rate is due to an accumulation of cells in the G2/M cell cycle phase, clearly distinct from the G1 transition blockage induced by NSAIDs. Moreover, in contradistinction to NSAIDs, curcumin failed to induce apoptosis.

Perillyl Alcohol

Perillyl alcohol, one of several hydroxylated derivatives of the monoterpene D-limonene, is found mostly in lavender and other natural foods such as cherries, mint or celery seeds. As a D-limonene, perillyl alcohol selectively inhibits the isoprenylation of small guanine-binding proteins such as the *ras* oncogene product. In addition, perillyl alcohol also inhibits tumor cell proliferation and promotes cell differentiation.

The chemopreventive properties of perillyl alcohol, studied mainly in CRC animal models, remain unclear. A recent study compared the incidence of azoxymethane-induced adenocarcinomas of the small intestine and colon in F-344 rats fed a diet with and without perillyl alcohol for 1 year [59]. The incidence and multiplicity of colonic adenocarcinomas were significantly suppressed in animals fed 1 g of perillyl alcohol/kg diet. The study also demonstrated a significant increase in the apoptotic index in colonic tumors of animals fed a diet containing perillyl alcohol when compared with controls.

Oltipraz

Oltipraz is a synthetic dithiolethione previously used to treat schistosomiasis. Natural dithiolethiones are found in large amounts in certain vegetables such as cabbage, cauliflower and broccoli. The decrease of CRC risk associated with a vegetable-rich diet is partly accounted for by dithiolethione-driven overexpression of a number of detoxication enzymes such as glutathione S-transferase and DT-diaphorase, which protect DNA from mutagen-induced damage.

Several tumor animal models have already demonstrated the preventive effect of oltipraz and large-scale studies in humans are currently under way. A recent study in 24 individuals at high risk for CRC demonstrated non-toxic doses of oltipraz (125 mg/m^2) to enhance glutathione S-transferase activity significantly, as well as the expression of CRC-protective genes such as DT-diaphorase and gamma-glutamylcysteine synthetase in colonic mucosa [60]. Additionally, modulation of gene expression in colonic mucosa correlated well with that noted in peripheral mononuclear cells, thereby identifying blood as an easily available alternative to sigmoidoscopic biopsy assessment of gene expression.

Selenium

The preventive potential of selenium in human CRC was noted in a multicenter randomized study in 1312 patients with a history of basal or squamous cell carcinoma of the skin [61]. A secondary endpoint was the incidence of prostate, lung and CRC.

With a total follow-up of 6.4 years, the investigators observed a significant reduction in the incidence of all three malignancies among individuals treated with 200 μg of selenium (in the form of brewer's yeast tablets) for 4.5 years when compared with those who received placebo.

Although not fully understood, the mechanisms by which selenium prevents colorectal carcinogenesis may include the inhibition of peroxidation, free radical scavenging, repair of molecular damage, and incorporation into detoxication enzymes such as glutathione peroxidase.

A study conducted in F-344 rats fed high- or low-fat diets supplemented with selenium, and subsequently challenged with the CRC-inducing chemical azoxymethane, demonstrated that the combination of selenium and a low-fat diet achieved the greatest reduction in both tumor incidence and multiplicity [62].

References

1. Guillem JG, Bastar AL, Ng J, Huhn JL, Cohen AM. Clustering of colorectal cancer in families of probands under 40 years of age. Dis Colon Rectum 1996;39:1004–1007.
2. Hall NR, Finan PJ, Ward B, Turner G, Bishop DT. Genetic susceptibility to colorectal cancer in patients under 45 years of age. Br J Surg 1994;81:1485–89.
3. Fearon ER, Vogelstein B. A genetic model for colorectal tumorigenesis. Cell 1990;61:759–67.
4. Kinzler KW, Vogelstein B. Lessons from hereditary colorectal cancer. Cell 1996;87:159–70.
5. Knudson AG, Hethcote HW, Brown BW. Mutation and childhood cancer: a probabilistic model for the incidence of retinoblastoma. Proc Natl Acad Sci U S A 1975;72:5116–20.
6. Howe JR, Guillem JG. The genetics of colorectal cancer. Surg Clin North Am 1997;77:175–95.
7. Burt RW, Petersen GM. Familial colorectal cancer: diagnosis and management. In: Young GP, Rozen P, Levin B, editors. Prevention and early detection of colorectal cancer. London: Saunders, 1996:171–94.
8. Guillem JG, Puig-La Calle J Jr, Cellini C, et al. Varying features of early age-of-onset "sporadic" and hereditary nonpolyposis colorectal cancer patients. Dis Colon Rectum 1999;42:36–42.
9. Laken SJ, Petersen GM, Gruber SB, et al. Familial colorectal cancer in Ashkenazim due to a hypermutable tract in APC. Nat Genet 1997;17:79–83.
10. Bodmer WF, Bailey CJ, Bodmer J, et al. Localization of the gene for familial adenomatous polyposis on chromosome 5. Nature 1987;328:614–16.
11. Pennisi E. How a growth control path takes a wrong turn to cancer. Science 1998;281:1438–41.
12. O'Sullivan MJ, McCarthy TV, Doyle CT. Familial adenomatous polyposis. From bedside to benchside. Am J Clin Pathol 1998;109:521–26.
13. He T-C, Sparks AB, Rago C, et al. Identification of c-Myc as a target of the APC pathway. Science 1998;281:1509–12.
14. Guillem J, Smith A, Puig-La Calle J Jr, Ruo L. Gastrointestinal polyposis syndromes. Curr Probl Surg 1999;36:217–324.
15. Isobe M, Emanuel BS, Givol G, Oren M, Croce CM. Localization of gene for human p53 tumour antigen to band 17p13. Nature 1986;320:84–85.
16. Grewal H, Guillem JG, Klimstra DS, Cohen AM. p53 nuclear overexpression may not be an independent prognostic marker in early colorectal cancer. Dis Colon Rectum 1995;38:1176–81.
17. Pricolo VE, Finkelstein SD, Wu TT, et al. Prognostic value of TP53 and K-ras-2 mutational analysis in Stage III carcinoma of the colon. Am J Surg 1996;171:41–46.
18. Belluco C, Guillem JG, Kemeny N, et al. p53 nuclear protein overexpression in colorectal cancer: a dominant predictor of survival in patients with advanced hepatic metastases. J Clin Oncol 1996;14:2696–701.
19. Fearon ER, Cho KR, Nigro JM, et al. Identification of a chromosome 18q gene that is altered in colorectal cancers. Science 1990;247:49–56.
20. Shibata D, Reale MA, Lavin P, et al. The DCC protein and prognosis in colorectal cancer. N Engl J Med 1996;335:1727–32.
21. Aaltonen LA, Peltomaki P, Leach FS, et al. Clues to the pathogenesis of familial colorectal cancer. Science 1993;260:812–16.
22. Ionov Y, Peinado MA, Malkhosyan S, Shibata D, Perucho M. Ubiquitous somatic mutations in simple repeated sequences reveal a new mechanism for colonic carcinogenesis. Nature 1993;363:558–61.
23. Thibodeau SN, Bren G, Schaid D. Microsatellite instability in cancer of the proximal colon. Science 1993;260:816–19.
24. Lynch HT, Smyrk TC, Watson P, et al. Genetics, natural history, tumor spectrum, and pathology of hereditary nonpolyposis colorectal cancer: an updated review. Gastroenterology 1993;104:1535–49.
25. Weber TK, Conlon W, Petrelli NJ, et al. Genomic DNA-based hMSH2 and hMLH1 mutation screening in 32 Eastern United States hereditary nonpolyposis colorectal cancer. Cancer Res 1997;57:3798–803.
26. Vogelstein B, Fearon ER, Hamilton SR, et al. Genetic alterations during colorectal tumor development. N Engl J Med 1988;319:525–32.
27. Goelz SE, Vogelstein B, Hamilton SR, Feinberg AP. Hypomethylation of DNA from benign and malignant human colon neoplasms. Science 1985;228:187–90.
28. Levin B and Murphy GP. Revision in American Cancer Society recommendations for the early detection of colorectal cancer. CA Cancer J Clin 1992;42:296–99.
29. Byers T, Levin B, Rothenberger D, Dodd GD, Smith RA. American Cancer Society guidelines for screening and surveillance for early detection of colorectal polyps and cancer: update 1997. CA Cancer J Clin 1997;47:154–60.
30. Hardcastle JD, Chamberlain JO, Robinson MHE, et al. Randomised controlled trial of faecal occult blood screening for colorectal cancer. Lancet 1996;348:1472–77.
31. Kronborg O, Fenger C, Olsen J, Jorgensen OD, Sondegaard O. Randomised study of screening for colorectal cancer with faecal occult blood test. Lancet 1996;348:1467–71.
32. Mandel JS, Bond JH, Church TR, et al. Reducing mortality from colorectal cancer by screening for fecal occult blood. N Engl J Med 1993;328:1365–71.
33. Allison JE, Tekawa IS, Ransom LJ, Adrain AL. A comparison of fecal occult blood test for colorectal cancer screening. N Engl J Med 1996;334:155–59.
34. Newcomb PA, Norfleet RG, Storer BE, Surawicz TS, Marcus PM. Screening sigmoidoscopy and colorectal cancer mortality. J Natl Cancer Inst 1992;84:1572–75.
35. Selby JV, Friedman GD, Quesenberry CP, Weiss NS. A case-control study of screening sigmoidoscopy and mortality from colorectal cancer. N Engl J Med 1992;326:653–57.

36. Winawer SJ, Zauber AG, Ho MN, et al. Prevention of colorectal cancer by colonoscopic polypectomy. N Engl J Med 1993;329:1977–81.

37. van Duijvendijk P, Vasen HFA, Bertario L, et al. Cumulative risk of developing polyps or malignancy at the ileal pouch–anal anastomosis in patients with familial adenomatous polyposis. J Gastrointest Surg 1999;3:325–30.

38. von Herbay A, Stern J, Herfarth C. Pouch–anal cancer after restorative proctocolectomy for familial adenomatous polyposis. Am J Surg Pathol 1996;20:995–99.

39. Vasen HFA, Mecklin J-P, Meera Khan P, Lynch HT. The International Collaborative Group on Hereditary Non-Polyposis Colorectal Cancer (ICG-HNPCC). Dis Colon Rectum 1991;34:424–25.

40. Rodriguez-Bigas MA, Boland CR, Hamilton SR, et al. A National Cancer Institute workshop on hereditary nonpolyposis colorectal cancer syndrome: meeting highlights and Bethesda guidelines. J Natl Cancer Inst 1997; 89:1758–62.

41. Rodriguez-Bigas MA, Vasen HF, Pekka-Mecklin J, et al. Rectal cancer risk in hereditary nonpolyposis colorectal cancer after abdominal colectomy: International Collaborative Group on HNPCC. Ann Surg 1997;225:202–207.

42. Rao CV, Rivenson A, Simi B, et al. Chemoprevention of colon carcinogenesis by sulindac, a nonsteroidal antiinflammatory agent. Cancer Res 1995;55:1464–72.

43. Tsujii M, Kawano S, Tsuji S, Sawaoka H, Hori M, DuBois RN. Cyclooxygenase regulates angiogenesis induced by colon cancer cells. Cell 1998;93:705–16.

44. Waddell WR, Ganser GF, Cerise EJ, Loughry RW. Sulindac for polyposis of the colon. Am J Surg 1989;157:175–79.

45. Giardiello FM, Hamilton SR, Krush AJ, et al. Treatment of colonic and rectal adenomas with sulindac in familial adenomatous polyposis. N Engl J Med 1993;328:1313–16.

46. Ishikawa H, Akedo I, Suzuki T, Narahara H, Otani T. Adverse effects of sulindac used for prevention of colorectal cancer. J Natl Cancer Inst 1997;89:1381.

47. Winde G, Schmid KW, Brandt B, Muller O, Osswald H. Clinical and genomic influence of sulindac on rectal mucosa in familial adenomatous polyposis. Dis Colon Rectum 1997;40:1156–69.

48. Taketo MM. Cyclooxigenase-2 inhibitors in tumorigenesis (Part I). J Natl Cancer Inst 1998;90:1529–36.

49. Taketo MM. Cyclooxigenase-2 inhibitors in tumorigenesis (Part II). J Natl Cancer Inst 1998;90:1609–20.

50. Karnes WE, Shattuck-Brandt R, Burgart LJ, et al. Reduced COX-2 protein in colorectal cancer with defective mismatch repair. Cancer Res 1998;58:5473–77.

51. Chan TA, Morin PJ, Vogelstein B, Kinzler KW. Mechanisms underlying nonsteroidal antiinflammatory drug-mediated apoptosis. Proc Natl Acad Sci USA 1998;95:681–86.

52. Lipkin M. Biomarkers of increased susceptibility to gastrointestinal cancer: new application to studies of cancer prevention in human subjects. Cancer Res 1988;48:235–45.

53. Bostick RM, Potter JD, Fosdick L, et al. Calcium and colorectal epithelial cell proliferation: a preliminary randomized, double blinded, placebo-controlled clinical trial. J Natl Cancer Inst 1993;85:132–41.

54. Armitage NC, Rooney PS, Gifford K-A, Clarke PA, Hardcastle JD. The effect of calcium supplements on rectal mucosa proliferation. Br J Cancer 1995;71:186–90.

55. Rooney PS, Clarke PA, Gifford K-A, Elliott LJ, Hardcastle JD, Armitage NC. A randomised trial of 1.5 g calcium in patients with colorectal adenomata. Gut 1995;36(suppl 1):A22.

56. Paganelli GM, Biasco G, Brandi G, et al. Effect of vitamin A, C and E supplementation on rectal cell proliferation in patients with colorectal adenomas. J Natl Cancer Inst 1992;84:47–51.

57. Greenberg ER, Baron JA, Tosteson TD, et al. A clinical trial of antioxidant vitamins to prevent colorectal adenoma. N Engl J Med 1994;331:141–47.

58. Hanif R, Qiao L, Shiff SJ, Rigas B. Curcumin, a natural plant phenolic food additive, inhibits cell proliferation and induces cell cycle changes in colon adenocarcinoma cell lines by a prostaglandin-independent pathway. J Lab Clin Med 1997;130:576–84.

59. Reddy BS, Wang C-X, Samaha H, et al. Chemoprevention of colon carcinogenesis by dietary perillyl alcohol. Cancer Res 1997;57:420–25.

60. O'Dwyer PJ, Szarka CE, Yao K-S, et al. Modulation of gene expression in subjects at risk for colorectal cancer by the chemopreventive dithiolethione oltipraz. J Clin Invest 1996;98:1210–17.

61. Clark LC, Combs JF Jr, Turnbull BW, et al. Effects of selenium supplementation for cancer prevention in patients with carcinoma of the skin: a randomized controlled trial. JAMA 1996;276:1957–63.

62. Reddy BS, Rivenson A, El-Bayoumy K, Upadhyaya P, Pittman B, Rao CV. Chemoprevention of colon cancer by organoselenium compounds and impact of high- or low-fat diets. J Natl Cancer Inst 1997;89:506–12.

4. The Role of Imaging in the Diagnosis and Staging of Primary and Recurrent Rectal Cancer

S. Sironi, C. Ferrero, L. Gianolli, C. Landoni, A. Del Maschio, F. Fazio and A.P. Zbar

Introduction

Malignant tumors of the rectum are most commonly detected by fecal occult blood testing, digital rectal examination, barium enema or lower gastrointestinal endoscopy (rigid sigmoidoscopy, flexible sigmoidoscopy or colonoscopy). The decision regarding appropriate treatment in the patient with rectal cancer depends on accurate imaging of the tumor in an effort to define tumor depth, the presence of involved mesorectal nodal involvement, and any evidence of distant metastases at the time of initial diagnosis. In the former instance, delineation of confinement of the tumor to the mucosa or submucosa would enhance decision making regarding local therapies such as local excision of distal lesions, transanal endomicrosurgery of small, more proximal tumors, photocoagulation or contact irradiation. Identification of transmural or serosal involvement, especially the presence of invasion into local structures, assists in defining patients who are suitable for preoperative neo-adjuvant chemoradiation, which has been shown to reduce locoregional recurrence and enhance survival in selected patients [1–3]. Clearly, the definition of contiguous pelvic visceral involvement in clinically tethered tumors also permits a selective approach towards radiotherapeutic downstaging as well as extending the range of palliative resection. Finally, accurate imaging in patients presenting with a primary rectal tumor will define those with visceral metastatic disease and/or peritoneal spread. In the postoperative setting, newer modalities have assisted in the distinction of pelvic recurrence from either post-surgical or post-irradiation fibrosis. Furthermore, positron emission tomography (PET) has shown tremendous potential for detecting small tumor deposits locoregionally and at distant sites.

It is still surprisingly somewhat debatable whether imaging designed to assess the local extent of spread is superior to careful digital examination performed by an experienced coloproctologist and whether it can influence overall surgical decision-making [4–6]. Despite numerous studies documenting that other tumor-related variables such as mucin production, ploidy and lymphovascular invasion are independent prognostic variables that influence recurrence and survival [7–10], stage of disease remains the most important feature influencing management and outcome. All efforts must be made to stage patients with rectal cancer accurately in order to direct therapy with the best oncologic result. This chapter outlines and critically reviews the role of clinical evaluation, contrast examination, endorectal ultrasound (ERUS), computed tomography (CT), magnetic resonance (MR) imaging (surface, pelvic phased-array or endoanal), PET and radioimmunoscintigraphy in the diagnosis and staging of primary and recurrent rectal cancer.

Diagnostic Imaging in the Staging of Primary Rectal Cancer

Clinical Evaluation

A number of rectal tumors can be detected by digital rectal examination. Results are often reported as "mobile", "tethered" or "fixed". Many tumors are obviously beyond the reach of the examining finger, making clinical staging impossible. The accuracy of clinical staging varies between examiners and is directly related to clinical experience [11]. Tumors that are large, fixed and contain bulky mesorectal lymph nodes are easily labeled "advanced"; however, it is the smaller tumors that can cause overstaging or understaging and may lead to inappropriate treatment. The palpation of extra-rectal metastases that are remote from the tumor, such as seen with a "palpable liver mass" indicative of metastases, obviously predict an unfavorable prognosis.

It is clear that current imaging modalities such as endorectal ultrasound are superior to that of digital rectal examination. The more frequent overstaging of small tumors is a major drawback of digital examination. The understaging of larger tumors is of minor importance because most will be removed by radical surgery. Nevertheless, the understaging of such lesions may distract the caregiver from employing neo-adjuvant therapy with its potential benefits of downstaging, increasing resectability and sphincter preservation. Mesorectal involvement is still met with uncertainty; it is crucial to delineate this when planning therapy. Digital examination seems to have little value in the detection of regional node metastases, except in far advanced tumors. The role of ERUS in delineating the presence of regional lymph nodes has been met with a high number of false positives as well as false negatives. It is commonplace today to employ an additional staging modality other than digital examination in the local staging of rectal cancer.

Contrast Examinations

A barium enema is an inexpensive, safe and effective way to diagnose colorectal neoplasms (Fig. 4.1). False-negative errors in interpreting the results of a barium enema are usually caused by perceptive lapses, technical problems or both [12]. The detection of such lesions depends on the quality and type of examination performed and the size of tumor present. An excellent review of the strengths and pitfalls of barium enema in the detection of colo-rectal neoplasms has been provided by Ott [12].

Nearly 50% of all large bowel neoplasms missed by single contrast barium enema are located in the rectum [13]. Despite improved detection offered by the double-contrast technique, it is still wise to perform either rigid (or preferably flexible) sigmoidoscopy prior to a contrast enema request in order to visualize this region adequately [14,15]. Rectal lesions may be polypoid (particularly in the rectal ampulla), annular (typically restosigmoid) or flat, therefore patient positioning may be required to assess fully these regions of the rectum. Polypoid lesions will appear as filling defects, typically located in dependent regions of the barium pool, whereas lesions near the angulated rectosigmoid junction are best seen by using cross-table lateral views with

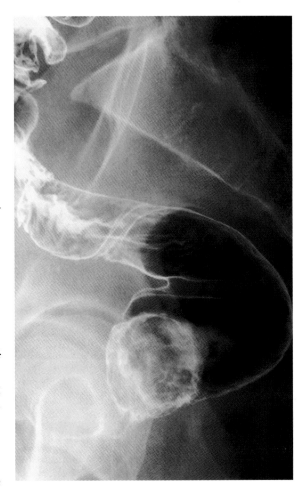

Fig. 4.1. Double contrast barium enema: 5 cm polypoid lesion of distal rectum and small polypoid lesion cranially. At pathological evaluation a pT1 adenocarcinoma in adenoma was found. The small polypoid lesions were hyperplastic polyps.

the patient screened prone. Lesions that are visible on only one projection can be obscured by contrast material and require a high degree of suspicion on the part of the radiologist.

Moreover, neoplasms that develop as a result of long-standing colitis, which are typically more plaque-like and infiltrative, associated with diffuse tapered narrowing of the lumen, relative gut rigidity on distension, and the effacement of normal mucosal folds, must be sought by dedicated positioning and screening. Small cloacogenic (basaloid) tumors originating in the transitional anal mucosa as well as secondary infiltrative malignancies (most notably carcinoid tumors and non-Hodgkin's lymphoma) will often be unassociated with a distinct mass effect, producing only secondary luminal distortion or a localized lack of normal rectal wall mobility [16]. It is common practice today to supplement a suspicious contrast enema with direct inspection of the rectal mucosa, especially in an effort to obtain tissue for diagnostic purposes. In the setting of a normal contrast enema in a patient in whom there is a heightened suspicion of rectal cancer, proctosigmoidoscopy should also be carried out. The suspicion of a rectal mass without a mucosal component should be evaluated with an additional imaging technique such as ERUS.

Endorectal Ultrasound

ERUS is currently a well-established method and appears to be the "gold standard" for the preoperative assessment of most rectal cancers [17,18]. Improvements in transducer technology have permitted the accurate identification of individual layers of the rectal wall [19], as well as the detection of involved pararectal lymph nodes within the field of view of the endoluminal probe. ERUS has the advantages of being relatively fast, minimally invasive, portable and rapidly interpretable. Currently, the accuracy of ERUS in evaluating perirectal neoplastic infiltration varies between 81% and 96%, while the accuracy in demonstrating perirectal lymph node involvement ranges between 60% and 83%. A number of additions to this procedure have emerged, such as color flow Doppler imaging as well as three-dimensional utility. Furthermore, the application of ultrasound techniques to evaluate rectal cancer and the pelvis/perineum have utilized transvaginal and transperineal approaches. These techniques are obviously operator dependent and results should be evaluated in relation to the experience of the operator.

In general, the rectum should be prepared by the patient prior to ERUS with a self-administered disposable enema. The transducer (10 MHz for the anal canal and 7.5 MHz for the rectum) rotates to provide a 360° display of the rectum and its immediate surrounds with the utilization of a hard protective plastic cone containing 40–60 ml of degassed water, providing excellent acoustic contact between the mucosa and the transducer.

The rectal wall has been shown to resolve sonographically into five main layers with variable (but reproducible) echogenicity. These consist of two hypoechoic circles interfaced with three hyperechoic circles. Evidence for histological layer confirmation has been achieved by in-vitro studies employing selective serial dissection and rescanning of rectal specimens [13].

The innermost white circle is represented by the transducer and cone and is reflected by the interface of the water, cone and sheath with the rectal mucosa. The middle hyperechoic region is formed between the mucosa (and submucosa) and the muscularis propria, while the outermost bright circle is the junction between the muscularis propria and the extrarectal fat. The innermost dark circle is represented by the combined mucosa, submucosa and internal anal sphincter and the outermost hypoechoic layer is formed by the muscularis propria. It is this latter landmark that is the key to the accurate diagnosis of serosal invasion using ERUS for the assessment of rectal cancer.

The position of the tumor will potentially provide pitfalls in endoluminal scanning [20,21]. High rectal lesions represent a particular difficulty with this technique since, at least in part, there may be relatively poor acoustic coupling of the probe against a portion of the tumor as well as a difficulty in negotiating the probe alongside the tumor leading edge. Bulky tumors that stenose the rectal lumen will also hamper accurate placement of the probe (or sufficiently distort the resulting image), preventing its use in up to 20% of scanned patients. For lesions that lie close to the anal verge, probe placement may be impossible because of persistent dislodgement or distortion of the balloon on inflation, resulting in a reverberating peritumoral artifact that obscures the image [22].

In general, rectal cancer appears hypoechoic, tending to disrupt the normal sonographic anatomy described above. The accuracy of ERUS for rectal cancer is generally reported as high (85–90%) [23–25] when using a modification of an ultrasonographically-derived staging system as originally described by Hildebrandt and Feifel [26]:

uT1 tumors are confined to the mucosa and submucosa, and consequently do not disrupt the middle bright interface.

uT2 tumors are confined to the rectal wall and distort the dark band comprising the muscularis propria. The outermost bridge echo in these tumors remains intact.

uT3 tumors penetrate the rectal wall and extend into perirectal fat, with interruption or distortion of the outermost normal echoes. Because this extent of spread may occur over a very short distance, very careful backwards and forwards scanning is needed to assess all areas of the muscularis propria and perirectal fat planes to confirm accurately that a tumor is in fact uT3. In the male, an empty bladder assists in the definition of the homogeneous hypoechoic edge of the prostate gland. This area too needs to be carefully assessed by the radiologist for focal invasion of the fascia of Denonvilliers by tumor. In the female, the vaginal vault appears as a darkened ellipse with a relatively echogenic edge. Invasion of the rectovaginal septum needs careful evaluation.

uT4 tumors invade adjacent pelvic viscera and appear locally fixed against probe movement.

The accuracy of ERUS is affected by tumor stage. ERUS has substantial limitations when used for rectal cancer staging. Most reported series have shown relative overstaging by ERUS of early rectal lesions (uT2 versus uT1), which will therefore not assist in decision making concerning local therapies. This has been considered to be secondary to inflammatory infiltrate around the tumor, which is sonographically indistinguishable from malignant tissue. Occasional uT2/uT3 overstaging will, however, result in patients receiving unnecessary preoperative radiotherapy [27]. Preoperative radiotherapy, of itself, may decrease the accuracy of T staging owing to increased echogenicity of the rectal wall.

The distinction between soft villous adenomas and early uT1 invasive carcinomas is generally possible by using ERUS because adenomas tend to maintain homogeneous echogenicity, whereas invasive neoplasms are more commonly echopoor [28]. The reported positive predictive value for ERUS in the detection of malignant foci within lesions is 67%; the negative predictive value is 89% [29].

With respect to mesorectal lymph nodes, increasing difficulty has arisen with improved histopathological examination of resected specimens using the fat clearance and radial margin assessment techniques [30,31]. Up to 20% of the lymph nodes examined are now reported to be <3 mm in maximal diameter, with 50% of metastatic nodes containing malignant deposits that are <5 mm in size [32,33]. These nodes are generally too small for ERUS to define their internal architecture, even when they are located within the field of view of the probe. When they are evident, however, metastatic lymph nodes are typically hypoechoic, usually comparatively larger than inflammatory nodes (i.e. frequently >4 mm in maximal diameter), and are irregular with sharply defined borders. The inflammatory node tends to contain multiple internal echogenic densities and, although frequently irregular, has a rough or typically fuzzy edge [34]. Further studies have demonstrated classic acoustic impedance patterns derived from malignant nodes close to the ERUS probe [35]. The reported accuracy for malignant node detection by ERUS varies from 53% to 86% [36,37].

Recent technical improvements in endoluminal transducers and available software have enabled high-resolution endoluminal scanning to be performed in conjunction with color Doppler imaging, with which Sudoakoff *et al.* and others have shown that rectal neoplasms tend to be hypervascular with relatively disorganized flow patterns when compared with normal controls [38,39]. This phenomenon is currently being evaluated in the postoperative rectum in an attempt to distinguish residual scar from recurrent disease. In the latter case, the presence of low-grade hypervascularity associated with an infiltrative hypoechoic leading edge would suggest the likelihood of recurrent tumor. This type of color flow imaging combined with pulsed Doppler will be a useful addition to conventional grey-scale ERUS when evaluating perirectal lymph nodes and may in the future be supplemented by three-dimensional ultrasound images, particularly when the primary tumor is bulky or potentially obstructive [40–42].

ERUS has been shown to be inaccurate in the assessment of patients (either preoperatively or postoperatively) who have been treated with radiotherapy. In this setting, interpretation of the rectal wall is difficult because of relative wall thickening and loss of layer interface. Primary rectal tumors are generally more heterogeneous after irradiation, consequent upon early scar formation [43].

Mesorectal nodes that are small tend to become hidden, whereas larger nodes develop hyperechoic patterns that resemble inflammatory glands [44]. The postoperative determination of local luminal recurrence after potentially curative resection when the patient has been irradiated is reported to be inaccurate when using ERUS as the only modality of staging [45–47].

To increase the value of ultrasound in the staging of stenotic rectal tumors, water enema transvaginal ultrasound was performed on 21 consecutive female patients with severely stenotic tumors [48]. Compared with the results of histologic examination, this modality correctly staged 19 or 21 tumors. In the detection of lymph node involvement, the sensitivity was 50% and the specificity was 78%.

ERUS is the most effective method of local tumor staging. It is highly effective and an accurate method for T staging, although it is least accurate for T2 and T4 tumors [49]. Lymph node staging is less accurate than T staging. ERUS remains a very accurate method for predicting the depth of tumor invasion, but it may not detect tumor extension or nodes that are outside the range of the transducer [49].

Computed Tomography

The potential role of CT scanning in patients with rectal carcinoma in twofold: The first is in assessing the local extent of the neoplasm and any involvement of regional lymph nodes or local extension, for

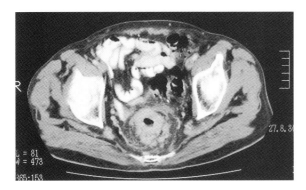

Fig. 4.2. CT scan of the pelvis: diffuse thickening of the rectal wall with irregularity of the perirectal fat and adjacent enlarged lymph nodes. At surgery a pT3/pN1 carcinoma was found.

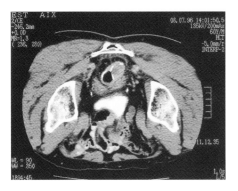

Fig. 4.3. CT scan of the pelvis: previous low anterior resection for rectal carcinoma; a 2.5 cm nodular lesion is visible close to the anastomotic site, which was suspicious for relapse and proved at pathological evaluation.

example to the genitourinary structures. The second is for the detection of the presence of metastatic disease outside the confines of the primary tumor. Many of the conclusions reached regarding the role of CT scanning in the detection of metastatic disease can be applied to both colon and rectal cancer (Figs 4.2 and 4.3). Information regarding the role of CT in assessing the depth of invasion of colon cancer is minimal, while its role in local staging of rectal cancer has been superseded by endorectal ultrasound.

On a CT scan, rectal cancer appears as a discrete mass or focal wall thickening, especially when it is asymmetric. Other than this non-specific finding, CT scanning fails to detect microscopic invasion of perirectal fat and is unable to depict the various layers of the bowel wall. Local extension of tumors is verified by direct involvement of adjacent muscle and spread to contiguous organs.

CT scanning is most useful in rectal cancer for defining the extent of local pelvic and extrapelvic

spread. It has a relatively poor capacity for the delineation of individual bowel wall layers. The initial reports on the use of CT for tumor staging in rectal cancer were encouraging, with accuracies between 77% and 100%. However, most patients in the early studies had advanced disease and the limitations of CT only became clear from later work. The sensitivity for the detection of advanced tumors (which are frequently obvious on clinical examination as a result of tethering or fixity) has been reported to be as high as 90%, with poor sensitivity in distinguishing T1 from early T2 tumors [50, 51]. Similarly, the accuracy of lymph node staging range between 22% and 73%.

There are several pitfalls when using CT scanning as the sole modality in staging rectal cancer. Tumors located low down in the rectum prove to be particularly difficult to stage because of the relative paucity of perirectal fat. There is also a recognized tendency for overstaging of the low rectal lesion, although the use of softcopy PACS workstation monitors (Picture Archive and Communication Systems; Lockheed Martin Medical Imaging System) enable CT images to be viewed in "stack" mode with a facility for rapid screen refreshing permitting cine-image viewing. The latter modality allows anatomical structures such as vessels and the levator ani muscle sling to be recognized more easily than when using conventional "tile" mode, limiting the effects of partial volume averaging and aiding in the discrimination of true perirectal spread from artifact [52].

The ability of CT to evaluate mesorectal nodes is, at best, 50%, with poor correlation between the number radiologically and pathologically detected glands. For both CT scanning and MR imaging there are no clear features apart from size that are predictive for nodal positivity (as there are described for ERUS) and it is not yet possible to analyze the internal architecture of very small nodes. Furthermore, the ability to distinguish mesorectal deposits by CT scanning is limited in bulky tumors, where involved nodes may be contiguous with the primary mass. Studies that compare CT with ERUS consistently show the latter to be more accurate for both tumor and lymph node staging.

There is a high degree of controversy regarding the optimal technique, if any, to assess the distant spread of tumor in patients with rectal carcinoma. It is estimated that up to 25% of those with colorectal carcinoma have metastatic disease at the time of diagnosis [53]. CT scanning is therefore used to determine if the primary neoplasm has metastasized to the liver, adrenal glands, ovaries, kidneys or lung. The liver is the most common site of extranodal metastasis. On CT scanning, colorectal liver metastases are readily identified after a bolus injection of contrast material; they produce a hyperdense pattern [53]. The accuracy of detection of liver metastases is 90%. CT with arterial portography is the most accurate means of detecting lesions in a normal-appearing lobe of the liver (usually lesions that are less than 1 cm in diameter). Other metastatic lesions such as peritoneal seeding are best visualized by helical CT scanning. Adrenal metastases appear as soft tissue masses. Bony metastases are depicted as areas of lytic destruction [53].

The lung represents the next most likely site after the liver for metastatic disease. CT of the chest is more sensitive than is chest radiography in detecting metastatic lung lesions. One hundred consecutive patients with negative chest radiography and potentially respectable hepatic colorectal metastases underwent chest CT [54]. Eleven of these had a positive CT scan, of which four demonstrated malignant change (three metastatic colorectal cancer).

CT scanning has not been found to be accurate in assessing the depth of rectal wall invasion and iden-

tifying lymph node metastases. A possible advantage of CT can be considered in assessing the lateral pelvic lymph nodes, pelvic wall invasion and involvement of levator ani muscle. CT remains an accurate modality in detecting distant adenopathy and distant metastases, and for staging patients with advanced disease. A normal CT scan in the setting of clinical suspicion or elevated tumor markers should direct one to employ other imaging modalities to detect undetermined metastases.

Magnetic Resonance Imaging

MR imaging, initially popularized in the late 1980s, has evolved into a useful tool in an effort to stage rectal cancer accurately (Fig. 4.4). Initial studies have shown accuracy rates similar to those obtained with ERUS and significantly better than those with standard MR, CT and clinical assessment. The use of

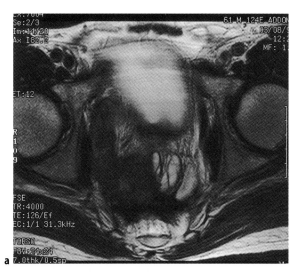

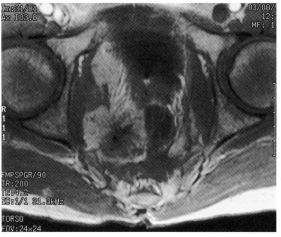

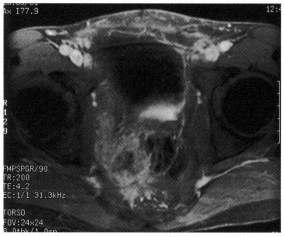

Fig. 4.4. MR image of the pelvis: previous rectal amputation for rectal cancer. **a** Plain axial image fast spin echo T2-weighted; **b** SP gradient echo T1-weighted; **c** SP gradient echo fat saturation T1-weighted after gadolinium infusion. Irregular enhancing solid tissue (6 cm) is clearly visible in the posterolateral pelvis, with infiltration of the seminal vesicle, and of the right pelvic floor structures. At pathologic evaluation a relapse was found.

MR imaging employing an endorectal surface coil has been extensively reported in the assessment of rectal cancer, and is the preferred modality for the definition of local pelvic spread and in identifying extrapelvic metastatic disease. In the former case, MR imaging compares favorably concerning the sensitivity of T staging with both CT scanning [55, 56] and ERUS [57]. In the latter situation, MR imaging appears to be significantly superior to CT scanning in the diagnosis of associated hepatic metastatic deposits [58]. It requires no patient preparation or sedation before the coil is put in place. However, a rectal examination should be performed to confirm that severe anorectal stenosis is not present.

MR will delineate three distinct layers in the normal rectum: an inner layer with an intermediate signal on T1 scans and a high signal on T2 scans is a combination of the mucosa and submucosa; a middle layer, which has low signal on both T1 and T2 sequences and corresponds to the muscularis propria; and an outer layer, which is composed of the subserosa, serosa and perirectal fat and has high signal on both T1 and T2 imaging sequences. Rectal tumors are focal masses with an intermediate signal on T1 and T2 imaging sequences. A large T1 tumor does not encroach on the muscularis propria; a stage T2 tumor extends into the muscularis propria, but not beyond it; a tumor is T3 if it extends into the perirectal fat; and a tumor is T4 if it invades other organs.

Reported sensitivities for the detection of the depth of tumor invasion ranges between 70% and 92%, while the accuracy for staging lymph node metastases appears to be comparatively worse in some series than CT scanning (about 40%). It shares the same size limitations on the likely preoperative diagnosis of nodal involvement as well as showing a considerable overlap of signal intensity between enlarged inflammatory and neoplastic mesorectal glands [59,60].

MR imaging appears to be slightly superior when compared with CT scanning in the diagnosis of recurrent pelvic tumors. Increases in T2 signal intensity are used as a guide to the presence of recurrent disease, particularly when radiotherapy has been previously employed [61–63]. In this setting, fibrous tissue present as a consequence of post-radiation reaction appears as a relatively low-intensity signal on both T1- and T2-weighted images, although this effect is not absolute if there is substantial tumor necrosis or extensive desmoplasia, or if the recurrent is particularly hypocelluar [64–66]. The recent use of thin-slice dedicated MR imaging has resulted in very high-resolution images showing excellent comparison with serial histologic

examination, both for tumor depth and for the demonstration of mesorectal deposits, provided the latter are of sufficient size. The sensitivity of this technique in the post-irradiated rectum is awaited [67].

MR imaging utilizing a body coil is unable to demonstrate distinct layers of the bowel wall. Recently we have evaluated endoanal MR imaging using an internal (endorectal) coil, which provides high-resolution images with superior soft-tissue contrast and which has proven value in complex and recurrent perirectal sepsis [68] as well as in defining the anatomy of external anal sphincter defects [69]. This technique of endoanal MR imaging using the specially designed internal coil has already been described [70,71]. A dedicated anal coil 12 mm in diameter and 90 mm in length is generally used. The coil is wound on an acetal homopolymer (Delrin) former and is designed to include the entire length of the anal sphincter. In order to prevent artifacts due to movement, it is supported by an external clamp attached to a baseplate held under the patient's thighs for scanning in the supine position.

Standard imaging using T1-weighted SE, T2-weighted SE and short-time inversion recovery (STIR) sequences provides high-resolution images of the normal sphincter with excellent separation of the subcutaneous, superficial and deep external sphincter muscles, best seen in oblique coronal images. In many patients, the longitudinal muscle is seen as a series of low-signal bands with a typically beaded appearance surrounded by high-signal fat and fibroelastic tissue that is best seen in transverse T1- and T2-weighted coronal views. The internal anal sphincter has a naturally high signal on all sequences, particularly on T2-weighting and STIR sequencing, possibly as a function of its inherent smooth muscle content and high vascularity. It is noted to be continuous with the longitudinal rectal muscle layer above and is either circular or crescentic in cross-section, being well delineated laterally by high-signal intersphincteric fat and enhancing strikingly after gadolinium-DTPA contrast [72]. The external anal sphincter also enhances, but to a much lesser degree. The layer definition appears to be superior to that achieved with standard phased-array imaging. A recent study using this technique in low rectal cancers (i.e. carcinomas located within 8 cm of the anal verge) has shown it to have similar accuracy in prediction of the T status of tumors when compared with CT [52] (Figs. 4.5–4.7).

The accuracy of endoluminal imaging of this type is greatest for T1 and T2 tumors confined to the bowel wall. There appears to be no advantage of this technique over surface imaging when digital examination is suggestive of tumor tethering [73]. One

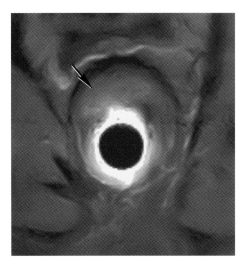

Fig. 4.5. Axial view of a submucosal rectal tumor = arrow inside levator ani complex.

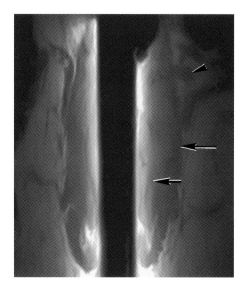

Fig. 4.7. Coronal view T2-weighted image of a rectal cancer invading the internal (short arrow) and external (long arrow) sphincters; a pathologic lymph node (arrow head) is shown above the levator ani.

should expect an overall accuracy when utilizing an endorectal coil for T staging to be between 66% and 91% and between 72% and 79% for N staging. An example of an endoanal MR image of a low cancer with sphincter invasion and a mesorectal deposit is shown in Fig. 4.7. As with any endoluminal facility, there will be tumors that are so stenotic that they will not properly admit placement of the coil, or whose rostral limit extends above the levator floor,

necessitating a supplementary pelvic phased-array multimodality approach. In each of these circumstances there does not appear to be any advantage to the patient in carrying out imaging.

Moreover, as for surface imaging, the accuracy of definition by the internal coil of the T status of a

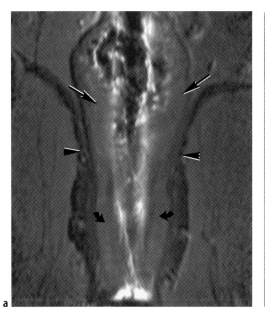

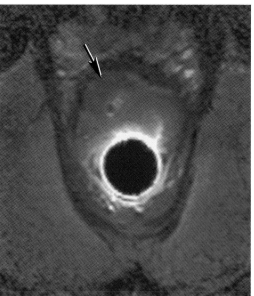

Fig. 4.6. **a** Sagittal view of a rectal cancer: long arrow = tumor; short arrow = invasion of the internal sphincter only; arrow head = intact external sphincter complex; **b** axial view of a submucosal rectal tumor = arrow inside levator ani complex.

tumor after radiotherapy needs to be established. Despite high-resolution images, endoanal MR imaging is not able sufficiently to distinguish those tumors that are suitable for local excision. As expected, endoanal MR imaging is not an advance in the detection of small neoplastic deposits in the mesorectum and appears inferior to ERUS [74], but equivalent to reported accuracies using external MR coils [75]. The identification of mesorectal deposits in the presence of an accompanying bulky pelvic tumor where involved nodes are contiguous with the primary mass however, better when compared with other forms of surface imaging. The accuracy of the internal coil in predicting the potential involvement of the lateral resection margins of a mesorectal excision specimen (as defined by Quirke et al. [76], see chapter 2) appears to be an advantage and needs further study. The coil has been universally successful in our hands in defining preoperatively those tumors with pelvic side-wall invasion that were also shown to have histologic involvement of the lateral resection margins. This information is quite distinct from the preoperative identification of tumors with extensive pelvic visceral involvement in which surface imaging alone may suffice in precluding initial surgery. The ability to resect the low or mid-rectal tumor with an undisturbed lymphovascular package has been emphasized by MacFarlane et al. [77] as being one of the principal technical determinants in the prevention of local recurrence after a low anterior resection for cancer. The identification before operation of patients in whom a pelvic residuum is likely, despite radical

surgery, will permit the selective utilization of preoperative radiotherapy, thus potentially diminishing overall perioperative radiotherapeutic morbidity by avoiding the blanket-style Swedish approach as advocated by Pahlman and Glimelius [78]. Imaging that accurately defines circumferential resection margins will also identify patients in whom pelvic exenteration is contraindicated.

The overstaging of lesions occurs because intramural lymph nodes and perirectal vessels simulating tumor extension. Understaging occurs as a consequence of the inability of MR to identify microscopic invasion. The major limitation of endorectal MR is in visualizing lesions that are high in the rectum.

Endorectal MR is a promising emerging technique for the accurate preoperative determination of the depth of invasion of rectal tumors. Overall, MR imaging appears to be inferior to ultrasonography for T and N staging. If there is a possibility of tumor extension into adjacent organs or the pelvic side wall, MR imaging is more accurate than CT scanning. MR imaging is unable to reveal small metastases in lymph nodes; however large lymph nodes remote from the primary tumor and not within reach of the sonic wave may prove detectable.

Positron Emission Tomography

The advent of PET has made it possible to demonstrate chemical and metabolic changes associated with various disease processes. PET will define

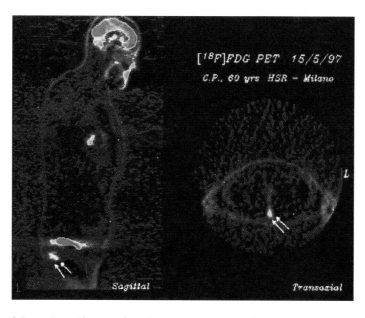

Fig. 4.8. PET-[18F]FDG study in a patient with operated rectal cancer, recent increase of CEA and residual tissue of uncertain nature in pelvis documented by CT. The presence of high FDG uptake within the lesion (white arrows) confirms tumor recurrence.

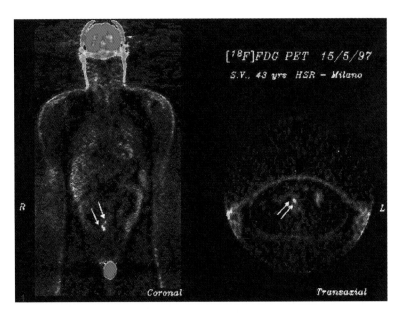

Fig. 4.9. PET-[18F]FDG study in a patient who had a colon resection for carcinoma 2 years earlier. High FDG uptake (white arrows) due to tumor involvement was observed in a unique 2-cm large lombo-aortic lymph node visible on abdominal CT.

fundamental differences in the metabolism of F-18-labeled-2-deoxyglucose (FDG) by malignant cells when compared with normal cells. In most cancers, dephosphorylation of FDG-6-phosphate (which is formed by hexokinase activity on intracellularly transported FDG) is intrinsically diminished in malignancy, with high tumor: background ratios noted several hours after intravenous FDG administration [79–81]. FDG PET has been widely used in patients with colorectal cancers. Most studies to date have focused on the role of PET in tumor recurrence.

For a typical tumor study, 3.7 B/kg body weight of FDG is administered (total dose ± 250–300 B on average), with the performance of a whole-body emission scan about 45 minutes after tracer administration. Whole-body acquisition results in a sequence of contiguous tomographic slices from the vertex to the pelvis using a 15 cm field of view with 5-minute bed positions. Semiquantitative tracer distribution analyses can then be performed with tomographic reconstruction as transaxial images, although coronal and sagittal reconstructions are also possible. Although quantitative approaches may be applied to analysis based on standardized uptake ratio [82], these images are typically interpreted qualitatively, comparing high-uptake areas with background activity [83–86].

Certain malignant tumors tend to use glucose at a higher rate than normal tissues. This phenomenon is based on the fact that malignant tumors have an exceptionally high rate of glycolysis compared with benign tissue. PET can sensitively detect cancers of increased glucose metabolism. In a recent study [83], PET scanning identified asymptomatic tumors in asymptomatic patients, of which three were colorectal cancers.

Although PET has acceptable sensitivity in the preoperative diagnosis of occult hepatic metastatic disease [87], it may find a specific use in patients in whom other surface images (CT scanning or MR imaging) are suggestive of recurrence. In these patients, the differentiation of pelvic recurrence from scar tissue (particularly in the irradiated patient) can be extremely difficult [88–93] (Fig. 4.8). Inflammatory masses may still cause confusion and both PET and MR imaging (the latter modality distinguishing recurrence from scar on T2-weighted images) still necessitate superimposed images as guidance for needle biopsy [94–96].

The role of PET in the primary diagnosis of rectal cancer and in staging remains as yet unproven, despite high reported accuracies for cancer diagnosis when compared with CT scanning [97]. Moreover, FDG-PET results appear to correlate with overall tumor grading and growth rate, this modality potentially functioning as a prognostic marker [99,100]. Difficulties still remain concerning the understaging of small lesions (<1 cm in maximal diameter), necrotic neoplasms with thin viable rims, and peritumoral inflammatory granulomas [101]. Because PET provides a functional image rather than a precise anatomical definition of the tumor, it lacks specificity and anatomical orientation. To date, there is no evidence of a role for PET in the preoperative staging of primary rectal cancer.

Radioimmunoscintigraphy

Radioimmunoscintigraphy is a functional examination that allows for the in-vivo imaging of abnormal pathologic processes such as infections, infarcts and malignant tumors. The recent production of murine and humanized monoclonal antibodies that specifically target well-characterized epitopes located on the tumor-associated antigen carcinoembryonic antigen (CEA), and which maintain their sensitivity and specificity after radionuclide conjugation, has permitted their use as diagnostic agents in radioimmunoscintigraphy (RIS) and in radioimmuno-guided surgery (RIGS).

These conjugates have been employed in the primary diagnosis of colorectal carcinoma and small-volume metastatic disease as well as in the detection of recurrence, particularly when conventional imaging has been negative. The value of RIS has been in its reported ability to upgrade colorectal cancer staging and to define extrahepatic metastatic disease, particularly when serum CEA levels are normal or borderline. In the development of this technology, the labeling of polyclonal broad anti-CEA antibodies was initially with radionuclides (most notably 131I and 123I) with images acquired by means of rectilinear scanners [102].

The introduction of monoclonal hybridoma technology permitted improved sensitivity and gave way to conjugation with radiometals (111In and 99mTc), which proved more suitable for gamma camera imaging and rapid image acquisition, and maintained basic antibody immunoreactivity after labeling [103–105].

In colorectal cancer the most frequent antibodies employed include B72.3 and IMMU-4 (both mouse IgG1 anti-TAG-72 antibodies), CYT-103, and PR1A3 (a murine IgG1 directed at a cell-based epitope of CEA) [106–109]. In general, sensitivity for the diagnosis of primary colorectal cancers using the technology is equivalent to CT scanning but it appears to be markedly less sensitive for the diagnosis of hepatic metastases, although it is dependent upon the circulation level of CEA and the heterogeneity of deposit of the tumor-associated antigen. Conventional RIS has recently been enhanced by the introduction of radionuclide single photon emission CT for primary diagnosis and for the detection of recurrence [110–112].

The main use of RIS appears to be in the preoperative detection of unsuspected advanced locoregional disease and distant metastases in the young patient, to guide preoperative neo-adjuvant therapy, and as a complement to CT or MR imaging in the follow-up of curative resections in equivocal cases where there is an elevated serum CEA level.

Most recently, antibody fragments (Fab, F(ab)′2 and single-chain Fv) have been used, showing more rapid clearance, faster image acquisition and higher tumor: background ratios [113–115]. Newer approaches, aimed at improving targeting and diminishing troublesome human anti-mouse antibody production with repeated scintigraphy, include regional antibody administration, antibody humanization and chirmaerization, novel radionuclide linkers and chelates, in-vivo pre-targeting of lesions using unconjugated antibodies and streptavidin/biotin conjugates with high affinity, and the use of antibody cocktails [116–119]. It remains to be seen whether these newer technologies prove to be cost-beneficial for patient management [120–122].

Monoclonal antibodies may also be employed for preoperative targeted use with a hand-held gamma-detecting probe, as first described by Martin and colleagues in 1984 [123]. Initial significant delays between injection and detection for background clearance and optimal tumor: normal ratios were reduced by pre-targeting using two-step and three-step approaches [124,125].

The overall sensitivity of RIGS in the detection of recurrent colorectal carcinoma appears to be greater than that experienced for the primary diagnosis [126–128] and, although there are many studies in the literature that suggest that the ability of RIGS guidance to re-stage patients intraoperatively as part of a decision-making algorithm may actually enhance cancer-related survival, the data are non-randomized [129,130]. The results of prospective randomized clinical trials using RIGS as the primary modality in recurrent tumors and the use of new techniques such as laparoscopically-guided RIGS are awaited [131].

It has been shown that various gastrointestinal tumors express substantial amounts of vasoactive intestinal peptide receptors. Previous investigators have demonstrated a promising clinical role for the visualization of primary and recurrent colorectal carcinomas. This modality has the potential to offer additional information to that obtained by conventional radiological imaging, especially for small cancers or suspected recurrences in the pelvis [132].

Diagnostic Imaging in the Diagnosis and Staging of Recurrent Rectal Cancer

The role of diagnostic imaging in the diagnosis of recurrent rectal cancer is also covered in Chapters 12 and 13. This discussion complements those chapters.

Ultrasound Techniques

In the patient who has undergone initial curative resection for rectal cancer, ultrasound techniques have been employed either transanally or transvaginally in an effort to determine the presence of local recurrence. Furthermore, at laparotomy, intraoperative ultrasound may aid in the detection of liver metastases not demonstrated by other preoperative imaging techniques.

In those who have undergone either a restorative proctectomy or transanal excision of a rectal tumor, endorectal ultrasound has been a useful tool in the assessment of local recurrence. Furthermore, in the female patient, transvaginal ultrasound has been employed, especially after abdominoperineal resection. In a recent study, 62 patients operated on for rectal cancer were prospectively enrolled in a follow-up program that involved ERUS, serial CEA levels, digital examination, colonoscopy and pelvic CT scanning. A total of 192 scans were performed, with a mean number of three per patient. Local recurrence occurred in 11 patients and was detected in all cases by ERUS. In two patients (18%) other techniques failed to detect recurrent disease [135]. The usefulness of postoperative ERUS has been confirmed in a number of prospective and retrospective studies reporting accuracy rates of 80–85% in detecting local neoplastic recurrence. The superiority of ERUS stems from the fact that the distinct ultrasound planes between organs are readily visualized sonographically. These results are similar to those seen with CT and ERUS; they should complement and not be an alternative to CT scanning.

Intraoperative ultrasound has been shown to be more accurate than either preoperative ultrasound, CT scanning with or without arterial portography, or surgical exploration in the detection of liver metastases from colorectal carcinoma. Laparoscopic ultrasound is also clearly indicated as a method of screening for these metastases. In patients with known liver malignancy, whether primary or metastatic, laparoscopic ultrasound has been effective in detecting previously unrecognized additional malignant foci within the hepatic parenchyma.

Computed Tomography

CT scanning has proved useful in assessing patients who may harbor metastatic disease from colorectal cancer. It is generally the modality of choice for imaging the postoperative patient. The CT scan features of recurrent colorectal tumors are similar to those described for primary tumors.

Unique to rectal cancer is the issue of local recurrence in the pelvis. Soft tissue masses can persist in the pelvis secondary to scar and fibrosis. Furthermore, in patients who have received adjuvant radiotherapy, post-radiation changes may produce diffuse thickening. Although very high sensitivity rates were initially reported for the CT and detection of locally recurrent tumors, accuracy is currently between 60% and 70%. Most errors result from a failure to detect microscopic invasion of perirectal fat, to detect metastatic foci in normal-sized lymph nodes, and to visualize anastomotic recurrence.

Magnetic Resonance Imaging

CT scanning has been widely utilized in the detection of extraluminal recurrences of rectal cancer. Nevertheless, the diagnosis of recurrent rectal cancer in the pelvis is often difficult owing to non-specific symptoms. In addition, scar tissue or fibrosis developing after surgery or radiation therapy can mimic tumor recurrence. However, studies with improved MR systems have demonstrated that this modality is superior on account of improved tissue discrimination (Figs 4.10 and 4.11). MR imaging has been reported to be highly accurate in distinguishing postoperative fibrosis from recurrence, based on the difference in signal intensity between these two types of tissue in T2-weighted images. In a study involving 25 consecutive patients with either suspected or verified local recurrence of rectal cancer, MR imaging was more accurate (87.5%) compared with CT scanning (76%) and

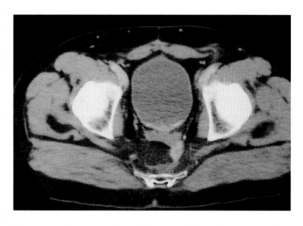

Fig. 4.10. Contrast-enhanced CT scan of the pelvis 3 years after abdominoperineal resection for rectal cancer. In the retrovesical fat, irregular nodular hyperdense tissue is visible, which is not dissociable from seminal vesicle. Relapsing cancer was proved by a CT-guided biopsy.

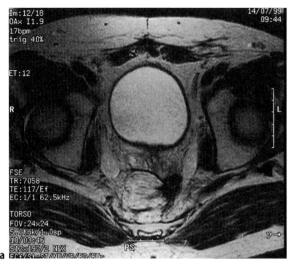

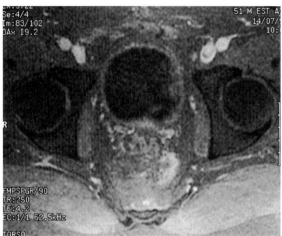

Fig. 4.11. **a** MR image (same patient of Fig. 4.5): axial fast spin echo T2-weighted image. In the retrovesical fat is a non-homogeneous nodular lesion with irregular margins; **b** axial gradient echo fat-saturated MR image after intravenous administration of contrast media (gadolinium-DTPA). The nodular lesion is partially enhanced as proof of the presence of vital tissue.

CEA scintigraphy (75%) [58]. Presacral masses developing after proctectomy are readily detected and staged with MR imaging [58–63].

Positron Emission Tomography and Immunoscintigraphy

Both PET and immunoscintigraphy with monoclonal antibodies demonstrate the presence of recurrent malignancy as areas of increased uptake. The differentiation of recurrent tumor from scar tissue in the presacral region is a difficult radiological problem. Two previous studies [91, 92] have suggested a role for FDG-PET in diagnosing recurrent rectal tumors. These employed semiquantitative techniques of FDG uptake into a region of interest to determine the likelihood of malignancy. The anatomic resolution of PET is inferior to CT scanning, so that a combination of these two modalities is needed for the exact localization of a mass. PET has shown some excellent preliminary results in detecting small tumor foci in metastatic lesions in lymph nodes, liver, adrenal gland and lung (Fig. 4.9). It can detect tumor in areas that are considered to be normal or of an equivocal nature by CT scanning or MR imaging. The use of monoclonal antibodies for detecting operable recurrent colorectal cancers is currently being evaluated.

Conclusions

There is increasing evidence to show enhanced cancer-specific survival for rectal malignancy when it is treated by a colorectal surgeon with specialist expertise in radical rectal resection techniques. This means that neo-adjuvant therapies aimed at reducing locoregional recurrence and improving overall survival must be tailored to the individual patient, based upon accurate preoperative staging [135].

Such staging should aim to define where possible the presence of serosal invasion, malignant perirectal lymphadenopathy, and extensive pelvic disease in which total mesorectal excision may potentially contain positive circumferential margins. In each of these scenarios, preoperative chemoradiotherapy has been shown to be advantageous to the long-term cancer-related outcome.

In this chapter, we have outlined the standard roles of conventional double-contrast studies and surface imaging (CT and MR) in the primary diagnosis of rectal cancer. The advantages of the latter techniques (and their new modifications) include the demonstration of visceral and soft-tissue extrarectal malignant deposits, the presence of which significantly affects management. Endoluminal staging modalities, although displaying individual bowel wall layers with high resolution, have not proved sufficient to identify candidates who are suitable for local resection. Although ERUS has spawned an extensive literature showing high accuracy for T staging, all endoluminal facilities suffer from limitations in the demonstration of extensive pelvic disease and micrometastatic mesorectal involvement. In this context, a multimodality approach combining accurate ERUS with pelvic phased-array MR or surface MR imaging will probably yield the best results. However, this technology is not uniformly available and has yet to be shown to be cost-effective. The nature of micrometastatic nodal disease implies that advances in such endoluminal technology are unlikely to assist further in defining candidates for neo-adjuvant treatment.

Both PEI and RIS have been outlined in this chapter, particularly in the setting of follow-up of the young patient after seemingly curative rectal resection and when conventional surface imaging is equivocal. It is hoped that improvements in the sensitivity and specificity of new monoclonal xenogeneic and humanized anti-CEA antibodies and their linkage to novel radiometal tracers will improve the accuracy of detection of nodal and small-volume metastatic disease.

References

1. Barrett MW. Chemoradiation for rectal cancer. Semin Surg Oncol 1998;15:114–19.
2. Pahlman L. Radiochemotherapy as an adjuvant treatment for rectal cancer. Recent Results Cancer Res 1998;146:141–51.
3. Habr-Gama A, deSouza PM, Ribeiro U, et al. Low rectal cancer: impact of radiation and chemotherapy on surgical treatment. Dis Colon Rectum 1998;41:1087–96.
4. Nicholls RJ, York Mason A, Morson BC, Dixon AK, Fry IK. The clinical staging of rectal cancer. Br J Surg 1982;69:404–409.
5. Beynon J, Mortensen NJ, Foy DM, Channer JL, Virjee J, Goddard P. Pre-operative assessment of local invasion in rectal cancer: digital examination, endoluminal sonography or computed tomography? Br J Surg 1986;73:1015–17.
6. Rafaelson SR, Kronborg O, Fenger C. Digital rectal examination and transrectal ultrasonography in staging of rectal cancer: a prospective blind study. Acta Radiol 1994;35:300–304.
7. Armitage NC, Robins RA, Evans DF, Turner DR, Baldwin RW, Hardcastle JD. The influence of tumor cell DNA abnormalities on survival in colorectal carcinoma. Br J Surg 1985;72:828–30.
8. Jones DJ, Moore M, Schofield PF. Prognostic significance of DNA ploidy in colorectal carcinoma: a prospective flow cytometric study. Br J Surg 1988;75:28–33.
9. Carlon CA, Fabris G, Arslan-Pagnini C, Pluchinotta AM, Chinelli E, Carniato S. Prognostic correlations of operable carcinoma of the rectum. Dis Colon Rectum 1985;28:47–50.
10. Fielding LP, Fenoglio-Preiser CM, Freedman LS. The future of prognostic factors in outcome prediction for patients with cancer. Cancer 1992;70:2367–77.
11. Nicholls RJ, Galloway DJ, Mason AY, Boyle P. Clinical local staging of rectal cancer. Br J Surg 1985;72(Suppl):S51–52.
12. Ott DJ. Barium enema: colorectal polyps and carcinoma. Semin Roentgenol 1996;31:125–41.
13. Rubesin SE, Levine MS, Laufer I, Herlinger H. Double-contrast barium enema examination technique. Radiology 2000;215:642–50.
14. Rex DK, Rahmani EY, Haseman JH, Lemmel GT, Kaster S, Buckley JS. Relative sensitivity of colonoscopy and barium enema for detection of colorectal cancer in clinical practice. Gastroenterology 1997;112:17–23.
15. Anderson N, Cook HB, Coates R. Colonoscopically detected colorectal cancer missed on barium enema. Gastrointest Radiol 1991;16:123–27.
16. Renard TH, Morton RL, Mathews R, Poulos E. Primary lymphoma of the rectum. Am Surg 1992;58:634–37.
17. Beynon J, Feifel G, Hildebrandt U, Mortensen NJMcC. An atlas of rectal ultrasonography. London: Springer-Verlag, 1991.
18. Saclarides TJ. Endorectal ultrasound. Surg Clin North Am 1998;78:237–49.
19. Beynon J, Foy DMA, Channer JL, Temple LN, Virjee J, Mortensen NJMcC. The endosonic appearances of normal colon and rectum. Dis Colon Rectum 1986;29:810–13.
20. Kruskal JB,. Kane TA, Sentovich SM, Esterbrook-Longmaid H. Pitfalls and sources of error in staging rectal cancer with endorectal ultrasound. Radiographics 1997;17:609–26.
21. Akasu T, Sugihara Y, Yoshihiro M, Fujita S. Limitations and pitfalls of transrectal ultrasonography for staging of rectal cancer. Dis Colon Rectum 1997;40(Suppl):S10–15.
22. Hulsmans FJH, Castelijns JA, Reeders J, Tytgat G. Review of artefacts associated with transrectal ultrasound: understanding, recognition and prevention of misinterpretation. J Clin Ultrasound 1995;23:489–94.
23. Beynon J, Roe AM, Foy DMA, Temple LN, Mortensen NJMcC. Endoluminal ultrasound in the assessment of local invasion in rectal cancer. Br J Surg 1986;73:474–77.
24. Nielsen MB, Qvitzau S, Pedersen JF, Christiansen J. Endosonography for preoperative staging of rectal tumors. Acta Radiol 1996;37:799–803.
25. Yanagi H, Kusunoki M, Shoji Y, Yamamura T, Utsonomiya Y. Preoperative detection of distal intramural spread of lower rectal carcinoma using transrectal ultrasonography. Dis Colon Rectum 1996;39:1210–14.
26. Hildebrandt U, Feifel G. Pre-operative staging of rectal cancer by intrarectal ultrasound. Dis Colon Rectum 1985;28:42–64.
27. Glaser F, Schlag P, Herfarth C. Endorectal ultrasonography for the assessment of invasion of rectal tumors and lymph node involvement. Br J Surg 1990;77:883–87.
28. Hulsmans FH, Tio TL, Mathus-Vliegen EM, Bosma A, Tytgat GN. Colorectal villous adenoma: transrectal US in screening for invasive malignancy. Radiology 1992;185:193–96.
29. Adams WJ, Wong WD. Endorectal ultrasonic detection of malignancy within rectal villous lesions. Dis Colon Rectum 1995;38:1093–96.
30. Scott KW, Grace RH, Gibbons P. Five-year follow-up study of the fat clearance technique in colorectal carcinoma. Dis Colon Rectum 1994;37:126–28.
31. Adam IJ, Mohamdee MO, Martin G, et al. Role of circumferential margin involvement in the local recurrence of rectal cancer. Lancet 1994;344:707–11.
32. Dwork O. Number and size of lymph nodes and node metastases in rectal carcinoma. Surg Endosc 1989;3:96–99.
33. Herrera-Ornelas L, Justiniano J, Castillo N, Petrelli NJ, Stulc JP, Mittelman A. Metastases in small lymph nodes from colon cancer. Arch Surg 1987; 122:1253–56.
34. Sinuochi K, Sakaguchi M, Higuchi Y, Namiki K, Muto T. Limitation of endorectal ultrasonography. What does a low echoic lesion more than 5 mm in size correspond to histologically? Dis Colon Rectum 1998;41:761–64.
35. Hildebrandt U, Klein T, Feifel G, Schwarz HP, Koch B, Schmitt RM. Endosonography of pararectal lymph nodes:in vitro and in vivo evaluation. Dis Colon Rectum 1990;33:863–68.
36. Beynon J, Mortensen NJMcC, Foy DMA, Channer JL, Rigby HS, Virjee J. Pre-operative assessment of meso-rectal lymph node involvement in rectal cancer. Br J Surg l989;76:276–79.
37. Katsura Y, Yamada K, Ishitzawa T, Yoshinaka H, Shimazu H. Endorectal ultrasonography for the assessment of wall

invasion and lymph node metastasis in rectal cancer. Dis Colon Rectum 1992;35:362–68.

38. Sudakoff GS, Gasparaitis A, Michelassi F, Hurst R, Hoffmann K, Hackworth C. Endorectal colour Doppler imaging of primary and recurrent rectal wall tumors: preliminary experience. AJR Am J Roentgenol 1996;166:55–61.

39. Henegan JP, Salem RR, Lange RC, Taylor KJW, Hammers LW. Transrectal sonography in staging rectal carcinoma: the role of grey-scale, color flow and Doppler imaging analysis. AJR Am J Roentgenol 1997;169:1247–52.

40. Krassimir DI, Diacov CD. Three-dimensional endoluminal ultrasound. New staging technique in patients with rectal cancer. Dis Colon Rectum 1997;40:47–50.

41. Hunerbein M, Schlag PM. Three-dimensional endosonography for staging of rectal cancer. Ann Surg 1997;225:432–38.

42. Hunerbein M, Dohmoto M, Haensch W, Schlag PM. Evaluation and biopsy of recurrent rectal cancer using three-dimensional endosonography. Dis Colon Rectum 1997;39:1373–78.

43. Beynon J, Mortensen NJMcC, Foy DMA, Rigby HS, Channer JL, Virjee J. The detection and evaluation of locally recurrent rectal cancer with rectal endosonography. Dis Colon Rectum 1989;32:509–17.

44. Hulsmans FH, Tio TL, Fockens P, Bosma A, Tytgat GN. Assessment of tumour infiltration depth in rectal cancer with transrectal ultrasonography: caution is necessary. Radiology 1994;190:715–20.

45. Napoleon B, Pujol B, Berger F, Valette PJ, Gerard JP, Souquet JC. Accuracy of endosonography in the staging of rectal cancer treated by radiotherapy. Br J Surg 1991;78:785–88.

46. Houvenaeghel G, Delpero JR, Giovannini M, et al. Staging of rectal cancer: a prospective study of digital examination and endosonography before and after preoperative radiotherapy. Acta Chir Belg 1993;93:164–68.

47. Alexander AA, Palazzo JP, Ahmad NR, Liu JB, Forsberg F, Marks J. Endosonographic and color Doppler flow imaging alterations observed within irradiated rectal cancer. Int J Radiat Oncol Biol Phys 1996;35:369–75.

48. Scialpi M, Rotondo A, Angelelli G. Water enema transvaginal ultrasound for local staging of stenotic rectal carcinoma. Abdom Imaging 1999;24:132–36.

49. Heriot AG, Grundy A, Kumar D. Preoperative staging of rectal carcinoma. Br J Surg 1999;86:17–28.

50. Thoeni RF, Moss AJ, Schnyuder P, Margulis AR. Detection and staging of primary rectal and rectosigmoid cancer by computed tomography. Radiology 1981;141:135–38.

51. Nicholls RJ, Mason AJ, Morson BC, Dixon AK, Fry IK. The clinical staging of rectal cancer. Br J Surg 1982;69:404–409.

52. Zbar AP, deSouza NM, Strickland N, Pignatelli M, Kmiot WA. Comparison of endoanal magnetic resonance imaging and computerized tomography in the preoperative staging of rectal cancer: a pilot study. Tech Coloproctol 1998;2:61–66.

53. Scharling ES, Wolfman NT, Bechfold RE. Computed tomography evaluation of colorectal carcinoma. Semin Roentgenol 1996;31:142–53.

54. Povoski SP, Fong Y, Sgouros SC, Kemeny NE, Downey RJ, Blumgart LH. Role of chest CT in patients with negative chest X-rays referred for hepatic colorectal metastases. Ann Surg Oncol 1998;5:9–15.

55. Hodgman CG, MacCarty RL, Wolff BG, et al. Preoperative staging of rectal carcinoma by computed tomography and 0.15T magnetic resonance imaging. Dis Colon Rectum 1986;29:446–50.

56. Guinet C, Buy JN, Ghossain MA, et al. Comparison of magnetic resonance imaging ,and computed tomography in the preoperative staging of rectal cancer. Arch Surg 1990;125:385–88.

57. Thaler W, Watzka S, Martin F, et al. Preoperative staging of rectal cancer by endoluminal ultrasound vs. magnetic resonance imaging: preliminary results of a prospective comparative study. Dis Colon Rectum 1994;37:1189–93.

58. Semelka RC, Shoenut JP, Ascher SM, et al. Solitary hepatic metastasis: comparison of dynamic contrast-enhanced CT and MR imaging with fat-suppressed T2-weighted, breath-hold-T1-weighted FLASH and dynamic gadolinium-enhanced FLASH sequences. J Magnet Reson Imaging 1994;4:319–23.

59. Guinet C, Buy JN, Sezeur A, et al. Preoperative assessment of the extension of rectal carcinoma: correlation of MR, surgical and histopathological findings. J Comput Assist Tomogr 1988;12:209–14.

60. McNicholas MMJ, Joyce Dolan J, Gibney RG, MacErlaine DP, Hyland J. Magnetic resonance imaging of rectal carcinoma; a prospective study. Br J Surg 1994;81:911–14.

61. Pema PJ, Bennett WF, Bova JG, Warman P. CT vs MRI in diagnosis of recurrent rectosigmoid carcinoma. J Comput Assist Tomogr 1994;18:256–61.

62. Krestin GP, Steinbrich W, Friedmann G. Recurrent rectal cancer: diagnosis with MR imaging versus CT. Radiology 1988;168:307–11.

63. deLange EE, Fechner RE, Spaulding CA, Edge SB. Rectal carcinoma treated by preoperative irradiation: MR imaging and histopathologic correlation. Radiology 1992;158:287–92.

64. Glazer HS, Lee JKT, Levitt RG, et al. Radiation fibrosis: differentiation from recurrent tumour by MR imaging. Radiology 1985;156:721–26.

65. Gomberg JS, Friedman AC, Radecki PD, et al. MRI differentiation of recurrent colorectal carcinoma from post-operative fibrosis. Gastrointest Radiol 1986;11:361–63.

66. Ebner F, Kressel HY, Mintz MC, et al. Tumour recurrence vs. fibrosis in the female pelvis: differentiation with MR imaging at 1.5T. Radiology 1988;166:333–40.

67. Brown G, Bourne MW, Williams GT, Radcliffe AG. MRI prediction of the circumferential resection margin involvement can influence preoperative adjuvant therapy and surgical strategy. Br J Surg 1999;86(Suppl 1):84–85.

68. Zbar AP, deSouza NM, Puni R, Kmiot WA. Comparison of endoanal magnetic resonance imaging with surgical findings in perirectal sepsis. Br J Surg 1998;85:111–14.

69. deSouza NM, Puni R, Zbar A, Gilderdale DJ, Coutts GA, Krausz T. MR imaging of the anal sphincter in multiparous females using an endoanal coil: correlation with in vitro anatomy and appearances in fecal incontinence. AJR Am J Roentgenol 1996;167:1465–71.

70. deSouza NM, Puni R, Gilderdale DJ, Bydder GM. Magnetic resonance imaging of the anal sphincter using an internal coil. Magnetic Res Q 1995;11:45–56.

71. Puni R, Hall AS, Coutts GA, deSouza NM. Development of an insertable surface coil for MRI of the anal sphincter. Proceedings of progress in Magnetic Resonance, British Institute of Radiology [abstract]. Radiology 1994;68(810):679.

72. Kmiot WA, Zbar AP, deSouza NM. MRI in anorectal disease. In: Nicholls RJ, Dozois RR, editors. Surgery of the colon and rectum. New York: Churchill Livingstone, 1997:135–49.

73. de Lange EE, Fechner RE, Edge SB. Preoperative staging of rectal carcinoma with MR imaging: surgical and histopathological correlation. Radiology 1990;176:623–28.

74. Joosten FBM, Jansen JBMJ, Joosten HJM, Rosenbusch G. Staging of rectal carcinoma using MR double surface coil, endorectal coil and intrarectal ultrasound: correlation with histopathologic findings. J Comput Assist Tomogr 1995;19:752–58.

75. McNicholas MMT, Joyce WP, Dolan J, Gibney RG, MacErlaine DP, Hyland J. Magnetic resonance imag-

ing of rectal carcinoma: a prospective study. Br J Surg 1994;81:911–14.

76. Quirke P, Durdey P, Dixon MF, Williams NS. Local recurrence of rectal adenocarcinorna due to inadequate surgical resection: histopathological study of lateral tumour spread and surgical excision. Lancet 1986;ii:996–99.

77. MacFarlane JK, Ryall RDH, Heald RJ. Mesorectal excision for rectal cancer. Lancet 1993;341:457–60.

78. Pahlman L, Glimelius B. Pre- and post-operative radiotherapy in rectal carcinoma: report from a randomized multicenter trial. Ann Surg 1990;211:187–95.

79. Monakhor NK, Niestadt EL, Shavlovskil MM, et al. Physicochemical properties and isoenzyme composition of hexokinase from normal and malignant human tissues. J Natl Cancer Inst 1978;61:27–34.

80. Flier JS, Mueckler MM, Usher P, Lodish HF. Elevated levels of glucose transport and transporter mRNA are induced by ras or src oncogenes. Science 1987;235:1492–95.

81. Beets G, Penninckx F, Schiepers C, et al. Clinical value of whole-body positron emission tomography with 18-F-fluorodeoxyglucose in recurrent colorectal cancer. Br J Surg 1994;81:1666–71.

82. DiChiro G, Books RA. PET quantitation: blessing and curse. J Nucl Med 1988;29:1603–604.

83. Conti PS, Lilien DL, Hawley K, Keppler J, Grafton ST, Bading JR. PET and (18F)-FDG in oncology: a clinical update. Nucl Med Biol 1996;23:717–35.

84. Som P, Atkins HL, Bandoypadhyay D, et al. A fluorinated glucose analog, 2-fluoro-2-deoxy-D-glucose (F-18): nontoxic tracer for rapid tumor detection. J Nucl Med 1980;21:670–75.

85. Wahl RL, Hutchins GD, Buschsbaum DJ, et al. 18F-2-deoxy-2-fluoro-D-glucose uptake in human tumour xenografts. Cancer 1991;67:1544–50.

86. Daenen F, Hustinx R, Paulus P, Demez P, Jacquet N, Rigo P. Detection of recurrent colorectal carcinoma with whole-body FDG-PET. J Nucl Med 1996;37:261.

87. Gupta NC, Falk PM, Frank AL, et al. Pre-operative staging of colorectal carcinoma using positron emission tomography. Nebraska Med J 1993;211:30–35.

88. Haberkorn U, Strauss LG, Dimitrakopoulou A, et al. PET studies of fluorodeoxyglucose metabolism in patients with recurrent colorectal tumors receiving radiotherapy. J Nucl Med 1991;32:1485–90.

89. Ito K, Kato T, Tadokoro M, et al. Recurrent rectal cancer and scar: differentiation with PET and MR imaging. Radiology 1992;182:549–52.

90. Pounds TR, Valk PE, Haseman MK, Myers RW, Lutrin CI. Whole-body PET-FDG imaging in diagnosis of recurrent colorectal cancer. J Nucl Med 1995;36:57.

91. Schiepers C, Penninckx F, DeVadder N, et al. Contribution of PET in the diagnosis of recurrent colorectal cancer: comparison with conventional imaging. Eur J Surg Oncol 1995;21:517–22.

92. Keogan MT, Lowe VJ, Baker ME, McDermott VG, Lyerly HK, Coleman RE. Local recurrence of rectal cancer: evaluation with F-18 fluorodeoxyglucose PET imaging. Abdom Imaging 1997;22:332–37.

93. Delbecke D, Vitola JV, Sandier MP, et al. Staging recurrent metastatic colorectal carcinoma with PET. J Nucl Med 1997;38:1196–201.

94. Butch RJ, Wittenberg J, Mueller PR, et al. Presacral masses after abdomino-perineal resection for rectal carcinoma: the need for needle biopsy. AJR Am J Roentgenol 1985;144:309–12.

95. Engehart R, Kimmig BN, Strauss LG, et al. Therapy monitoring of presacral recurrences after high dose irradiation: PET, CT, CEA and pain score. Strahlenther Onkol 1992;168:203–12.

96. Larsen SM, Cohen AM, Cascade MBA. Clinical application and economic implications of PET in the assessment of colorectal cancer recurrence: a retrospective study. Inst for Clinical PET Meeting May 1994: Fairfax, VA, USA.

97. Falk PM, Gupta NC, Thorson AG, et al. Positron emission tomography for preoperative staging of colorectal carcinoma. Dis Colon Rectum 1994;37:153–56.

98. Sweeney MJ, Ashmore J, Morris HP, et al. Comparative biochemistry of hepatomas. IV: Isotope studies of glucose and fructose metabolism in liver tumours of different growth rates. Cancer Res 1963;23:995–1002.

99. Komblith PL, Cummins CJ, Smith GH, Brooks RA, Patronas NJ, diChiro G. Correlation of experimental and clinical studies of metabolism by PET scanning. Prog Exp Tumor Res 1984;27:170–78.

100. Alavi JB, Alavi A, Chawluk J, et al. Positron emission tomography in patients with glioma. A predictor of prognosis. Cancer 1988;62:1074–78.

101. Akhurst T, Scott AM, Berlangieri SU, et al. Validation of F-18-fluorodeoxyglucose-PET with surgical pathology in the detection of recurrent colorectal cancer. J Nucl Med 1996;37:131P.

102. McCardle RJ, Harper PV, Spur IL, Bale WF, Andros G, Jimenez F. Studies with Iodine-131 labeled antibody to human fibrinogen for diagnosis and therapy of tumors. J Nucl Med 1966;7:833–47.

103. Kohler G, Milstein C. Continuous cultures of fused cells secreting antibody of predefined specificity. Nature 1975;256:495–97.

104. Goldenberg DM, DeLand F, Kim E, et al. Use of radiolabeled antibodies to CEA for the detection and localization of diverse cancers by external photoscanning. N Engl J Med 1978:298:184–88.

105. Mather SJ, Ellison D. Reduction-mediated Tc-99m labeling of monoclonal antibodies. J Nucl Med 1990;31: 692–97.

106. Johnson VJ, Schlom J, Paterson AJ, Bennett J, Magnani JL, Colcher D. Analysis of a human tumor-associated glycoprotein (TAG-72) identified by the monoclonal antibody B72.3. Cancer Res 1986;46:850–57.

107. Patt YZ, Podoloff DA, Curley S, et al. Tc-99m-labeled-IMMU-4: a monoclonal antibody against CEA for imaging of occult recurrent colorectal cancer in patients with, rising serum CEA levels. J Clin Oncol 1994;12:488–95.

108. Doerr RJ, Herrera L, Abdel-Nabi H. In-111-CYT-103 monoclonal antibody imaging in patients with suspected recurrent colorectal cancer. Cancer 1993;71:4241–47.

109. Granowska M, Jass JR, Britton KE, Northover JMA. A prospective study of the use of 111-In-labelled monoclonal antibody against CEA in colorectal cancer and some biological factors affecting its uptake. Int J Colorectal Dis 1989;4:97–108.

110. Kramer EL, Noz ME, Sanger JJ, Megibow AJ, Maguire GO. OT-SPECT fusion to correlate radiolabeled monoclonal antibody uptake with abdominal CT findings. Radiology 1989;172:861–65.

111. Maguire LC, Kaplan IL. Image fusion in medicine: an overview using the CT-SPECT model. J Nucl Med Technol 1989;17:31–35.

112. Scott AM, Macapinlac HA, Divgi CR, et al. Clinical validation of SPECT and CT/MRI image registration in radiolabeled monoclonal antibody studies of colorectal carcinoma. J Nucl Med 1994;35:1976–84.

113. Buchegger F, Haskell CM, Schringer M, et al. Radiolabeled fragments of monoclonal antibodies against CEA for localization of human colon cancer grafted into nude mice. J Exp Med 1983;158:413–27.

114. Moffat FL, Pinsky CM, Hammersharib L, et al. Clinical utility of external immunoscintigraphy with IMMU-4 Tc-99m Fab' antibody fragment in patients undergoing surgery for carci-

noma of the colon and rectum: results of a pivotal phase III trial. J Clin Oncol 1996;14:2295–305.

115. Behr TM, Becker WS, Bair HJ, et al. Comparison of complete versus fragmented technetium-99m-labeled anti-CEA monoclonal antibodies for immunoscintigraphy in colorectal cancer. J Nucl Med 1995;36:430–41.

116. Goldenberg DM, Larson SM. Radioimmunodetection in cancer identification. J Nucl Med 1992;33:803–14.

117. McKearn TJ. Radioimmunodetection of solid tumours: future horizons and applications for radioimmunotherapy. Cancer 1993;71:4302–13.

118. Hnatowich DJ, Virzi F, Rusckowska M. Investigations of avidin and biotin for imaging applications. J Nucl Med 1987;28:1294–302.

119. Paganelli G, Pervez S, Siccardi AG, et al. Intraperitoneal radiolocalization of tumours pretargeted by biotinylated monoclonal antibodies. Int J Cancer 1990;45:1184–89.

120. Begent RHJ, Keep PA, Searle F, Green AJ, Mitchell HID, Jones BE. Radioimmunolocalization and selection for surgery in recurrent colorectal cancer. Br J Surg 1986;73:64–67.

121. Tempero M. Pitfalls in antibody imaging in colorectal cancer. Cancer 1993;71(12 Suppl):4248–51.

122. Lunniss PJ, Skinner S, Britton KE, Granowska M, Northover JMA. Effect of radioimmunoscintigraphy on the management of recurrent colorectal carcinoma. Br J Surg 1998;86:244–49.

123. Martin DT, Aitkin D, Thurston M, et al. Successful experimental use of a self-contained gamma-detecting device. Curr Surg 1984;41:193–94.

124. Sung C, Van Osdol WW. Pharmacokinetic comparison of direct antibody targeting with pre-targeting protocols based on streptavidin-biotin binding. J Nucl Med 1995;36:867–76.

125. Paganelli G, Magnani P, Zito F, et al. Three-step monoclonal antibody tumour targeting in CEA-positive patients. Cancer Res 1991:51:5960–66.

126. Schneebaum S, Ritter DC, Burak WE. Radioimmunoguided surgery: primary clinical trials and applications. Semin Colon Rectal Surg 1995;6:217–25.

127. Burak WE, Schneebaum S. Radioimmunoguided surgery: recurrent clinical trials and applications. Semin Colon Rectal Surg 1995;226–35.

128. Schneebaum S, Papo J, Graif M, Bavatz M, Baron J, Skornik Y. Radioimmunoguided surgery: benefits for recurrent colorectal carcinoma. Ann Surg Oncol 1997;4:371–76.

129. Arnold MW, Young DC, Hitchcock CA, et al. Radioimmunoguided surgery in primary colorectal carcinoma: an intraoperative prognostic tool and adjuvant to traditional staging. Am J Surg 1995;170:315–18.

130. Butsch DJ, Burak WE, Young WC, et al. Radioimmunoguided surgery improves survival for patients with recurrent colorectal carcinoma. Surgery 1995;118:6340–39..

131. Ahtab F, Stoldt HS, Testori A, et al. Radioimmunoguided surgery and colorectal cancer. Eur J Surg Oncol 1996;22:381–96.

132. Raderer M, Kurtaran A, Hejna M, et al. 123I labelled vasoactive intestinal peptide receptor scintigraphy in patients with colorectal cancer. Br J Cancer 1998;78:1–5.

133. Rotondano G, Esposito P, Pellecchia L, Novi A, Romano G. Early detection of locally recurrent rectal cancer by endosonography. Br J Radiol 1997;70:567–72.

134. Kolecki R, Schirmer B. Intraoperative ultrasound and laparoscopic ultrasound. Surg Clin North Am 1998;78:251–71.

135. Hawley PR. Commentary: does rectal endosonography influence rectal cancer treatment? Int J Colorect Dis 1986;1:224–26.

5. Neo-adjuvant Therapy

B.D. Minsky, C.-H. Köhne and C. Greco

Introduction

A number of advances have been made in the adjuvant management of resectable rectal cancer. In patients with clinically resectable disease, pelvic radiation therapy decreases local recurrence and, in the preoperative setting, increases the chance of sphincter preservation. The addition of systemic chemotherapy further enhances local control and improves survival. The potential additional benefits of preoperative radiation therapy (with or without chemotherapy) include enhanced sphincter preservation and less toxicity.

This chapter will examine the results and selected controversies in the treatment of patients with clinically resectable rectal cancer who undergo neo-adjuvant (preoperative) therapy. This will include a discussion of the development and results of ongoing and recently completed randomized trials as well as the design of innovative Phase I/II programs. The role of preoperative therapy in patients with locally advanced/unresectable disease [1] has previously been reviewed and will not be discussed. Likewise, the results of postoperative combined modality therapy are reviewed in a separate chapter.

Preoperative Therapy

Rationale

Preoperative therapy (most commonly radiation therapy combined with systemic chemotherapy) has been gaining acceptance as a standard adjuvant therapy. The potential advantages of delivering adjuvant therapy in the preoperative setting include: decreased tumor seeding, less acute toxicity, increased radiosensitivity owing to more oxygenated cells, and enhanced sphincter preservation [2–7].

The primary disadvantage of preoperative radiation therapy is possibly overtreating patients with either early stage (T1–2N0) or metastatic disease. However, imaging techniques such as computed tomography [8], magnetic resonance imaging with a phased-array [9] or an endorectal coil [10], endorectal ultrasound [11], ultrasound guided pararectal lymph node biopsy [12], and positron emission tomography [13] allow more accurate selection, thereby decreasing the number of patients who are overtreated. The most accurate method of predicting T stage is endorectal ultrasound. In the preoperative setting its accuracy is as high as 90%. However, it is less accurate when performed after preoperative radiation [14].

Predictors of Response to Preoperative Therapy

In patients who receive preoperative therapy, it would be helpful to identify clinicopathologic features that could predict those tumors that will respond favorably. Based on the data showing that rapidly dividing cells are more sensitive to radiation, Willett et al. analyzed the proliferative index in patients with locally advanced/unresectable disease who underwent preoperative radiation therapy with or without 5-fluorouracil (5-FU) [15]. Tumors with a higher proliferation index had a higher response rate to preoperative therapy and, after radiation, there was a corresponding reduction in the proliferative index [16]. Desai and colleagues reported a higher incidence of recurrence in proliferating cell nuclear antigen (PCNA)-positive rectal cancers but noted a decreased likelihood of downstaging in PCNA-positive cancers [17]. By multivariate analysis, Neoptolemos and associates showed that this index did not add to the prognostic value of the Dukes' staging system [18]. Although the proliferative index may be useful in predicting the response to preoperative therapy, more experience is needed.

Additional tumor markers have been examined for their ability to predict downstaging. Rich and colleagues treated 50 patients with preoperative combined modality therapy and reported that tumors with a low spontaneous apoptosis index and positive BCL-2 staining had lower rates of downstaging. In 167 patients treated with preoperative radiation, there was a significant increase in downstaging in well-differentiated cancers [19]. Using residual tumor cell density rather than stage as a measure, this difference did not reach statistical significance. By univariate analysis, patients with a pathologic complete response had a non-significant improvement in survival. Berger and associates found that well-differentiated tumors had a greater degree of downstaging compared with moderately or poorly differentiated tumors [20].

The data suggest that, although some biologic or genetic markers may be more predictive than others, the decision to use preoperative therapy should not be made solely on their presence or absence. The development of predictive markers remains an active area of investigation.

Results of Preoperative Therapy

Non-randomized trials of preoperative radiation therapy with or without chemotherapy have shown improved local control and possibly survival [21–24]. It should be emphasized that some trials include patients with early stage (T1–2N0) or metastatic disease. These patients are excluded from the postoperative adjuvant therapy trials, therefore a randomized trial is necessary in order to compare accurately the results of preoperative and postoperative therapies.

To date, the only randomized trial is the Uppsala Trial, in which 471 patients were randomized to receive either a short intensive course of preoperative radiation (25.5 Gy in 1 week) or postoperative radiation (60 Gy split course) [25,26]. Patients with stage T1–2N0 disease who were randomized to the postoperative arm did not receive radiation and underwent observation only.

Preoperative radiation significantly decreased local recurrence (13% versus 22%; $p = 0.02$), however there was no difference in 5-year survival (42% versus 38%). Although there was no increase in postoperative mortality, there was a significant increase of perineal wound sepsis in the preoperative group (33% versus 18%; $p < 0.01$). Despite

the increased incidence of acute toxicity with preoperative radiation therapy, the long-term toxicity was decreased. The incidence of small bowel obstruction was 5% in the preoperative group and 11% in the postoperative group ($p = 0.01$). The incidence of grade 3+ toxicity was 20% for the preoperative group and 41% for the postoperative group. The high incidence of complications associated with short intensive course preoperative radiation therapy will be discussed later.

The first reported randomized trial of preoperative combined modality therapy was from the European Organization for Research on Treatment of Cancer (EORTC) [27]. Patients received preoperative radiation plus 5-FU (375 mg/m^2 bolus days 1–4) versus radiation alone. Overall, combined modality therapy decreased survival (46% versus 59%; $p = 0.06$). 5-FU was not employed as a systemic therapy with monthly cycles and the radiation techniques were unconventional, therefore it is difficult to interpret the results of this trial.

Given the advantage of chemotherapy in the postoperative setting, a variety of Phase I/II preoperative combined modality treatment programs have been developed. Retrospective data suggest that preoperative combined modality therapy increases pathologic downstaging compared with preoperative radiation therapy [28] and is associated with a lower incidence of acute toxicity compared with postoperative combined modality therapy [2]. The question of whether preoperative combined modality therapy is more effective than preoperative radiation therapy is being addressed in an ongoing randomized trial from the EORTC. The trial will determine if bolus 5-FU/leucovorin, either preoperatively and/or postoperatively, is superior to preoperative radiation therapy alone. The results are pending at this time.

Selected trials of preoperative combined modality therapy that were limited to patients with clinically resectable disease are listed in Table 5.1. The trials from Chari et al. [29] and Grann et al. [5] used bolus 5-FU-based chemotherapy, whereas the trials from Stryker et al. [30] and Rich et al. [31,32] used continuous infusion 5-FU-based chemotherapy.

On combining the four series, the incidence of grade 3+ toxicity during the combined modality segment was 21–25%, the pathologic complete response rates were 9–29%, and the incidence of local recurrence was 0–5%. The limited data do not allow a valid comparison of bolus versus continuous infusion 5-FU.

There have been 11 modern randomized trials carried out on preoperative radiation therapy (without chemotherapy) for resectable rectal cancer [27,33–44]. All used low to moderate doses of radia-

Table 5.1. Selected series of preoperative combined modality therapy for T3 clinically resectable rectal cancer

Series	No. Pts	Clinical[a] stage	Adjuvant therapy		% Acute grade 3+ toxicity[b]	Median F/U (months)	% Local failure	% Actuarial survival
			Preoperative	Postoperative				
Stryker et al. [30] (Northwestern University)	30	T3[c] and/or N+	45.0–50.4 Gy Bolus MMC CI 5-FU	43% had 5-FU	23	39	4	85 5-y
Rich et al. [31,32] (MD Anderson Hospital)	77	T1–3 (75% had T3)	45 Gy CI 5-FU	43% had CI 5-FU	N/A	27	4	83 3-y
Chari et al. [29] (Duke University)	43	T2–3	45 Gy Bolus 5-FU + CDDP × 2	None	21	25	5	93 5-y
Grann et al. [5] (MSKCC)	32	T3	50.4 Gy Bolus 5-FU/LV × 2	Bolus 5-FU/LV	25	24	0*	100 2-y[d]

[a] Determined by endorectal ultrasound.
[b] Total grade 3+ toxicity during the preoperative combined modality segment.
[c] 50% underwent transrectal ultrasound.
[d] Limited to the 15 patients with a minimum follow-up of 1 year or developed failure prior to 1 year.
 F/U, Follow-up; MMC, mitomycin-C; 5-FU, 5-fluorouracil; CI, continuous infusion; N/A, data not available in manuscript; CDDP, *cis*-diamine dichloroplatinum; MSKCC, Memorial Sloan-Kettering Cancer Center; LV, leucovorin.

tion. The second Medical Research Council Trial, which revealed a significant improvement in local control, distant control and disease-free survival, is excluded from this analysis because these patients had fixed or partially fixed (T4) disease [45].

Overall, some of the trials show a decrease in local recurrence; in five this difference reached statistical significance. A retrospective analysis of the trials reported prior to 1988 suggests that there may be a dose-response effect favoring preoperative radiation compared with postoperative radiation [46]. Although in some trials a subset analysis has revealed a significant improvement in survival [27,34,40], until the Swedish Rectal Cancer Trial was carried out none has reported a survival advantage for the total treatment group.

Intensive Short Course Preoperative Radiation

The Swedish Rectal Cancer Trial was the first randomized trial of preoperative radiation therapy to reveal a significant improvement in survival by intention to treat. A total of 1168 patients with clinically resectable rectal cancer were randomized to 25 Gy in 1 week followed by surgery 1 week later versus surgery alone [44]. With a median follow-up of 75 months, patients who were randomized to preoperative radiation had a significant decrease in local recurrence (12% versus 27%; $p < 0.001$) and an

improvement in 5-year survival (58% versus 48%; $p = 0.004$).

The survival benefit is intriguing. Furthermore, compared with postoperative combined modality therapy, this approach offers increased patient convenience and lower cost. For example, patients receive only five fractions (1 week) compared with 28 fractions (6 weeks) of radiation and do not require 6 months of chemotherapy. If the 1-week course of preoperative radiation improves survival significantly, then why not adopt it as standard therapy?

First, given that the other ten randomized trials of preoperative radiation therapy did not demonstrate a survival benefit, these data clearly need to be confirmed by additional studies. Secondly, even if future trials confirm a survival benefit, there are other equally important endpoints in rectal cancer that need to be addressed. These include acute toxicity, sphincter preservation and function, and quality of life.

Although prior trials of intensive short course radiation have revealed a significant increase in mortality [47], these differences were not reported in the Swedish Rectal Cancer Trial. This may have been related to the use of multiple field techniques.

Conventional radiation techniques include the use of multiple fields rather than simple anterior/posterior fields, computerized treatment planning and customized blocking. These techniques allow the delivery of higher doses of radiation while sparing the surrounding normal tissues such as the small intestine. As previously discussed in the Uppsala trial [25,26] the anterior/posterior radiation techniques commonly used with the other intensive short course radiation therapy trials are associated with an increase in toxicity.

The absence of an increase in mortality in the Swedish trial may have been related to the fact that 91% of patients received radiation using the more sophisticated multiple field radiation techniques. As reported in patients who receive conventional doses administered by techniques of preoperative combined modality therapy [2], the volume of small bowel in the radiation field may be the dose-limiting organ with radiation therapy [48]. In this trial, those patients who received radiation utilizing multiple fiel [48]d techniques had a significant decrease in postoperative mortality compared with those who received treatment with an anterior/posterior technique (3% versus 15%; $p < 0.001$). The postoperative mortality with surgery alone was 12%. However, the incidence of postoperative morbidity for the total group of patients receiving radiation (regardless of the technique) was still significantly higher when compared with the surgery control arm (44% versus 34%; $p = 0.001$). This is consistent with other trials of intensive short course preoperative radiation [49].

It should be emphasized that, even when multiple field techniques are used, data from the Stockholm I and II trials suggest that there is still a significant increase in postoperative mortality (4% versus 1%) when patients receive intensive short course radiation [47]. These high complication rates have not been reported in patients who receive conventional doses and techniques of preoperative radiation.

Sphincter Preservation with Preoperative Radiation

A major goal of preoperative radiation therapy is sphincter preservation. A variety of treatment approaches have been used and their selection depends on factors such as tumor histology, size, location, mobility, anatomic constraints and the technical expertise of the surgeon and radiation oncologist.

An analysis of 1316 patients treated in two previously published Scandinavian trials of intensive short courses of radiation reveals that downstaging was most pronounced when the interval between the completion of radiation and surgery was at least 10 days [50]. However, none of the randomized trials of intensive short course preoperative radiation addressed one of the most important controversies with preoperative therapy, which is whether the degree of downstaging is adequate to enhance sphincter preservation.

From the viewpoint of sphincter preservation, the advantage of preoperative therapy is to decrease the volume of the primary tumor. When the tumor is located in close proximity to the dentate line, this decrease in tumor volume may allow the surgeon to perform a sphincter conserving procedure that would not otherwise be possible. However, it should be emphasized that patients whose tumors directly invade the anal sphincter are unlikely to undergo sphincter preservation, even after a complete response.

In general, when sphincter preservation is the goal of therapy, the use of preoperative radiation therapy should be limited to patients who are not technically able to undergo a local excision owing to tumor size and/or anatomic constraints. For example, if the tumor is close to the anal sphincter, a full-thickness local excision with negative margins may require partial removal of the sphincter, resulting in compromised function.

Two surgical techniques have been used after preoperative therapy: local excision and a low anterior resection with or without a coloanal anastomosis. The use of a local excision has been limited to patients who are medically or technically unable to undergo a conventional operation [51], therefore this discussion will be limited to those who undergo a low anterior resection with or without a coloanal anastomosis.

When the goal of preoperative therapy is sphincter preservation, conventional doses and techniques of radiation are recommended. These include multiple field techniques to a total dose of 45–50.4 Gy at 1.8 Gy/fraction. Surgery should be performed 4–6 weeks after the completion of radiation. Unlike the intensive short course of radiation, this conventional design allows for recovery from the acute side effects of radiation and enhances tumor downstaging.

Preoperative Prospective Clinical Assessment

The most accurate method by which to determine if preoperative therapy has enhanced sphincter preservation is to perform a prospective clinical assessment. In this setting, the operating surgeon examines the patient prior to the commencement of preoperative therapy and declares the type of operation required. It must be emphasized that this assessment is based on an office examination and may not accurately reflect the assessment when the patient is relaxed under general anesthesia. The only method by which to account for this potential bias is to perform a randomized trial of preoperative versus postoperative therapy. With this randomized design, the accuracy of the assessment is determined because half of the patients are randomized to undergo surgery prior to postoperative therapy.

Clinical Experience with Sphincter Preservation

There are only five series that have reported results in patients with clinically resectable rectal cancer who underwent a prospective clinical assessment by their surgeon prior to the start of preperative therapy and were declared to need an abdominoperineal resection (Table 5.2). All used conventional doses and techniques of radiation therapy. Two of the series are from the Memorial Sloan-Kettering Cancer Center (MSKCC). The initial approach to sphincter preservation at the MSKCC was preoperative radiation therapy alone; the results of this prospective Phase I/II trial have been reported by Wagman et al. [4]. The more recent approach at the MSKCC has been the use of preoperative combined modality therapy, which has been reported by Grann and associates [5]. A trial of preoperative radiation therapy (without chemotherapy) was reported by Rouanet et al. from the Montpellier Cancer Institute [6]. The remaining two trials used combined modality therapy. Hyams and colleagues reported an interval analysis of the ongoing National Surgical Adjuvant Breast and Bowel Project (NSABP) R-03 Phase III randomized trial of preoperative versus postoperative combined modality therapy [7]. The remaining trial was reported by Maghfoor and colleagues from the Ellis Fischel Cancer Center [3].

There are other series in which patients have received preoperative radiation therapy followed by sphincter preserving surgery. For example Papillon and Gerard from the Centre Leon Berard [52] have reported their results and there is considerable experience with preoperative radiation therapy from the Thomas Jefferson University [16,23]. However, because patients did not undergo a prospective clinical assessment by their surgeon, the impact of the preoperative radiation therapy on enhancing sphincter preservation cannot be determined in these trials.

Preoperative Radiation Therapy

In an update of the MSKCC series by Wagman et al., 36 patients with clinically resectable disease underwent a prospective clinical assessment by their surgeon and were declared to require an abdominoperineal resection owing to the tumor's proximity to (but not invasion of) the anal sphincter [4]. By transrectal ultrasound, the clinical stage was T2 in five patients and T3 in 31 patients. The median distance from the anal verge was 4 cm and the median tumor size was 3.8 cm. Patients received 50.4 Gy followed by surgery 4–5 weeks later. Although no chemotherapy was delivered concurrently with radiation, patients with pathologically positive pelvic nodes or metastatic disease received postoperative 5-FU-based chemotherapy. A diverting colostomy was performed in all patients, which was reversed 2–4 months postoperatively. Sphincter function monitoring was performed by using a tele-

Table 5.2. Results of preoperative therapy in patients prospectively declared to require an abdominoperineal resection

	Wagman et al. [4] (MSKCC)	Grann et al. [5] (MSKCC)	Rouanel et al. [6] (Montpellier)	Hyams et al. [7] (NSABP R-03)	Maghfoor et al. [3] (Ellis Fischel)
No. enrolled	36	32	37	59	29
No. declared to need an APR	36	20	37	22	29
No. who underwent surgery	35	20	27	22	29
No. with T-3 disease (%)	31 (86)	20 (100)	12 (32)	22 (100)	25 (86)
No. who underwent LAR ± coloanal anastomosis (%)	27 (77)	17 (85)	17 (63)	16 (23)	22 (76)
No. who underwent local excision (%)	0	0	4 (15)	0	0
Local failure %	17	0	8	N/A	3
Survival %	64 5-y	100 2-y	83 2-y	N/A	87[a]
No. evaluable for sphincter function analysis (%)	27 (77)	N/A	14 (52)	N/A	N/A
Sphincter function %	85% Good to excellent	N/A	71% Perfect	N/A	N/A

[a] Disease-free survival with a median follow-up of 12 months.
MSKCC, Memorial Sloan Kettering Cancer Center; APR, abdominoperineal resection; LAR, low anterior resection; N/A, data not reported in the manuscript.

phone survey and utilizing the the MSKCC anal sphincter function scale [53]. Definitions of this scale include: excellent = 1–2 bowel movements per day, no soilage; good = 3–4 bowel movements per day and/or mild soilage; fair = episodic >4 bowel movements per day and/or moderate soilage; and poor = incontinence.

Of the 35 patients who underwent surgery, 27 (77%) were able to undergo a low anterior resection/coloanal anastomosis and the pathological complete response rate was 14%. With a median follow-up of 56 months, the 17% cumulative local failure rate as a component of failure was crude; the 5-year actuarial rate was 21%. The 5-year actuarial disease-free survival was 60% and overall survival was 64%. Of the 27 patients who were eligible for analysis, sphincter function was: excellent in 59%, good in 26%, fair in 15%, and poor in 0%. Therefore, 85% had good or excellent sphincter function. The median number of bowel movements was 2 per day (range: 0–8).

A similar approach was reported by Rouanet and associates [6]. A total of 37 patients (T2 in 15 patients and T3 in 12) received 40 Gy preoperatively. Further treatment was based on the primary tumor response. If at 3 weeks after the completion of radiation there was a ≥30% response, an additional 20 Gy was delivered and a low anterior resection/coloanal anastomosis was performed 2–4 weeks later. If there was a <30% response, patients proceeded directly to surgery. Of the 27 patients who were brought to surgery, 17 (63%) underwent a low anterior resection/coloanal anastomosis and four (15%) underwent a transanal local excision, resulting in a total of 78% of patients who were able to undergo sphincter preserving surgery. Of the 14 patients available for sphincter function analysis, 71% had "perfect continence", 86% had ≤2 bowel movements per day, and 14% had urgency.

Preoperative Combined Modality Therapy

Extrapolating from data that show a decrease in local recurrence and an increase in survival with postoperative combined modality therapy [54], most patients with clinically resectable T3 disease receive preoperative combined modality therapy rather than radiation therapy alone. The preliminary results of the MSKCC experience have been reported by Grann et al. [5]. A total of 32 patients with transrectal ultrasound-staged T3 rectal cancers received preoperative combined modality therapy with the concurrent 5-FU/low-dose leucovorin regimen. Patients underwent surgery 4–5 weeks later, and received a median of two monthly cycles of postoperative 5-FU and leucovorin. All patients underwent surgery, 75% (24/32) with sphincter preserving surgery (a low anterior resection with or without a coloanal anastomosis). Of the 20 patients who on prospective clinical assessment were declared to require an abdominoperineal resection, 17 (85%) were able to undergo sphincter preserving surgery. The outcome analysis was limited to the 15 patients with a minimum follow-up of 1 year or who developed failure prior to 1 year. With a median follow-up of 24 months there were no local recurrences; the 2-year actuarial disease-free survival was 86% and the overall 2-year survival was 100%.

An analysis of the first 116 patients enrolled on the NSABP R-03 randomized trial of preoperative versus postoperative combined modality therapy has been presented by Hyams and colleagues [7]. It should be noted that this is an interim analysis of an ongoing trial; therefore the results should be interpreted with caution. A prospective clinical assessment was performed on the 59 patients who received preoperative combined modality therapy, which identified 22 who were judged to require an abdominoperineal resection. Of the 22, 16 actually required an abdominoperineal resection. Therefore, the preoperative therapy converted only 27% of these patients from an abdominoperineal resection to a low anterior resection/coloanal anastomosis. The reason for the low rate of sphincter preservation in the NSABP trial is unclear. It is to be hoped that future research will address this issue.

Since half the patients were randomized to undergo surgery prior to the postoperative therapy, the accuracy of the office assessment to predict the type of operation required could be determined. Of the 57 patients randomized to the postoperative combined modality arm, 26 were declared clinically to require an abdominoperineal resection and all 26 underwent this procedure. Therefore, the data suggest that the office assessment is an accurate method by which to predict the type of operation required. The incidence of postoperative complications was similar in both the preoperative and postoperative arms (33% and 30% respectively). Functional results were not presented.

In the preliminary report from Maghfoor and colleagues [3], 29 patients with T3 (n = 25) or T4 (n = 4) disease who were judged clinically to require an abdominoperineal resection received continuous infusion 5-FU concurrently with 54 Gy. The pathologic complete response rate was 14% and 22 patients (76%) were able to undergo sphincter preserving surgery. With a median follow-up of 12 months, the disease-free survival was 87% and the local failure rate was 3%. Sphincter function data were not presented.

Sphincter preservation without adequate function is meaningless. A well-functioning colostomy may be more desirable than a poorly-functioning sphincter. The effect on sphincter function is most likely related to the cumulative impact of the three components of therapy (surgery, radiation and chemotherapy). Not only is there a lack of prospective, randomized data examining functional results, but most series use subjective assessment tools such as telephone and mail surveys. One series has reported that the detrimental effect on sphincter function seen with postoperative radiation therapy [55,56] may not be so problematic with preoperative radiation therapy. Birnbaum and colleagues have examined prospectively the short-term [57] and long-term [58] impact of preoperative radiation therapy on sphincter function. Patients received conventional doses and techniques of radiation and were assessed objectively by anal manometry with or without transrectal ultrasound. In the 20 patients assessed for short-term and 10 patients assessed for long-term results, radiation therapy had a "minimal" effect on sphincter function.

In summary, the data suggest that preoperative combined modality therapy, albeit less intense than postoperative therapy, may affect sphincter function adversely. This potential morbidity needs to be weighed against the benefits of adjuvant therapy.

Given the suggestion of decreased acute toxicity and enhanced sphincter preservation with preoperative radiation therapy, randomized trials are needed. Three randomized trials of preoperative versus postoperative combined modality therapy for clinically resectable, T3 rectal cancer have been developed. Two are from the USA (INT 0147; NSABP R0-3) and one from Germany (CAO/ARO/AIO 94). All three use conventional doses and techniques of radiation therapy and concurrent 5-FU-based chemo-

therapy. Both the INT 0147 and the NSABP R-03 trials require a preoperative clinical assessment declaring the type of operation required. Unfortunately, low accrual has resulted in the closure of the INT 0147 trial and may also jeopardize the NSABP R-03 trial. Although sphincter preservation is an endpoint of the German CAO/ARO/AIO 94 trial, it does not require a preoperative clinical assessment (Fig. 5.1 [59]). Therefore, although the German trial will address the issue of toxicity and efficacy of preoperative versus postoperative combined modality therapy, it will not clearly answer the question of sphincter preservation.

Is Adjuvant Therapy Necessary in Patients Undergoing a Total Mesorectal Resection?

Some physicians contend that adjuvant therapy is not necessary if patients undergo more extensive surgery. In one series, total mesorectal excision, which involves sharp dissection around the integral mesentery of the hind gut, decreased the local recurrence rate to 5% [60]. However, these data must be interpreted with caution because this procedure allows the identification and exclusion of patients with more advanced disease when compared with patients treated in the adjuvant trials in which more conventional surgery is performed. This results in a clear selection bias. In addition, some patients with T3 and/or N1–2 disease received radiation therapy with or without chemotherapy (i.e. 28% in the series

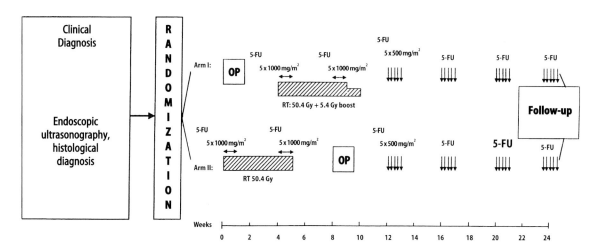

Fig. 5.1. German CAO/ARO/AIO 94 randomized trial of preoperative versus postoperative combined modality therapy (redrawn from Minsky 1998 [59]).

from Enker, et al. [61] and 18% in the series by Haas-Kock et al. [62]. Furthermore, total mesorectal excision may also be associated with higher complication rates. In the Basingstoke Hospital experience of 219 patients who underwent a total mesorectal resection, 11% had major and 6% had minor anastomotic leaks [63]. In the series from Aitken, operative deaths were excluded from the analysis [64].

The Dutch CKVO 95-04 trial is examining the role of intensive short course preoperative radiation therapy in patients who undergo total mesorectal excision. Patients are randomized to the administration of 25 Gy in 1 week versus surgery alone. Postoperative radiation is reserved for patients in the surgery-only arm who do not undergo a curative resection. Investigator participation is limited to surgeons who have demonstrated proficiency in performing a total mesorectal excision. The trial is open to accrual and the results are not yet available.

The use of total mesorectal excision has increased awareness of the importance of surgical technique. Careful surgical techniques are central to the successful management of rectal cancer. However, they should be considered as a valuable component of therapy, not in competition with adjuvant therapy. The relative benefits and risks of total mesorectal excision (focusing on endpoints such as local control, survival, sphincter preservation and function, surgical morbidity and mortality, and quality of life) need to be more carefully documented.

Investigational Approaches

Although there have been advances in adjuvant therapy, the development of innovative treatment techniques needs to continue. Selected approaches include radiation fractionation schemes and new chemotherapeutic agents. Some of these techniques have been developed in patients with advanced disease and have not yet been used in the adjuvant setting.

Altered Radiation Fractionation Schemes

Various fractionation programs have evolved with the goal of enhancing tumor cell damage by radiation without increasing normal tissue injury [65]. The repair of subcellular injury, regeneration, cell cycle redistribution, and reoxygenation are all factors operating at the cellular level that contribute to differences in how various normal tissues and tumors respond to fractionated radiation. The use of hyperfractionation and accelerated fractionation schedules take advantage of some of these factors. A Phase I trial from Lausanne of postoperative accelerated hyperfractionation (1.6 Gy b.i.d. to 48 Gy) demonstrated acceptable acute toxicity [66]. A follow-up report from the same group suggests that b.i.d. radiation is better tolerated when delivered preoperatively compared with postoperatively [67]. Although the late effects should be the same as or, more likely, less than conventional fractionation schemes, the major limitation of accelerated hyperfractionation is acute normal tissue toxicity.

In a randomized trial of patients receiving radiation therapy for pelvic malignancies, three-dimensional conformal radiation therapy decreased the volume of normal tissue in the radiation field; however, it did not decrease acute toxicity [68]. Other techniques such as neutron beam radiation [69], hyperthermia [70,71] radiosensitizers [72], radioprotectors [73,74], altered radiation fractionation schemes [66,67], and proton and three-dimensional treatment planning [75,76] are encouraging, but remain experimental.

New Chemotherapeutic Agents

Selected new chemotherapeutic agents having activity in colorectal cancer, which are in either in development or have been approved, include CPT-11, tomudex, trimetrexate, oxaliplatin and UFT [77–80]. Clinical trials examining the combination of some of these agents with pelvic radiation are under way [82,82]. In patients with unresectable disease, Marsh and associates have combined chronobiologically shaped 5-FU infusion with preoperative radiation therapy [83].

Summary

For patients who have clinically resectable disease, the decision to use preoperative rather than postoperative therapy is based on a number of issues. The most important one is the assessment of the type of surgery required. If the tumor is proximal enough in the rectum such that it is able to be removed with a low anterior resection, then most physicians would recommend surgery. If the tumor is T3 and/or N1-2, this would be followed by postoperative combined modality therapy. If sphincter preserving surgery is not technically possible then the preoperative approach should be used. The decision of whether to use preoperative radiation therapy or preoperative combined modality therapy is based on the results of the endorectal ultrasound. If it reveals T2 disease, the patient may have pathologic T2N0M0 disease, when the sole reason for preoperative therapy would be sphincter preservation. Therefore, preoperative radiation therapy alone is recommended. If positive mesorectal and/or pelvic lymph nodes are identified at the time of surgery, adjuvant postoperative 5-FU-based chemotherapy is for 6 months recommended. There are two potential disadvantages to this approach. First, the ultrasound may understage approximately 10% of patients who have pathologic stage T3 disease. Secondly, because preoperative radiation downstages pelvic lymph nodes, the true incidence of node-positive disease is unknown. Obviously, these disadvantages need to be weighed against the risk of overtreating these patients with combined modality therapy.

In contrast, patients with transrectal ultrasound-staged T3 disease who clinically require an abdominoperineal resection should receive preoperative combined modality therapy followed by surgery and postoperative 5-FU-based chemotherapy. This recommendation is based on extrapolation of the significant improvement in local control and survival in patients with T3 and/or N1-2 disease who receive adjuvant postoperative combined modality therapy. Trials in progress will help to determine if the preoperative approach is superior to the postoperative approach.

References

1. Minsky BD. Management of locally advanced/unresectable rectal cancer. Radiat Oncol Invest 1995;3:97–107.
2. Minsky BD, Cohen AM, Enker WE, et al. Combined modality therapy of rectal cancer: decreased acute toxicity with the pre-operative approach. J Clin Oncol 1992;10:1218–24.
3. Maghfoor I, Wilkes J, Kuvshinoff B, et al. Neoadjuvant chemoradiotherapy with sphincter-sparing surgery for low lying rectal cancer [sbstract]. Proc ASCO 1997;16:274.
4. Wagman R, Minsky BD, Cohen AM, Guillem JG, Paty PB. Sphincter preservation with pre-operative radiation therapy (RT) and coloanal anastomosis: long term follow-up [abstract]. Int J Radiat Oncol Biol Phys 1997;39:167.
5. Grann A, Minsky BD, Cohen AM, et al. Preliminary results of pre-operative 5-fluorouracil (5-FU), low dose leucovorin, and concurrent radiation therapy for resectable T3 rectal cancer. Dis Colon Rectum 1997;40:515–22.
6. Rouanet P, Fabre JM, Dubois JB, et al. Conservative surgery for low rectal carcinoma after high-dose radiation. Functional and oncologic results. Ann Surg 1995;221:67–73.
7. Hyams DM, Mamounas EP, Petrelli N, et al. A clinical trial to evaluate the worth of preoperative multimodality therapy in patients with operable carcinoma of the rectum. A progress report of the National Surgical Adjuvant Breast and Bowel Project protocol R0-3. Dis Colon Rectum 1997;40:131–39.
8. Koehler PR, Feldberg MAM, van Waes PFGM. Preoperative staging of rectal cancer with computerized tomography. Accuracy, efficacy, and effect on patient management. Cancer 1984;54:512–16.
9. Hadfield MB, Nicholson AA, MacDonald AW, et al. Preoperative staging of rectal carcinoma by magnetic resonance imaging with a pelvic phased-array coil. Br J Surg 1997;84:529–31.
10. deSouza NM, Hall AS, Puni R, Gilderdale DJ, Young IR, Kmiot WA. High resolution magnetic resonance imaging of the anal sphincter using a dedicated endoanal coil. Comparison of magnetic resonance imaging with surgical findings. Dis Colon Rectum 1996;39:926–34.
11. Hunerbein M, Schlag PM. Three-dimensional endosonography for staging of rectal cancer. Ann Surg 1997;25:432–38.
12. Milsom JW, Czyrko C, Hull TL, Strong SA, Fazio VW. Preoperative biopsy of pararectal lymph nodes in rectal cancer using endoluminal ultrasonography. Dis Colon Rectum 1994;37:364–68.
13. Falk PM, Gupta NC, Thorson AG, et al. Positron emission tomography for preoperative staging of colorectal carcinoma. Dis Colon Rectum 1994;37:153–56.
14. Bernini A, Deen KI, Madoff RD, Wong WD. Preoperative adjuvant radiation with chemotherapy for rectal cancer: its impact on stage of disease and the role of endorectal ultrasound. Ann Surg Oncol 1996;3:131–35.
15. Willett CG, Warland G, Coen J, Shellito PC, Compton CC. Rectal cancer: the influence of tumor proliferation on response to preoperative irradiation. Int J Radiat Oncol Biol Phys 1995;32:57–61.
16. Willett CG, Warland G, Hagan MP, et al. Tumor proliferation in rectal cancer following preoperative irradiation. J Clin Oncol 1995;13:1417–24.
17. Desai GR, Meyerson RJ, Higashikubo R, et al. Carcinoma of the rectum: possible cellular predictors of metastatic potential and response to radiation therapy. Dis Colon Rectum 1996;39:1090–96.
18. Neoptolemos JP, Oates GD, Newbold KM, Robson AM, McConkey C, Powell J. Cyclin/proliferation cell nuclear antigen immunohistochemistry does not improve the prognostic power of Dukes' or Jass' classifications for colorectal cancer. Br J Surg 1995;82:184–87.
19. Rich TA, Sinicrope F, Stephens C, et al. Downstaging of T3 rectal cancer after preoperative infusional chemoradiation is correlated with spontaneous apoptosis index and BCL-2 staining [abstract]. Int J Radiat Oncol Biol Phys 1996;36:259.
20. Berger C, de Muret A, Garaud P, et al. Preoperative radiotherapy (RT) for rectal cancer: predictive factors of tumor downstaging and residual tumor density (RTCD): prognostic implications. Int J Radiat Oncol Biol Phys 1997;37:619–27.
21. Zlotecki RA, Mendenhall WM, Copeland EM, et al. Preoperative radiotherapy for resectable rectal cancer: improved local control is prognostic for distant metastasis occurrence and survival [abstract]. Int J Radiat Oncol Biol Phys 1996;36:261.
22. Myerson RJ, Michalski JM, King ML, et al. Adjuvant radiation therapy for rectal carcinoma: predictors of outcome. Int J Radiat Oncol Biol Phys 1995;32:41–50.
23. Bannon JP, Marks GJ, Mohiuddin M, Rakinic J, Nong-Zhou J, Nagle D. Radical and local excisional methods of sphincter-sparing surgery after high-dose radiation for cancer of the distal 3 cm of the rectum. Ann Surg Oncol 1995;2:221–27.
24. Bosset JF, Pavy JJ, Hamers HP, et al. Determination of the optimal dose of 5-fluorouracil when combined with low dose d,l-leucovorin and irradiation in rectal cancer: results of three consecutive Phase II studies. Eur J Cancer 1993;29:476–86.
25. Pahlman L, Glimelius B. Pre- or postoperative radiotherapy in rectal and rectosigmoid carcinoma: report from a randomized multicenter trial. Ann Surg 1990;211:187–95.

26. Frykholm GJ, Glimelius B, Pahlman L. Preoperative or post-operative irradiation in adenocarcinoma of the rectum: final treatment results of a randomized trial and an evaluation of late secondary effects. Dis Colon Rectum 1993;36:564–72.

27. Boulis-Wassif S, Gerard A, Loygue J, Camelot D, Buyse M, Duez N. Final results of a randomized trial on the treatment of rectal cancer with preoperative radiotherapy alone or in combination with 5-fluorouracil, followed by radical surgery. Cancer 1984;53:1811–18.

28. Minsky BD. Multidisciplinary management of resectable rectal cancer. Oncology 1996;10:1701–14.

29. Chari RS, Tyler DS, Anscher MS, et al. Preoperative radiation and chemotherapy in the treatment of adenocarcinoma of the rectum. Ann Surg 1995;221:778–87.

30. Stryker SJ, Kiel KD, Rademaker A, Shaw JM, Ujiki GT, Poticha SM. Preoperative "chemoradiation" for Stages II and II rectal carcinoma. Arch Surg 1996;131:514–19.

31. Rich TA, Skibber JM, Ajani JA, et al. Preoperative infusional chemoradiation therapy for stage T3 rectal cancer. Int J Radiat Oncol Biol Phys 1995;32:1025–29.

32. Rich TA. Infusional chemoradiation for operable rectal cancer: post-, pre-, or nonoperative management? Oncology 1997;11:295–315.

33. Gerard A, Buyse M, Nordlinger B, et al. Preoperative radiotherapy as adjuvant treatment in rectal cancer. Ann Surg 1988;208:606–16.

34. Cedermark B, Johansson H, Rutqvist LE, Wilking N. The Stockholm I trial of preoperative short term radiotherapy in operable rectal carcinoma. Cancer 1995;75:2269–75.

35. Higgins GA, Humphrey EW, Dwight RW, Roswit B, Lu LE Jr, Keehn RJ. Preoperative radiation and surgery for cancer of the rectum: Veterans Administration Surgical Oncology Group trial II. Cancer 1986;58:352–59.

36. Rider WD, Palmer JA, Mahoney LJ, Robertson CT. Preoperative irradiation in operable cancer of the rectum: report of the Toronto Trial. Can J Surg 1977;20:335–38.

37. Roswit B, Higgins GA Jr, Keehn R. Preoperative irradiation for carcinoma of the rectum and rectosigmoid colon: report of a national Veterans Administration randomized study. Cancer 1975;35:1597–602.

38. Duncan W. Adjuvant radiotherapy in rectal cancer: the MRC trials. Br J Surg 1985;72:S59–S62.

39. Reis Neto JA, Quilici FA, Reis JA Jr. A comparison of non-operative vs preoperative radiotherapy in rectal carcinoma: a 10 year randomized trial. Dis Colon Rectum 1989;32:702–10.

40. Cedermark B. The Stockholm II trial on preoperative short term radiotherapy in operable rectal carcinoma: a prospective randomized trial [abstract]. Proc ASCO 1994;13:198.

41. Swedish Rectal Cancer Trial. Initial report from a Swedish multicentre study examining the role of preoperative irradiation in the treatment of patients with resectable rectal cancer. Br J Surg 1993;80:1333–37.

42. Swedish Rectal Cancer Trial. Local recurrence rate in a randomized multicentre trial of preoperative radiotherapy compared to surgery alone in resectable rectal cancer. Eur J Surg 1996;162:397–402.

43. Goldberg PA, Nicholls RJ, Porter NH, Love S, Grimsey JE. Long-term results of a randomized trial of short-course low-dose adjuvant pre-operative radiotherapy for rectal cancer: reduction in local treatment failure. Eur J Cancer 1994;30A:1602–606.

44. Swedish Rectal Cancer Trial. Improved survival with pre-operative radiotherapy in resectable rectal cancer. N Engl J Med 1997;336:980–87.

45. Medical Research Council Rectal Cancer Working Party. Randomized trial of surgery alone versus radiotherapy followed by surgery for potentially operable, locally advanced rectal cancer. Lancet 1996;348:1605–609.

46. Glimelius B, Isacson U, Jung B, Pahlman L. Radiotherapy in addition to radical surgery in rectal cancer: evidence for a dose–response effect favoring preoperative treatment. Int J Radiat Oncol Biol Phys 1997;37:281–87.

47. Holm T, Rutqvist LE, Johansson H, Cedermark B. Post-operative mortality in rectal cancer treated with or without preoperative radiotherapy: causes and risk factors. Br J Surg 1996;83:964–68.

48. Frykholm GJ, Isacsson U, Nygard K, et al. Preoperative radiotherapy in rectal carcinoma: aspects of acute adverse effects and radiation technique. Int J Radiat Oncol Biol Phys 1996;35:1039–48.

49. Holm T, Singnomklao T, Rutqvist LE, Cedermark B. Adjuvant preoperative radiotherapy in patients with rectal carcinoma. Adverse effects during long term follow-up of two randomized trials. Cancer 1996;78:968–76.

50. Graf W, Dahlberg M, Osman MM, Holmberg L, Pahlman L, Glimelius B. Short-term preoperative radiotherapy results in down-staging of rectal cancer: a study of 1316 patients. Radiother Oncol 1997;43:133–37.

51. Mohiuddin M, Marks J, Bannon J. High-dose preoperative radiation and full thickness local excision: a new option for selected T3 distal rectal cancer. Int J Radiat Oncol Biol Phys 1994;30:845–49.

52. Papillon J, Gerard JP. Role of radiotherapy in anal preservation for cancers of the lower third of the rectum. Int J Radiat Oncol Biol Phys 1990;19:1219–20.

53. Minsky BD, Cohen AM, Enker WE, Paty P. Sphincter preservation with preoperative radiation therapy and coloanal anastomosis. Int J Radiat Oncol Biol Phys 1995;31:553–59.

54. National Institutes of Health Consensus Conference. Adjuvant therapy for patients with colon and rectal cancer. JAMA 1990;264:1444–50.

55. Kollmorgen CF, Meagher AP, Pemberton JH, Martenson JA, Ilstrup DM. The long term effect of adjuvant postoperative chemoradiotherapy for rectal cancer on bowel function. Ann Surg 1994;220:676–82.

56. Paty PB, Enker WE, Cohen AM, Minsky BD, Friedlander-Klar H. Long-term functional results of coloanal anastomosis for rectal cancer. Am J Surg 1994;167:90–95.

57. Birnbaum EH, Dreznik Z, Myerson RJ, et al. Early effect of external beam radiation on anal sphincter; a study using anal manometry and transrectal ultrasound. Dis Colon Rectum 1992;35:757–61.

58. Birnbaum EH, Meyerson RJ, Fry RD, Kodner IJ, Fleshman JW. Chronic effects of pelvic radiation therapy on anorectal function. Dis Colon Rectum 1994;37:909–15.

59. Minsky BD. Adjuvant therapy for rectal cancer: results and controversies. Oncology 1998;12:1129–39.

60. MacFarlane JK, Ryall RD, Heald RJ. Mesorectal excision for rectal cancer. Lancet 1993;341:457–60.

61. Enker WE, Thaler HT, Cranor ML, Polyak T. Total meso-rectal excision in the operative treatment of carcinoma of the rectum. J Am Coll Surg 1995;181:335–45.

62. Haas-Kock DFM, Baeten CGMI, Jager JJ, et al. Prognostic significance of radial margins of clearance in rectal cancer. Br J Surg 1996;83:781–85.

63. Karanjia ND, Corder AP, Bearn P, Heald RJ. Leakage from stapled low anastomosis after total mesorectal excision for carcinoma of the rectum. Br J Surg 1995;81:1224–26.

64. Aitken RJ. Mesorectal excision for rectal cancer. Br J Surg 1996;83:214–16.

65. Withers HR. Biological basis for altered fractionation schemes. Cancer 1985;55:2086–95.

66. Coucke PA, Cuttat JF, Mirimanoff RO. Adjuvant post-operative accelerated hyperfractionated radiotherapy in

rectal cancer: a feasibility study. Int J Radiat Oncol Biol Phys 1993;27:885–89.

67. Coucke PA, Sartorelli B, Cuttat JF, Jeanneret W, Gillet M, Mirimanoff RO. The rationale to switch from postoperative hyperfractionated accelerated radiotherapy to preoperative hyperfractionated accelerated radiotherapy in rectal cancer. Int J Radiat Oncol Biol Phys 1995;32:181–88.

68. Tait DM, Nahum AE, Meyer LC, et al. Acute toxicity in pelvic radiotherapy; a randomised trial of conformal versus conventional treatment. Radiother Oncol 1997;42:121–36.

69. Duncan W, Arnott SJ, Jack WJL, Orr JA, Kerr GR, Williams JR. Results of two randomized trials of neutron therapy in rectal adenocarcinoma. Radiother Oncol 1987;8:191–98.

70. Ichikawa D, Yamaguchi T, Yoshioka Y, Sawai K, Takahashi T. Prognostic evaluation of preoperative combined treatment for advanced cancer in the lower rectum with radiation, intraluminal hyperthermia, and 5-fluorouracil suppository. Am J Surg 1996;171:346–50.

71. Ohno S, Tomoda M, Tomisaki S, et al. Improved surgical results after combining preoperative hyperthermia with chemotherapy and radiotherapy for patients with carcinoma of the rectum. Dis Colon Rectum 1997;40:401–406.

72. Liu T, Liu Y, He S, Zhang Z, Kligerman MM. Use of radiation with or without WR-2721 in advanced rectal cancer. Cancer 1992;69:2820–25.

73. Stelzer KJ, Koh WJ, Kurtz H, Greer BE, Griffin TW. Caffeine consumption is associated with decreased severe late toxicity after radiation to the pelvis. Int J Radiat Oncol Biol Phys 1994;30:411–17.

74. Rhomberg W, Eiter H, Hergan K, Schneider B. Inoperable recurrent rectal cancer: results of a prospective trial with radiation therapy and razoxane. Int J Radiat Oncol Biol Phys 1994;30:419–25.

75. Tatsuzaki H, Urie MM, Willett CG. 3-D comparative study of proton vs X-ray radiation therapy for rectal cancer. Int J Radiat Oncol Biol Phys 1991;22:369–74.

76. Isacsson U, Montelius A, Jung B, Glimelius B. Comparative treatment planning between proton and X-ray therapy in locally advanced rectal cancer. Radiother Oncol 1997;41:263–72.

77. Pitot HC, Wender DB, O'Connell MJ, et al. Phase II trial of irinotecan in patients with metastatic colorectal carcinoma. J Clin Oncol 1997;15:2910–19.

78. Cunningham D, Zalcberg JR, Rath U, et al. Final results of a randomised trial comparing "Tomudex" (raltitrexed) with 5-fluorouracil plus leucovorin in advanced colorectal cancer. Ann Oncol 1996;961:961–65.

79. Saltz LB, Leichman CG, Young CW, et al. A fixed-ratio combination of uracil and ftorafur (UFT) with low dose leucovorin. Cancer 1995;75:782–85.

80. Gorlick R, Metzger R, Danenberg K, et al. Higher levels of thymidylate synthase gene expression are observed in pulmonary as compared with hepatic metastases of colorectal adenocarcinoma. J Clin Oncol 1998;16:1465–69.

81. Botwood N, James R, Vernon C, Price P. A Phase I study of "Tomudex" (raltitrexed) with radiotherapy (RT) as adjuvant treatment in patients (pt) with operable rectal cancer [abstract]. Proc ASCO 1998;17:277.

82. Rich TA, Kirichenko AV. Camptothecin radiation sensitization: mechanisms, schedules, and timing. Oncology 1998;12:114–19.

83. Marsh RW, Chu NM, Vauthey JN, et al. Preoperative treatment of patients with locally advanced unresectable rectal adenocarcinoma utilizing continuous chronobiologically shaped 5-fluorouracil infusion and radiation therapy. Cancer 1996;78:217–25.

6. Restorative Procedures

J.W. Milsom and H.-J. Cho

Introduction

Rectal cancer is a common malignancy in the USA and, by itself (apart from cancer of colon), ranks sixth among intestinal malignancies [1]. Despite expanding interest in chemotherapy and radiation therapy for the management of rectal cancer, surgical efforts remain the foundation of nearly all curative therapy. Applying the most advanced surgical principles, the surgeon now has the opportunity to excise completely most rectal cancers and give the majority of patients the possibility of anal sphincter preservation and relatively normal bowel and pelvic function.

Restorative procedures (anterior resection, low anterior resection and coloanal anastomosis) are performed more frequently than ever before. Complete abdominoperineal resection of the lower rectum and anal canal with permanent colostomy remains an important procedure and benchmark for curative treatment but, in the hands of most experts, it is used only when the rectal tumor directly or nearly directly invades the anal sphincters [2].

The purpose of this chapter is to define the role of major surgical resections in the treatment of rectal carcinoma. We hope to provide the reader with insights into the relevant anatomy, the factors influencing the choice of operation, and some of the controversies surrounding rectal cancer surgery, including use of laparoscopic techniques. Important concepts regarding sphincter salvage and pelvic nerve preservation together with maintenance of sound oncologic principles also are highlighted.

Relevant Anatomy of the Rectum and Perirectal Tissues

By surgical convention, the rectum is divided into thirds. Because of variations in body habitus and length of the anal canal, it is difficult to assign precise lengths to each third of the rectum but, in general, the upper third extends from the sacral promontory distally to the anterior peritoneal reflection, making it lie approximately 10–15 cm above the anal verge on proctologic examination. This part of the rectum is easily resected and demonstrates oncologic behavior similar to the sigmoid colon. The middle third of the rectum begins at the anterior peritoneal reflection (10–11 cm from the anal verge) and extends to 5 or 6 cm above the anal verge. The lower third of the rectum begins 5 or 6 cm from the verge and ends at the top of the anal sphincters (top of the surgical anal canal). The upper portion of the "surgical" anal canal begins at the top of the anal sphincters and extends to the anal verge, which is denoted grossly by the junction of hair- and non-hair-bearing skin seen at this location.

The literature on sphincter saving rectal cancer surgery is rife with confusion about precisely where tumors are located, primarily because most surgeons reporting on tumor location do so with reference to distance from the anal verge. The problem with this convention in tumors of the middle and lower rectum is that the length of the surgical anal canal is highly variable (Fig. 6.1) and may range from 2 to 7 cm depending on sex and body habitus. Thus, a tumor with its lower margin at 8 cm from the anal verge in a thin woman may lie well within the mid-rectum, with 5 or 6 cm of clearance above the anal sphincters. In a heavily muscled man with a tumor at the same distance above the verge, this tumor may lie only 1 or 2 cm above the sphincters. The surgical implications of this kind of difference are tremendous; thus a profound understanding of these anatomic variations is crucial in providing expert care in rectal cancer management.

The plentiful blood supply of the rectum and pelvic tissues ensures, in nearly all instances, that major portions of the rectum and its blood supply

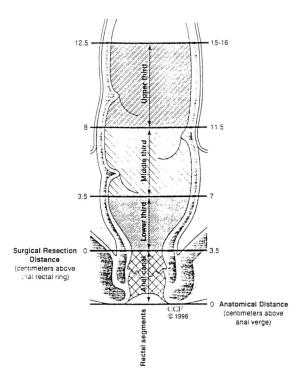

Fig. 6.1. Surgical and purely anatomical regions of the rectum as they relate to the anal sphincters and pelvic floor.

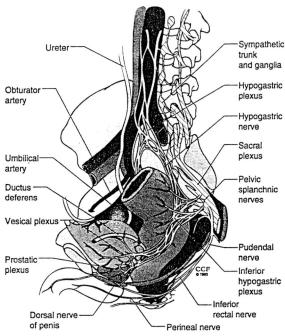

Fig. 6.2. Pelvic innervation (lateral view).

may be removed, yet the remainder of the organ will survive. Superiorly, the inferior mesenteric artery (IMA) is the major source of vascular inflow to the upper rectum by way of the superior rectal (hemorrhoidal) artery, which represents the terminal branch of the IMA. Anterolaterally, in the region of the mid-rectum, the middle rectal arteries branch from the internal iliac vessels to supply the rectum at this level. These vessels are often diminutive, and may be absent in 50% or more of patients. Inferiorly, branching from the internal pudendal vessels are the inferior rectal arteries. These supply the anal sphincters and lower rectum by passing up through the pelvic floor and along the wall of the rectum. They are the important vascular supply to the distal rectal segment in instances of sphincter sparing surgery.

An understanding of the innervation of the rectum and adjacent pelvic structures is also crucial to the performance of safe and effective rectal cancer surgery. The rectum is surrounded by both the sympathetic and parasympathetic components of the autonomic nervous system. The sympathetic nerves cascade as a plexus from the pre-aortic region, just posterior to the IMA, bifurcating at the sacral promontory and then running laterally and inferiorly down the pelvic side walls. The parasympathetic nerves branch from sacral nerve roots two to four (S2–S4) and, intertwined with the sympathetic nerves, form the lateral stalk of the rectum, imparting to it the tough, fibrous consistency that leads this region of pelvis to be called the lateral "ligaments" (Fig. 6.2). As is discussed later, these nerves govern important motor and sensory functions to the pelvic organs; their disruption at surgery leads to postoperative bladder and sexual dysfunction after proctectomy.

The lymphatic drainage of the rectum is especially complex because, unlike other portions of the intestinal tract, this is through the portal (mesenteric) as well as the systemic (internal iliac) circulations. Drainage follows the course of the vascular supply, as described earlier. Thus, the spread of rectal cancer may occur along the inferior mesenteric vessels as well as to the lateral pelvic wall (along the middle rectal and internal iliac vessels).

In performing proctectomy, several fascial planes around the rectum are of surgical significance. The mesorectum, surrounding the posterior one-half or more of the rectum is enveloped by a thin, fibrous covering called the fascia propria (or visceral pelvic fascia). This forms an important oncologic barrier to primary and lymphatic spread to extrarectal pelvic tissues and should be preserved intact in rectal dissection. It is positioned immediately anterior to the fascia propria of the sacrum (or parietal pelvic fascia). The potential space between these layers should represent the posterior extent of dissection for proctectomy. The surgical significance of this is discussed later. At the level of approximately S3, the rectosacral (Waldeyer's) fascia attaches itself to the presacral fascia, then travels inferiorly to the region of the anorectal junction. This fascia must usually be intentionally divided to mobilize the rectum safely and thoroughly to the pelvic floor. Anteriorly, the plane between the rectum and the prostate and seminal vesicles contains another important fascial layer, Denonvillier's fascia. This also may represent an important boundary to tumor growth anteriorly and must often be incised purposefully in the performance of complete rectal mobilization and safe separation of the rectum from the seminal vesicles and prostate.

There are many other aspects of important surgical anatomy that the surgeon performing proctectomy for rectal cancer will encounter. These are highlighted in the section on "Technical details".

Surgical Options in Restorative Procedures

Surgery for rectal cancers can be divided broadly into local procedures and radical extirpative operations. The latter can be divided into resectional procedures with permanent stoma (abdominoperineal resection and Hartmann's procedure) and sphincter saving restorative procedures (anterior resection, low anterior resection, coloanal anastomosis, and colonic J-pouch procedures). Local procedures and abdominoperineal resection are described elsewhere in the text. This chapter focuses on sphincter saving resectional procedures, each of which is briefly defined in this section. The low anterior resection is distinguished from the anterior or "high" anterior resection in that the latter applies to lesions of the upper rectum (11–16 cm from the anal verge), typically located above the peritoneal reflection of the rectum. The anterior resection does not differ significantly from the sigmoid resection, therefore this procedure will not be discussed in this chapter. Mobilization of the rectum for low anterior resection is identical to that for abdominoperineal resection and involves the following:

1. Complete circumferential opening of the pelvic peritoneum around the rectum
2. Division of the lateral ligaments (pelvic neurovascular pedicles) of the rectum
3. Elevation of the rectum posteriorly out of the presacral space, nearly always to the anorectal ring

4. Dissection of the anterior attachment of rectum to the prostate or the vagina

Because most of the blood supply to the sigmoid colon is also sacrificed in low anterior resection, the sigmoid colon as well as the rectum is resected (proctosigmoidectomy) before anastomosis of the descending colon to the rectum. Complete mobilization of the splenic flexure is also usually required to fashion a tension-free anastomosis deep within the pelvis.

In coloanal anastomotic procedures, the entire rectum is mobilized as in low anterior or abdominoperineal resection and is removed just above the level of the anorectal ring. In the method originally described by Parks in 1966 [3], the anal mucosa from the dentate line cephalad to the transection line is then excised transanally. By Parks' description, the well-mobilized descending colon is then brought down through the anorectal remnant and anastomosed to the dentate line, usually by a hand-suturing technique "through the anal canal, which is held open by retractors or sutures". The anastomosis is usually protected temporarily with a diverting stoma.

The colonic reservoir (or colonic J-pouch) involves folding the distal 8–10 cm segment of the terminus of the descending colon on itself after proctosigmoidectomy and forming a J-shaped reservoir, the most dependent part of which is anastomosed to the anal sphincter in a circular stapled or hand-sewn side-to-end fashion. The addition of a "pouch" may improve the functional results of very low anterior or coloanal anastomotic procedures.

The ability of laparoscopic instrumentation to mobilize bowel segments completely and perform intraperitoneal or pelvic bowel resection in cadaver and animal models has been demonstrated [4–7]. The rectum can be mobilized completely to the pelvic floor using laparoscopic guidance and this type of surgery is increasingly being utilized in patients with rectal carcinoma. (Details of this procedure are described in Ch. 9.)

Less commonly used over the last decades are the so-called pull-through techniques for preservation of the anal sphincters and bowel continuity. These procedures involve rectal mobilization and transection similar to that in a coloanal procedure, but the descending colon is pulled through the anal orifice and sutured primarily to an everted anal canal (Bacon technique) or allowed to protrude through the anus for up to 7–10 days, at which time excess colon is trimmed away and a coloanal anastomosis is fashioned (as described by Turnbull and Cuthbertson [8], Cutait and Figliolini [9], and others). Functional outcome after these operations has been inferior to that with primary coloanal anastomosis; they are rarely used in modern surgery. Their limited role, however, is described later in this chapter.

The use of combined abdominal–transsacral procedures has been described for removal of the rectum and more direct visualization of the lower rectum and anal sphincters for lower colorectal and coloanal anastomosis. Abdominosacral approaches require the healing of an extra (i.e. sacral) incision; they can injure the pelvic floor and sphincters, and they can be complicated by anastomotic leaks, leading to a troublesome fecal fistula. These procedures are rarely, if ever, required if adequate transabdominal and transperineal approaches are used. They are not discussed further in this chapter.

Preoperative Evaluation and Patient Preparation

Surgical treatment for rectal cancer ranges from local, transanal procedures performed by a single surgeon on an outpatient basis to major extirpative operations requiring a complex multidisciplinary approach. When confronted with rectal cancer, the surgeon has many therapeutic options from which to choose. A thorough preoperative evaluation allows the surgeon and the patient to choose a proper course of action based on the patient's condition and the extent of the tumor. The preoperative evaluation is designed to answer the following questions:

1. Is the patient fit for a major pelvic operation?
2. What is the exact location of the tumor? This location is best judged in relation to the top of the anorectal ring, not the anal verge.
3. How large is the tumor, what are its histologic features, what is its stage, and is there evidence of local or distant spread?
4. What is the status of the bowel proximal to the lesion?
5. What is the functional status of the sphincter?

The evaluation begins with the taking of a thorough history. Excision of a rectal cancer low in the pelvis is a major surgical endeavor and warrants a careful assessment of the overall medical condition of the patient. Cardiac, pulmonary, renal and hematologic status must be suitable to allow for 2–4 hours of general anesthesia with a reasonable expectation for postoperative recovery and healing of the surgical wounds. In general, the higher the operative risk the more flexible the surgeon must be in choosing the appropriate therapy. A thorough

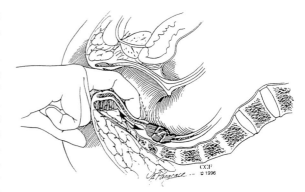

Fig. 6.3. The height of a rectal tumor above the anorectal ring (the top edge of the anal sphincters) is the most relevant factor in assessing a patient for a sphincter saving operation.

history of bowel movement frequency and anal continence should be taken, especially if a sphincter saving procedure is contemplated. A standard abdominal examination is performed with special attention paid to the liver edge, the inguinal and supraclavicular lymph nodes, the presence of jaundice, the overall size of the patient, and the relative size of the pelvis. A careful digital examination of the rectum is most important. With the examining finger, the surgeon palpates the sphincters and assesses the resting and maximal squeeze pressures generated by the patient. Next, the height of the tumor above the anorectal ring (the top edge of the sphincters) is noted, as well as the tumor size and extent (Fig. 6.3). Approximate staging and fixation are determined as well as the relationship to adjacent organs (vagina, cervix and uterus in women and the prostate in men) and musculoskeletal components of the pelvis. In women, a bimanual pelvic examination must be performed to evaluate the pelvis thoroughly.

During rigid sigmoidoscopy, the distance of the tumor from the anal verge is noted, the gross morphologic features (e.g. if it is sessile or pedunculated, and the extent of circumferential involvement) are recorded, and the lesion is biopsied. At least one of the samples should be taken from the edge of the tumor so that those characteristics of the advancing edge of the growth can be evaluated. "Palpation" with the sigmoidoscope may also aid in assessing fixation in tumors that are proximal to the examining fingers. The height of the tumor with regard to the surgical procedure being contemplated should not be assessed with the flexible sigmoidoscope because this is unreliable.

Of patients with rectal cancer, 2–8% harbor a more proximal synchronous carcinoma, and 30–40% have a proximal polyp. For this reason, all patients without significant obstruction should undergo an evaluation of the proximal bowel with either a barium enema or preferably a colonoscopy. Colonoscopy is preferred because of its sensitivity and accuracy in identifying lesions as well as its therapeutic potential. In the face of a nearly obstructing lesion, an intraoperative evaluation of the proximal bowel can be made by palpation and gentle colonoscopy after the anastomosis is completed.

Anorectal manometry is used to evaluate and quantitate anorectal sphincter pressures at rest and with maximal squeeze effort. When considering a sphincter saving procedure in a patient complaining of minor incontinence, a normal manometric examination may reassure the surgeon that these complaints are secondary to secretions caused by the tumor or the pressure of a pelvic mass. Conversely, manometric studies indicating a very weak sphincter, substantiated by electromyographic studies showing denervation of the sphincters, would argue against a restorative procedure.

Once the surgeon has ascertained that the patient is a suitable candidate for bowel resection, then certain preoperative and intraoperative maneuvers should be undertaken to maximize safety and operative results. Although more than 90% of patients undergoing elective surgery can undergo outpatient mechanical bowel preparation, those with significant underlying medical conditions or an obstructing tumor that might preclude thorough bowel cleansing, or any patient judged to be unreliable, should be admitted the day before surgery. A 48–72-hour clear liquid diet combined with a gentle laxative (citrate of magnesia, 5–10 ounces orally every 4–6 hours) is used if significant obstruction is present. In the unobstructed patient, we use a mechanical preparation of clear liquids for 24 hours before surgery, then polyethylene glycol (4 l) or sodium phosphate (3 ounces plus added liquid) to purge the intestinal tract thoroughly of food. If there is concern about bowel preparation because of the obstruction, after hospital admission some gentle tap water enemas (300–500 ml) can also be administered to cleanse the distal bowel.

Preoperative planning for a temporary or permanent stoma must also be considered. This means that potential sites on the right and left sides of the abdomen should be marked. An enterostomal therapy nurse may be of major assistance, both in choosing satisfactory sites and in counseling patients before surgery. Bilateral stoma marks are important because temporary diversion with colorectal anastomosis may be preferable using a loop ileostomy. The rationale for this is as follows. If a locally advanced tumor is found that precludes anastomosis, a permanent (left-sided) colostomy

may be preferable. Temporary diversion in concert with colorectal anastomosis using a left-sided colostomy is undesirable because the marginal artery of the colon (leading to the anastomosis) may be jeopardized. A right-sided loop colostomy for temporary diversion is often large and foul smelling, and liquid stool is no easier for the patient to deal with than the smaller and relatively odorless loop ileostomy. The loop ileostomy also seems technically easier to close than the right-sided colostomy, mainly because of its smaller size.

Oncologic Principles in Rectal Surgery

Extent of Resection

The general principles of oncologic colorectal surgery have become well established over the last century. These include proximal ligation of the vascular pedicle, thorough regional lymphadenectomy, and wide en bloc resection of tumor-bearing soft tissue and mesentery. However, the exact extent of resection necessary during a rectal cancer operation still generates considerable discussion.

High Versus Low Ligation of the Inferior Mesenteric Artery

A "high" versus "low" ligation of the IMA continues to stir up controversy, yet the literature on the subject is quite clear: no good evidence exists to support the concept that a high ligation (ligation proximal to the left colic artery) improves survival. Miles [10], in his initial description of the abdominoperineal resection, proposed ligating the IMA below the left colic artery. In that same year, 1908, Moynihan [11] championed a radical concept of ligating the IMA flush with the aorta, based on the concept that oncologic surgery is related directly to the "anatomy of the lymphatic system". Cuthbert Dukes and colleagues substantiated this concept by demonstrating that lymphatic extension of rectal carcinoma was remarkably constant, nearly always following the path of the IMA to the aorta [12,13]. Goligher, in a study examining the blood supply of the sigmoid colon and mesentery, reported that the distance between the IMA's origin at the aorta and the take-off of the left colic artery averaged 4 cm, and that as many as 10 lymph nodes could be retrieved from this margin [14]. Subsequent studies reported an 11–22% incidence of positive nodes between the origin of the left colic artery and the IMA [15,16]. There would seem to be obvious value in resecting these involved lymph nodes, but a number of studies have shown this not to be the case. Bacon and associates reported a 5% increase in survival with high ligation in their series, but statistical significance was not reached. Grinnell and Hint, early advocates of high ligation [17], reversed their opinion on the value of high ligation in 1965 when they were unable to show increased survival after this procedure [18]. More recently, in a large study from St Mark's Hospital involving over 1300 resections, no difference in crude or age-corrected 5-year survival rate for any Dukes' classification could be demonstrated after high ligation [19]. Further analysis of data from St Mark's confirmed that the level of ligation has no effect on patient survival [20].

Two pathologic features of rectal cancer probably explain the failure of high ligation to improve survival: the lymphatic and hematogenous drainage of the rectum is through multiple vessels coursing through the pelvis along the inferior mesenteric and internal iliac vessels, and even through inguinal routes; and the involvement of nodes at the base of the IMA suggests that cancer cells have already spread elsewhere in the lymphatics, outside the reach of surgery.

Despite the fact that it does not appear to influence survival, high ligation of the IMA does have some technical merit in that it allows for a more complete mobilization of the left colon, which facilitates a tension-free low pelvic or anal anastomosis. Ischemia of the left colon after high ligation is of some concern, especially in patients with known or suspected atherosclerotic disease. It may also lead to a higher morbidity rate. Our approach to proximal ligation is as follows: a high ligation of the IMA is attempted if safe and if disease appears to be localized to the pelvis. If a high ligation could be hazardous or unduly prolong the operation (as with evidence or suspicion of mesenteric vascular disease, obesity or major underlying medical problems), ligation and division of the IMA distal to the left colic artery is logical because this is unlikely to affect long-term survival adversely. We prefer to ligate the inferior mesenteric vein (IMV) at the inferior edge of the pancreas or adjacent to the IMA. A high ligation of the vein also frees the colon to move caudally to the pelvis for a low anastomosis.

Distal Margin of Resection

The historical shift from radical abdominoperineal resection for all rectal tumors to the use of sphincter saving techniques in most patients has resulted primarily from a better understanding of what constitutes an adequate distal resection margin. Mayo, in 1916, recommended abdominoperineal resection for any rectal cancer [21]. Dixon showed, 32 years later, that a low morbidity and mortality as well as a high 5-year survival (63.7%) could be achieved after a sphincter saving low anterior resection [22]. In 1949, Best and Blair demonstrated that the use of a 3.5 cm distal margin was oncologically safe in treating nearly all rectal cancers [23]. In 1951, Goligher and colleagues reported on a pathologic review of 1500 rectal cancer specimens. They found distal intramural spread in only 6.5% and spread of more than 2 cm in less than 2% [24]. Based on these data, the somewhat arbitrary "5 cm distal margin" concept was developed. In the 1980s Williams and colleagues [25] and Pollett and Nicholls [26] proposed that perhaps even a 2 cm distal resection margin was justifiable. In Williams and colleagues' report on 50 patients with rectal cancer, 76% had no intramural spread and an additional 14% had distal spread of less than 1 cm. Of the five patients with distal spread greater than 1 cm, all had poorly differentiated Dukes' C tumors and all had distant metastatic disease within 3 years of operation. A 5 cm distal margin did not affect survival favorably. Pollett and Nicholls, in their review of 334 patients treated for rectal cancer at St Mark's Hospital, were also unable to show any survival advantage or reduction in local recurrence rates when distal resections greater than 5 cm were compared with those less than 2 cm.

The literature regarding the distal resection margin is somewhat problematic in that authors measure the margin in various ways. Weese and colleagues determined that a 5 cm margin in situ became 2.4 cm in the "fixed, unpinned" state in 10 rectal cancer specimens [27]. We prefer to ascertain the distal resection margin in the following manner: the rectum is completely mobilized to the pelvic floor when proctectomy is undertaken. When a sphincter saving operation is attempted, the 2 cm margin distal to the tumor is estimated using the distance of "two fingersbreadth" on the unstretched rectum in situ. Electrosurgery is used to mark the rectal wall at this point and a complete mesorectal excision down to this level is undertaken. After resection, we routinely open the specimen on the back table of the operating room and measure the distal margin. If there is less than 2 cm in a given area, a frozen section of the area in question will be taken to rule out the possibility of intramural extension, especially if unfavorable histology was documented on preoperative biopsy. Unfavorable histology and a margin of less than 2 cm would lead to an abdominoperineal resection in most patients.

If the tumor is exophytic or a villous lesion and seems well encompassed by the resection, even a 1 cm margin on gross examination of the specimen is acceptable. The use of preoperative radiation for a low-lying lesion (<5 cm from the top of the anal sphincters) might justify the acceptance of a margin of 1–2 cm because the periphery of an irradiated lesion would be less likely to contain malignant cells. Based on a 2 cm distal margin, sphincter saving operations can be justified in most patients, with recurrence rates identical to those after abdominoperineal resection [20,23].

Radial Margin and Complete Mesorectal Resection

Obtaining an adequate distal margin of resection is of little value if the lateral margins are not clear. Clear margins must be obtained circumferentially around the tumor. The wide variation in local recurrence rates (2–50%) may be explained on the basis of inadequate lateral or radial margins of resection [28–31]. During the 1980s and 1990s, a fundamental change in operative technique has taken place. Conventional surgery, which is performed using a blunt technique, has given way to sharp dissection along definable planes. The technique, known as total mesorectal excision (TME), produces complete resection of an intact package of the rectum and its surrounding mesorectum, enveloped within the visceral pelvic fascia with uninvolved circumferential margins. Quirke and colleagues [32], Heald and associates [33], and Hojo et al. [34] have been responsible for emphasizing this important concept. Quirke and colleagues studied the degree of lateral spread in rectal cancer in a group of 52 patients, 23 of whom underwent an abdominoperineal resection; 29 were treated by sphincter saving operations. They noted spread of cancer to the lateral margin in 13 patients. Local recurrence was present in 11 of these patients and in only one patient who had negative lateral or radial margins. Exacting surgical technique (avoiding "coning in" on the rectum) is the critical technical component in achieving clear lateral margins. In nearly all cases of curative rectal cancer surgery the lateral dissection is flush with the endopelvic fascia of the pelvic side wall. Heald and coworkers maintain that local recurrence results from spread into the mesorectum. Their pathologic studies have demonstrated microscopic foci of tumor cells in the mesorectum 2 cm distal to the tumor [33]. Reporting a local recurrence rate of 2–3% and an 85% survival at 9 years in one series, Heald and Ryall argue emphatically that complete mesorectal excision is a key in obtaining good results with sphincter saving operations [35]. Our experience with 162 lower rectal cancer patients treated with wide pelvic clearance and complete mesorectal excision and colorectal anastomosis supports these concepts. At 5-year follow-up we found an 8% incidence of isolated local pelvic recurrence; 5-year disease-free survival rates were 70.5% [36].

Between the parietal and visceral layers of pelvic fascia, a layer of areolar tissue surrounds the entire anatomic unit of the rectum and the mesorectum from the sacral promontory to the anal outlet via the levator ani muscles. Dissecting along this plane ensures excision of the complete and intact mesorectal package. Conventional surgery fails to identify this areolar plane and also fails to maintain the dissection along this pathway. Violation of the mesorectum is commonly associated with blunt or even forceful dissections. Sharp dissection, using scissors, cautery etc., under direct vision, along this strictly defined plane, is a reproducible technique that respects the boundaries of the visceral pelvic fascia, producing a resectable package of this "regional" unit, ensuring the resection of all regional disease spread.

Several authors have suggested extending the lateral resection to the internal iliac nodes beneath the endopelvic fascia [34,37]. We have not routinely practiced this type of dissection and believe that there is little evidence to support its use.

En Bloc Resection (Resection of Adjacent Structures with the Tumor)

The presence of a locally advanced (Stage T4) tumor with direct invasion into other organs or structures is seen in 5–20% of patients with rectal cancer. This fixation does not necessarily preclude a curative operation if the tumor is localized [38–41]. The major morbidity of wide excisional surgical procedures in the pelvis (as high as 39% in some series [36]) must, however, be balanced against the long-term cure rate.

When history and physical examination suggest invasion of adjacent pelvic structures, careful preoperative staging is undertaken. Computed tomographic scans of the pelvis and abdomen are typically used. We have also found endorectal ultrasonography to be accurate in detecting adjacent organ involvement. Adjacent structures most commonly involved include the pelvic side wall (89%), the vagina (81%), the small intestine (20–30%), and the uterus (24%) [39].

If preoperative staging suggests a Stage T4 lesion, we recommend preoperative external beam radiation therapy over a period of 4–6 weeks to a dose of 40–50 Gy. This may downstage a rectal cancer and may convert a lesion from fixed to mobile. Often, 5-fluorouracil is given at the beginning and end of the radiotherapy to enhance the effects of the radiation.

After a suitable recovery period (4–6 weeks) patients undergo surgery. If involvement of the urinary tract is suspected, a urologist should be consulted and the patient advised about the possible need for urinary diversion. At operation, if a thorough abdominal and pelvic exploration reveals localized disease, contiguous organ involvement is an indication for en bloc resection. Any adhesions between the tumor and adjacent organs should be assumed to be malignant and excision with 1–2 cm of adjacent normal tissue undertaken. The bladder and vagina are easily managed in this fashion. Involvement of the bladder trigone is usually an indication for cystectomy and urinary diversion. Five-year survival rates for node-negative disease under these circumstances may be as high as 50–90%. Positive nodes reduce the likelihood of survival to 20–29% at 5 years [38–40].

Sacral resection is warranted when localized sacral involvement is present and the patient is a good operative risk. The sacrum may be safely excised up to the S2–S3 junction without fear of bony instability [42]. Sugarbaker has reported survival in excess of 3 years in four of six patients undergoing partial sacrectomy and en bloc resection [43]. Consideration of sacral resection should prompt consultation with an orthopedic surgeon skilled in pelvic bony surgery.

Autonomic Nerve Preservation

Conventional low anterior resection and abdominoperineal resections for rectal cancer are associated with a significant incidence of sexual and urinary dysfunction. The presumed mechanism for these morbidities is damage to the pelvic autonomic (parasympathetic and/or sympathetic) nerves during surgery. These injuries are most commonly related to blunt dissection or to the degree of lateral dissection. In TME, the rectum is mobilized circumferentially using sharp dissection under direct vision along the parietal pelvic fascia. This technique, together with an awareness of the pelvic autonomic nerve pathways, makes it possible to identify and preserve the pelvic autonomic nerves, therefore minimizing sexual and urinary dysfunction.

Final Preparations for the Restorative Procedures

Certain preoperative and intraoperative strategies help to ensure the smooth conduct of an operation and good results. Medical conditions such as cardiopulmonary disease or diabetes are evaluated before surgery with the help of appropriate medical consultation. Physiologic parameters are optimized before and during surgery. It is helpful to plan for invasive intraoperative monitoring if it may be needed. Preoperative nutritional status should not be ignored; patients with significant weight loss should be considered for nutritional supplementation. A thorough preoperative staging work-up allows for the appropriate preoperative administration of adjuvant therapy. This allows the surgeon to plan the operation with the patient, it minimizes intraoperative surprises, and it maximizes the chance for a good outcome.

The patient is placed on the operating table in the supine position. With induction of anesthesia, broad-spectrum antibiotics are administered (we usually use a third generation cephalosporin with metronidazole). After suitable general anesthesia is achieved, pneumatic sequential compression stockings for deep vein thrombosis prophylaxis are applied and the legs are placed in special padded lithotomy stirrups (OR Direct Stirrups, Acton, MA). These stirrups support the foot and lower calf but place no pressure on the peroneal nerve at the fibular head. Thus, a neuropraxia, even after an extended operation, is highly unlikely. The foot of the table is dropped and the buttocks are pulled to the end of it so that the anus is accessed easily. A towel roll is occasionally used to elevate the sacrum. The lower extremities are abducted only enough to allow access to the perineum. With the knee flexed, the hips are flexed only slightly so that the legs do not encroach on the abdominal field. A bladder catheter is put in place and taped over the right thigh at the inguinal crease.

A rectal washout is then gently performed using warm saline through a large mushroom catheter connected to a 3-liter irrigation bag. When the rectal effluent is clear, a final digital examination and rigid sigmoidoscopy are carried out to reassess the relationship of the tumor to the anal sphincters. The rectal tube is then replaced and 60–100 ml of povidone-iodine 4% are instilled into the rectum. A bag is secured to the tube and it is left in place to drain the rectum.

The entire abdomen, genitalia and perineum are then prepared and draped into the field with a separate drape covering the perineum/pelvis. The abdomen is entered through a long mid-line incision and a thorough and systemic exploration is carried out away from the pelvis. Suspect areas are sampled and sent for frozen section analysis. A careful bimanual palpation of liver is performed and intraoperative ultrasonography is used to investigate any suspicious liver lesions. If a laparoscopic procedure is being performed, liver ultrasonography may be carried out laparoscopically [44,45]. The distal sigmoid colon is then encircled with a woven tape and tied down to isolate the proximal colon from the lumen of the rectum. The colon is palpated and the pelvis is surveyed. For tumors above the peritoneal reflection, the operative course can usually be outlined at this time. For tumors below the peritoneal reflection, final operative decision making is deferred until the pelvic dissection is complete.

Technical Details

Proctosigmoidectomy

General Concepts
If the rectal tumor appears to be resectable, the preliminary steps of any operation to remove the rectum are nearly identical, whether performing a low anterior resection with colorectal anastomosis, a coloanal anastomosis, or an abdominoperineal resection. Thus, the early part of this section focuses on the mobilization and vascular ligation phases of rectal resection. Special aspects of the anastomotic preparation (low anterior resection, coloanal anastomosis, colonic J-pouch) are dealt with in individual subsequent sections.

Step 1: Vascular Isolation and Ligation After ligating the sigmoid colon with a heavy tape (as described earlier), the small bowel is reflected cephalad and to the right. The base of the sigmoid mesentery, specifically the inferior mesenteric pedicle, is grasped by the surgeon's non-dominant hand and the peritoneum encircling the IMA and IMV is incised from just to the right of the origin of the IMA to the sacral promontory. The surgeon's fingertips are swept posterior to these vessels, and the hypogastric (sympathetic) nerve plexus is bluntly dissected posteriorly away from the IMA and IMV, leaving it in situ. Further sharp dissection at the base of the IMA should allow for preservation of most of the pre-aortic sympathetic nerve fibers traveling to the pelvis. By mobilizing the sigmoid colon from its retroperitoneal attachment, this may allow for identification of the left ureter and gonadal vessels. These structures should be clearly identified and swept clear of the IMA and inferior mesenteric vein to allow for safe ligation of the vessels.

Each vessel is isolated and doubly ligated with size 0 or 2–0 ligatures. If the IMA is calcified, it may be wise to suture-ligate it after initial tying. "High ligation", above the left colic artery, is performed in nearly all patients for oncologic reasons (see the previous section on high versus low ligation of the IMA), as well as to allow the left colon to extend completely without tethering of the mesentery by the connected left colic artery. In a clinical situation in which vascular insufficiency from the middle colic artery is possible, preservation of the left colic artery is advisable.

Step 2: Mobilizing the Descending and Sigmoid Colon After mobilizing the sigmoid colon from the sacral promontory to the lateral aspect of the iliac fossa, the anterior aspect of Gerota's fascia is carefully separated from the posterior portion of the sigmoid and descending colon mesentery. This allows for easy elevation of the left colon away from its lateral peritoneal attachments up to the splenic flexure. If exposure of the splenic flexure becomes tedious, either the abdominal wall incision should be extended or the dissection should continue by detaching the omentum from the left portion of the transverse colon. After this, the transverse and descending colon may be grasped simultaneously (the omega maneuver) to enhance exposure and ultimate takedown of the splenic flexure. Extreme care must be taken in detaching the posterior mesenteric attachment of the splenic region because the marginal vessels of the left colon are at risk for injury during this dissection. These vessels are the lifeline of the mobilized bowel, bringing blood from the middle colic vasculature to the left colon.

Step 3: Mobilizing the Rectu Down to the Pelvic Floor with Autononomic Nerve Preservation After vascular ligation/division and left colon mobilization, the pelvic dissection commences. Frequently, at this point, the inferior vascular pedicle is divided on its left (lateral) edge all the way to the bowel at the junction between the sigmoid and descending colon, then the bowel is occluded with clamps and also divided.

The concept of TME allows the operating surgeon to identify and preserve the main components of the pelvic autonomic nervous system, which control urinary and sexual functions. The sympathetic functions (bladder filling and sphincter excitation, emission and lubrication, some components of orgasm and resolution) result from innervation by the hypogastric nerves, which are identified at the sacral promontory, approximately 1 cm lateral to the midline and 2 cm medial to each ureter. The hypogastric nerve lies posterior to the peritoneum and directly anterior to the visceral pelvic fascia. It continues caudally and laterally, following the course of the ureter and the internal iliac artery along the pelvic wall. Parasympathetic nerve functions (bladder contraction and sphincter relaxation, erection or vulvar engorgement, and bulbocavernosus spasm) are mediated by the anterior sacral nerve roots of S2, S3 and S4. The splanchnic branches of the sacral nerves may be identified at the sacral foramina. The splanchnic nerves run laterocaudad and anteriorly along the pelvic wall over the piriformis muscle. The hypogastric nerve and the sacral splanchnic nerves join laterally on the pelvic wall to form the pelvic autonomic nerve plexus (at the "lateral ligament" of the rectum). The pelvic autonomic nerve plexus is a rhomboid plaque of nervous tissue from which the final nerve pathways are directed to the genitourinary visceral compartment [46].

The rectum is mobilized and freed from surrounding structures, first by incising the lateral peritoneal reflections just below the sacral promontory, then by mobilizing it posteriorly from the sacral hollow. This is accomplished by sharp dissection in the plane between the fascia propria of the rectum (visceral pelvic fascia) and the presacral fascia (parietal pelvic fascia). Inadvertent dissection too posteriorly (usually when blunt dissection of the rectum is attempted) risks tearing of the presacral veins. These veins drain directly through the sacral periosteum and connect to the basivertebral venous system; they may bleed profusely. Because of this, sharp dissection for the entire posterior mobilization is recommended. Control of presacral bleeding, should it occur, is usually best accomplished by fingertip pressure, then by placement of a thumbtack-like device directly into the sacral bone, over the bleeding vessel. This usually results in rapid control of the hemorrhage. It is possible that, if there is no direct involvement of the tumor posteriorly, the presacral hypogastric nerves may be separated from the fascia propria of the rectum and preserved, because they lie just on top of the presacral fascia.

The ligamentous lateral stalks of the rectum are approached after posterior dissection down to the pelvic floor. Lighted, long, narrow pelvic retractors (Brite Trac 10 × 1.5 inch blades; Codman, New Brunswick, NY) are of great assistance in supplying traction on the pelvic side walls. Electrosurgical dissection is used to divide these nerve-laden structures bilaterally because very few blood vessels are actually present within them. With a posterior-to-anterior approach, much of the nerve tissue supplying the pelvic organs other than the rectum may be preserved and swept laterally (unless the primary tumor is located at or just adjacent to the lateral stalks). Under direct vision, the lateral stalks must be dissected close to the pelvic side wall if the tumor is in proximity to them. The contralateral nerves may then be preserved by a dissection closer to the rectal wall, but still encompassing the visceral pelvic fascia. After adequate dissection bilaterally, the anterior plane is dissected using strong anterior retrac-

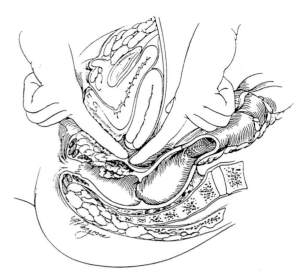

Fig. 6.4. Careful bimanual palpation of pelvic structures may be warranted. The surgeon should place an extra sterile glove or sleeve over the palpating hand, passed transvaginally or transrectally. Proper tissue planes for dissection can be more fully appreciated using this technique (from Wanebo HJ. Colorectal cancer. St Louis, MO: Mosby Year Book, 1993).

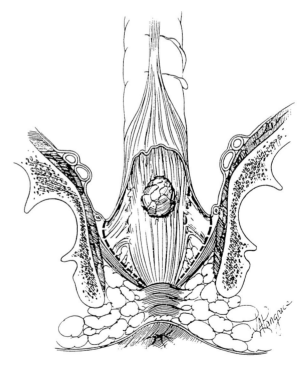

Fig. 6.5. Lateral dissection along the pelvic side wall entails avoidance of "coning in" on the rectum during pelvic dissection (from Wanebo HJ. Colorectal cancer. St Louis, MO: Mosby Year Book, 1993).

tion with a narrow retractor and equally forceful posterior and upward traction on the rectum. This dissection may be assisted by having a perineal surgeon to supply pressure between the ischial tuberosity by using a fist or, in women, intravaginally using a sponge stick. The dissection is complete when the anorectal ring is reached. Careful bimanual palpation of pelvic structures by the surgeon may be warranted to define the anterior planes (Fig. 6.4). An anteriorly placed tumor may invade the vagina, the space between the rectum and Denonvillier's fascia, or the bladder. These structures must then be considered for en bloc resection. Once the complete, circumferential dissection to the pelvic floor has been attained, carefully avoid-ing "coning in" on the rectum during dissection (Fig. 6.5), a final decision regarding a sphincter sparing operation (low anterior resection with a circular stapled anastomosis, proctectomy with coloanal anastomosis) versus abdominoperineal excision must be made.

Any evidence for sphincter or pelvic floor involvement of the primary tumor mandates complete proctectomy with a permanent colostomy. If mobilization has permitted more than 2 cm of rectal wall clearance between the lower edge of the tumor and the top of the anal sphincters, then it may be rea-

sonable to consider a sphincter saving operation (Fig. 6.6).

Low Anterior Resection

The low anterior resection is the optimal procedure for tumors lying at or slightly below the peritoneal reflection (the mid-rectum) in a patient with good anal sphincter function and acceptable operative risk factors. Certain small tumors in the upper portion of the low rectum (3–4 cm above the anal sphincters) may also be amenable to this type of operation, but complete circumferential mobilization of the rectum must be achieved. This thorough freeing of the rectum may provide an additional 2–3 cm elevation of the tumor above the pelvic floor.

The distal margin of the tumor may be estimated at the time of induction of anesthesia and placement of the patient in the modified lithotomy position, but the final judgement must rest after full rectal mobilization, often with the surgeon using bimanual palpation of the tumor to estimate clearance above the pelvic floor. If a 2 cm distal margin can be achieved below the tumor, then low anterior resection may be a reasonable option.

Concept of Distal Rectal Washout

Although there is no definite proof that the rectum should be irrigated with a cytotoxic solution before the formation of a distal rectal anastomosis, at our institution we prefer to do this because it is theoretically appealing, inexpensive and takes relatively little time. To accomplish this, long, narrow pelvic retractors are placed deep in the pelvis anterior to the rectum and a right-angled bowel clamp is placed 2 cm below the cancer and then closed. An assistant, working from between the patient's legs, gently places an irrigating syringe transanally and irrigates the rectum thoroughly with a cytotoxic agent. We use 40% ethanol, followed by a saline washout to avoid any risk of igniting the alcohol with electrosurgery. If it is possible to pass a 30 mm linear stapler below the bowel-occluding clamp, this is done, and a double-stapled anastomosis is performed. If this is not feasible, then the rectum is divided with electrosurgery just below the bowel clamp and a size 0 polypropylene purse-string suture is placed. This is accomplished carefully, using strategically placed long, narrow pelvic retractors and perineal pressure. As the rectum is gradually divided, the leading edge is grasped with a long Babcock clamp so that the rectal wall, usually under considerable tension, does not recede from the surgeon's view as the purse-string suture is placed.

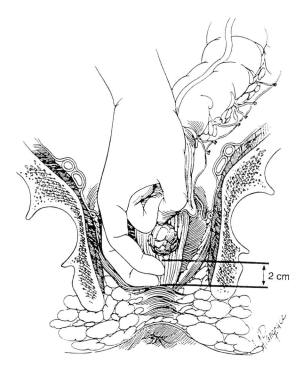

Fig. 6.6. Placing two fingers below the tumor is a reasonable means of estimating a 2 cm margin of clearance between the lower edge of a rectal cancer and the pelvic floor (from Wanebo HJ. Colorectal cancer. St Louis, MO: Mosby Year Book, 1993).

Anastomosis

After distal rectal management and specimen removal, the proximal colon also is prepared for anastomosis with a similar purse-string suture placement, then the center rod and anvil of the largest possible circular stapler (nearly 31 mm: Premium CEEA; United States Surgical Corp., Norwalk CT) is placed into the bowel lumen and the purse-string securely tied. The stapler is thoroughly lubricated and gently passed transanally. If any anal stenosis is present, dilation using two fingertips is recommended before trying to pass the instrument. This lessens any risk of rectal injury by forceful dilation of the anal sphincter with the stapler, which can then rapidly "pop" through the sphincters and inadvertently tear the rectum. The stapler head can be quickly recognized in the rectum by the operating surgeon. Once the top of the remainder of the rectum is reached by the stapler head, the instrument's wing nut is unscrewed counterclockwise, causing the center shaft to protrude up through the rectum. If the rectum has been closed with the linear stapler, then a sharp spike on the center shaft should protrude through the rectum just adjacent to the staple line (preferably posteriorly). Once the center shaft is fully extended, the plastic spike is removed from the shaft and the center post protruding from the proximal bowel is securely placed into it. If a purse-string has been placed, this is tied about the center rod; the two ends of the stapler are joined and the instrument is fully tightened down over the bowel ends using clockwise screwing of the instrument's wing nut. The stapler is fired and the wing nut is again used to loosen the anvil slightly from the stapler head. The instrument is gently rotated and removed from the rectum.

Anastomotic integrity is assessed by: directly palpating the anastomosis transanally; evaluating the "completeness" of each tissue "donut" (on the stapler center shaft) removed from the rectum and colon anastomotic sites; and direct visualization with a rigid proctoscope, which is also used to insufflate air into the rectum after filling the pelvis with warm saline. The surgeon then looks for air bubbles emanating from the anastomosis. The absence of any such air bubbles is a reliable predictor of good anastomotic healing, but there is at least a 4% false-negative rate [47].

If any question remains about tissue integrity, including concern over irradiated tissue, steroid use, diabetes, excessive intraoperative bleeding, instability of the patient, and so forth, it is wise to consider the use of a diverting, loop ileostomy placed through the rectus sheath in the right lower quadrant. This can usually be closed 2–3 months after the patient has achieved medical stability and a healed anastomosis.

Special Consideration: Coloanal Anastomosis

This technique uses a primary endoanal suturing technique and has been appropriately termed a "pull-to" procedure [3]. When it becomes apparent, after complete rectal mobilization, that adequate distal rectal clearance is not possible without excision of the entire rectum above the pelvic floor, then this procedure is an option.

The perineal phase of this anastomotic technique begins by effacing the anus with six to eight heavy sutures placed at the lower edge of the anal sphincters or by using a self-retaining retractor (Lone Star, Houston, TX). An abdominal surgery assistant tucks a laparotomy pad behind the rectum all the way down to the anorectal junction, then the anus and rectum are irrigated with a cytotoxic solution. To minimize bleeding during the transanal dissection, the anal submucosa is infiltrated with an epinephrine-containing solution (at a dilution of 1:200 000). Dissection of the mucosa begins at the dentate line and is continued cephalad for 5–10 mm. This dissection is then deepened so that it goes entirely through the muscularis propria into the surrounding perirectal tissues for 1–2 cm. This lower rectal segment is then closed with sutures, using a running absorbable stitch. A cytotoxic solution is again used to irrigate this area; then dissection is carried further cephalad, circumferentially, until the rectum is entirely disconnected from the pelvic tissues.

The specimen is removed, the pelvis is irrigated, and a long Babcock clamp is passed transanally up into the pelvis to grasp the end of the mobilized left colon and carefully pull it down into the anal canal. This end of the colon has usually been closed with a linear stapling device; thus, when it presents at the anal orifice, it is opened and sequentially sutured anteriorly, laterally and posteriorly. Additional sutures are placed so that four or five per quadrant are in place on completion of the anastomosis. Palpation is used to verify anastomotic integrity and then the anal retraction sutures are removed and a temporary loop ileostomy is created in the right lower quadrant.

When is a classically described "pull-through" operation performed? These techniques [8,9,48] are carried out in our practice only when there is an urgent need to complete the operation without taking time to create the coloanal anastomosis. The distal rectum is transected by everting the anorectum, then by pulling the specimen (rectum) through the anus. The proximal colon, still attached to the specimen, is drawn through the anus, so that 2–3 cm of it protrudes beyond the everted anus. The specimen is transected at this point and the proximal bowel sutured rapidly to the everted anus. This segment may be secured further with a gauze stent wrapped around the colon [8,48]. One week to 10 days later, assuming the patient is in a good medical condition, he or she is returned to the operating room and the excess intestine is trimmed and a primary coloanal anastomosis created. The anus either retracts spontaneously or it may be reduced by gentle massage at the second procedure.

Special Consideration: Colonic Reservoir (J-Pouch)

One of the main drawbacks to the very low colorectal or coloanal anastomosis may be a poor functional outcome, with fecal urgency or soilage that may remain for many months or even permanently. These troubling sequelae of the low anastomosis may be caused by the operative anal manipulation, loss of the rectal reservoir capacity, and the postoperative radiation therapy. In the late 1980s, a colonic J-shaped reservoir was proposed to ameliorate some of the functional deficiencies of the low anastomosis [49].

This should be a rapid modification of the coloanal procedure, wherein the distal 6–10 cm of the preserved left colon is folded on itself, then a J-pouch is created using a linear cutting stapler or by a hand-sewn technique (using a length of 6 cm or longer). The anastomosis is performed either by a circular stapler or by a hand-sewn technique. This anastomosis should be protected in nearly all instances with a diverting loop ileostomy. Anastomosis and pouch

integrity are ensured at 2–3 months after surgery with a water soluble enema before stoma closure.

Outcome After Low Anterior Resection Versus Abdominoperineal Resection

Although the abdominoperineal resection maintains an important place in the surgical management of rectal cancer, most of these patients can be treated with sphincter saving procedures, the low anterior resection being used most commonly. There has been reluctance among some surgeons to recommend the widespread use of low anterior resection, which is based on the fear that, in preserving the distal rectum, anal canal and sphincters, a less than adequate oncologic operation is performed. Whether a low anterior resection compromises long-term outcome compared with abdominoperineal resection will probably never be addressed in a prospective, randomized trial because of informed consent issues, but there are numerous retrospective and uncontrolled prospective studies reported in the literature that address this issue (Table 6.1 [2,25,28,36,50–56]) Williams and colleagues reported no significant difference in local recurrence (14% versus 18%) or in 5-year survival when comparing low anterior resection and abdominoperineal resection in 133 patients with rectal tumors located 3–12 cm from the anal verge [25]. Heimann and coworkers reported similar rates (16% versus 17%) of local recurrence in their series of 320 patients undergoing either low anterior or

Table 6.1. Incidence of local recurrence after abdominoperineal resection (APR) compared with low anterior resection (LAR) (or restorative procedures)

Authors	Year	No. patients		Local recurrence (%)	
		APR	LAR	APR	LAR
Morson et al. [51]	1963	1596	177	9.7	7.3
McDermott et al. [52]	1982	107	310	17	19
Rich et al. [53]	1983	110	28	31	29
Phillips et al. [28]	1984	478	370	12	18
Williams and Johnston [54]	1984	83	71	8	11
Williams et al. [25]	1985	100	33	19	14
Heimann et al. [50]	1986	118	202	17	16
Amato et al. [55]	1991	69	78	10	12
Dixon et al. [56]	1991	61	150	5	4
Heald et al. [2]	1997	15	85	33	1
Lavery et al. [36]	1997	99	162	11	8

abdominoperineal resection for middle and upper rectal tumors [50]. A report from the University of Chicago also noted no difference in local recurrence rates between the two methods [57]. Finally, Heald and colleagues reported extremely low rates of local recurrence (<5%) after low anterior resection [2,58].

Laparoscopic Rectal Cancer Surgery

While the use of laparoscopic techniques in benign colorectal surgery has expanded over the last several years, controversy continues to surround the use of laparoscopic resection in patients with rectum and colon carcinoma. For benign diseases, diagnostic laparoscopy, the creation of stomas, and limited resections are all becoming reasonable indications. In patients with malignancy, resection either through a conventional incision or a laparoscope must adhere to the same defined surgical oncologic principles. Current randomized trials comparing open to laparoscopic resection have begun to address these concerns [59]. Port-site metastasis remains a leading hindrance to the widespread acceptance of laparoscopic resection for colorectal carcinoma, although it may be a rare phenomenon. In the subsequent chapter on laparoscopic resection, we will discuss the applications of laparoscopic surgery for rectal cancer. Further research in this area, combined with advances in laparoscopic technology, will be critical to the future successful application of laparoscopic surgery for colorectal carcinoma.

Conclusions

The modern development of rectal cancer surgery, barely more than a century old, was initially concerned with radical tumor extirpation combined with attempts to keep operative mortality to a minimum. Function was rationally sacrificed in favor of survival in the earliest surgical endeavors. Abdominoperineal excision was and is a valued procedure in the treatment of rectal cancer, yet the frequency of its use has diminished markedly with improvements in rectal mobilization, dissection, the use of the circular stapler, and in the understanding of pelvic anatomy and pelvic floor function. Proctosigmoidectomy with sphincter preservation should not be considered a less radical approach to rectal cancers that lie 2–3 cm (or more) above the top of the anal sphincters. Distal intramural spread of rectal cancers beyond 2 cm occurs only in rare instances. The functional results after low colorectal

anastomosis seem to be highly satisfactory and there is evidence that new techniques in function preservation are improving outcomes after rectal cancer surgery (the colonic J-pouch and pelvic nerve preservation).

When compared with conventional surgery, the use of laparoscopic techniques offers several advantages to patients requiring rectal resection. Future study will be likely to confirm the reduced postoperative pain, earlier return of gastrointestinal function, and quicker resumption of normal activities seen in previous reports. The most recently reported investigations with follow-up of up to 2 years have not demonstrated reduced survival. The fear of port-site recurrence is the leading concern IN the laparoscopic resection of rectal cancer, although more recent studies have documented recurrence rates similar to conventional surgery. Future laboratory and clinical trials will be likely to confirm the validity of the laparoscopic approach. Advances in instrumentation and surgical techniques will also probably demonstrate the feasibility of a laparoscopic oncologic resection of the rectum with autonomic nerve preservation in the majority of these patients.

Effective surgical technique stands as the most potent therapy for nearly all patients with rectal cancer. The special challenges presented by rectal cancer require a profound knowledge of the intricacies of pelvic anatomy, an understanding of the biologic behavior of these tumors, and critical attention to the details of restorative surgery. If this can be accomplished, the vast majority of these patients will be free of disease and enjoy nearly normal bladder, sexual and rectal function. Thus, the surgeon who chooses to treat rectal cancer patients must be the central co-ordinator of their care.

References

1. Böhm B, Parker SL, Tong T, Bolden S. Cancer statistics 1997. CA Cancer J Clin 1997;47:5.
2. Heald RJ, Smedh RK, Kald A, Sexton R, Moran BJ. Abdominoperineal excision of the rectum: an endangered operation. Dis Colon Rectum 1997;40:747.
3. Parks AG. Benign tumors of rectum. In: Rob C, Smith R, Morgan CN, editors. Clinical surgery: abdomen and rectum and anus. 2nd ed. London: Butterworths, 1966:541.
4. Böhm B, Milsom JW, Kitago K, Brand M, Fazio VW. Laparoscopic oncologic total abdominal colectomy with intraperitoneal stapled anastomosis in a canine model. J Laparosc Surg 1994;4:23.
5. Böhm B, Milsom JW, Kitago K, Brand M, Stolfi VM, Fazio VW. Use of laparoscopic techniques in oncologic right colectomy in a canine model. Ann Surg Oncol 1995;2:6.
6. Milsom JW, Böhm B, Decanini C, Fazio VW. Laparoscopic oncologic proctocosigmoidectomy with low colorectal anastomosis in a cadaver model. Surg Endosc 1994;8:1117.

7. Decanini C, Milsom JW, Böhm B, Fazio VW. Laparoscopic oncologic abdominoperineal resection. Dis Colon Rectum 1994;37:552.
8. Turnbull RB, Cuthbertson A. Abdominorectal pull-through resection for cancer and for Hirschsprung's disease. Cleve Clin Q 1961;28:109.
9. Cutait DE, Figliolini FJ. A new method of colorectal anastomosis in abdominoperineal resection. Dis Colon Rectum 1961;4:335.
10. Miles WE. A method of performing abdomino-perineal excision for carcinoma of the rectum and of the terminal portion of the pelvic colon. Lancet 1908;ii:1812.
11. Moynihan BGA. The surgical treatment of cancer of the sigmoid flexure and rectum. Surg Gynecol Obstet
12. Gordon WC, Dukes C. The treatment of carcinoma of the rectum with radium with an introduction in the spread of cancer of the rectum. Br J Surg 1930;17:643.
13. Gabriel WB, Dukes C, Bussey FU. Lymphatic spread of cancer of the rectum. Br J Surg 1935;23:395.
14. Goligher JC. The blood supply of the sigmoid colon and rectum. Br J Surg 1949;37:157.
15. Bacon HF, Dirbas F, Myers TB, et al. Extensive lymphadenectomy and high ligation of the inferior mesenteric artery for carcinoma of the left colon and rectum. Dis Colon Rectum 1958;1:457.
16. Sugarbaker PH, Corlew S. Influence of surgical techniques on survival in patients with colorectal cancer: a review. Dis Colon Rectum 1982;25:545.
17. Grinnel RS, Hint RB. Ligation of inferior mesenteric artery at the aorta in resection for carcinoma of the sigmoid and rectum. Surg Gynecol Obstet 1952;94:526.
18. Grinnel RS. Results of ligation of the inferior mesenteric artery at the aorta in resections of carcinoma of the descending and sigmoid colon and rectum. Surg Gynecol Obstet 1965;120:1031.
19. Pezim ME, Nicholls RJ. Survival after high or low ligation of the inferior mesenteric artery during curative surgery for rectal cancer. Ann Surg 1984;200:729.
20. Surtees P, Ritchie JK, Phillips RKS. High versus low ligation of the inferior mesenteric artery in rectal cancer. Br J Surg 1990;77:618.
21. Mayo WJ. The radical operation for cancer of the rectum and rectosigmoid. Trans Am Surg Assoc 1916; 34:261.
22. Dixon CF. Anterior resection for malignant lesions of the upper part of the rectum and lower part of the sigmoid. Ann Surg 1948;128:425.
23. Best RR, Blair JB. Sphincter preserving operations for rectal carcinoma as related to the anatomy of the lymphatics. Ann Surg 1949;128:425.
24. Goligher JC, Dukes CE, Bussey HJR. Local recurrence after sphincter saving excisions for carcinoma of the rectum and rectosigmoid. Br J Surg 1951;39:119.
25. Williams NS, Durdey P, Johnston D. The outcome following sphincter-saving, resection and abdomino-perineal resection for low rectal cancer. Br J Surg 1985;72:595.
26. Pollett WG, Nicholls RJ. The relationship between the extent of distal clearance and survival and local recurrence rates after curative anterior resection for carcinoma of the rectum. Ann Surg 1983;198:159.
27. Weese JL, O'Grady MG, Ottery FD. How long is the five centimeter margin? Surg Gynecol Obstet 1986;163:101.
28. Phillips RKS, Hittinger R, Blesovsky L, Fry JS, Fielding LP. Local recurrence following "curative" surgery for large bowel cancer: II. The rectum and rectosigmoid. Br J Surg 1984;71:17.
29. Pilipshen RJ, Heiliveil M, Quan SHQ, Sternberg SS, Enker WE. Patterns of pelvic recurrence following definitive resections of rectal cancer. Cancer 1984;53:1354.
30. Rao AR, Kazan AR, Chan PM, Gilbert HA, Nusebaum H, Hintz BL. Patterns of recurrence following curative resection alone for adenocarcinoma of the rectum and sigmoid colon. Cancer 1981;48:1492.
31. Case AW, Millior RR, Pfaff WW. Patterns of recurrence following surgery alone for adenocarcinoma of the colon and rectum. Cancer 1976;37:2861.
32. Quirke P, Dundey P, Dixon MF, Williams NW. Local recurrence of rectal adenocarcinoma due to inadequate surgical resection. Lancet 1986;i:996.
33. Heald RJ, Husband EM, Ryall RDH. The mesorectum in rectal cancer surgery: the clue to pelvic recurrence? Br J Surg 1982;69:613.
34. Hojo K, Savada T, Moriya Y. An analysis of survival, voiding and sexual function after wide ileopelvic lymphadenectomy in patients with carcinoma of the rectum, compared with conventional lymphadenectomy. Dis Colon Rectum 1989;32:128.
35. Heald RJ, Ryall RDH. Recurrence and survival after total mesorectal excision for rectal cancer. Lancet 1986;i:1479.
36. Lavery IC, Lopez-Kostner F, Fazio VW, Fernandez-Martin M, Milsom JW, Church JM. Chances of cure are not compromised with sphincter-saving procedures for cancer of the lower third of the rectum. Surgery 1997;122:779.
37. Enker WE, Heiliveil ML, Hertz REL, et al. En bloc pelvic lymphadenectomy and sphincter preservation in the surgical management of rectal cancer. Ann Surg 1986;203:426.
38. Pittman MR, Thornton H, Ellis H. Survival after extended resection for locally advanced carcinomas of the colon and rectum. Ann R Coll Surg Engl 1984;66:81.
39. Orkin BA, Dozois RIZ, Beart RW, et al. Extended resection for locally advanced primary adenocarcinoma of the rectum. Dis Colon Rectum 1989;32:286.
40. Boey J, Wong I. Pelvic exenteration for locally advanced colorectal carcinoma. Ann Surg 1982;195:513.
41. Bonfanti G, Bozzetti F, Fori R, et al. Results of extended surgery for cancer of the rectum and sigmoid. Br J Surg 1982;69:305.
42. Wanebo HJ, Gaber DL, Whitehall R, Morgan RF, Constable WC. Pelvic recurrence of rectal cancer: options for curative resection. Ann Surg 1987;205:482.
43. Sugarbaker PH. Partial sacrectomy for en bloc excision of rectal cancer with posterior fixation. Dis Colon Rectum 1982;26:208.
44. John TG, Garden OJ. Laparoscopic ultrasonography: extending the scope of diagnostic laparoscopy. Br J Surg 1994;81:5.
45. Marchesa P, Milsom JW, Hale JC, O'Malley CM, Fazio VW. Intraoperative laparoscopic liver ultrasonography for staging of colorectal cancer. Initial experience. Dis Colon Rectum 1996;39:S73.
46. Havenga K, DeRuiter MC, Enker WE, Welvaart K. Anatomical basis of autonomic nerve-preserving total mesorectal excision for rectal cancer. Br J Surg 1996;83:384.
47. Beard JD, Nicholson ML, Sayers RD, Lloyd D, Everson NW. The intraoperative air testing of colorectal anastomosis: a prospective randomized trial. Br J Surg 1990;77:1095.
48. Bacon BE. Evolution of sphincter muscle preservation and reestablishment of continuity in the operative treatment of rectal and sigmoid cancer. Surg Gynecol Obstet 1945;181:113.
49. Lazorthes F, Fages P, Chiotasso P, Lemozy J, Bloom E. Resection of the rectum with construction of a colonic reservoir and coloanal anastomosis for carcinoma of the rectum. Br J Surg 1976;73:136.
50. Heimann TM, Szporn A, Bolnick K, Aufses AH Jr. Local recurrence following surgical treatment of rectal cancer: comparison of anterior and abdominoperineal resection. Dis Colon Rectum 1986;29:862.

51. Morson BC, Vaughn EG, Bussey HJR. Pelvic recurrence after excision of rectum for carcinoma. BMJ 1963;ii:13.

52. McDermott F, Hughes E, Pihl E, Milne J, Price A. Long term results of restorative resection and total excision for carcinoma of the middle third of the rectum. Surg Gynecol Obstet 1982;154:833.

53. Rich T, Gunderson L, Galdibini JJ, Cohen AM, Donaldson G. Patterns of recurrence of rectal cancer after potentially curative surgery. Cancer 1983;52:1317.

54. Williams NS, Johnston D. Survival and recurrence after sphincter saving resection and abdominoperineal resection for carcinoma of the middle third of the rectum. Br J Surg 1984;71:278.

55. Amato A, Pescatori M, Butti A. Local recurrence following abdominal/perineal excision and anterior resection for rectal carcinoma. Dis Colon Rectum 1991;34:317.

56. Dixon AR, Maxwell WA, Thornton Holmes J. Carcinoma of the rectum: a 10-year experience. Br J Surg 1991;78:308.

57. Michelassi F, Vannucci L, Ayala JJ, et al. Local recurrence after curative resection of colorectal adenocarcinoma. Surgery 1990;108:787.

58. Macfarlane JK, Ryall RDH, Heald RJ. Mesorectal excision for rectal cancer. Lancet 1993;341:457.

59. Milsom JW, Böhm B, Hammerhofer KA, Fazio VW, Steiger E, Elson P. A prospective, randomized trial comparing laparoscopic versus conventional techniques in colorectal cancer surgery: a preliminary report. J Am Coll Surg 1998;187:46.

7. Abdominoperineal Resection

D.J. Schoetz, Jr. and P.L. Roberts

Introduction

Cancer of the rectum continues to present technical challenges to the surgeon. One can only imagine how difficult it was for surgeons attempting to excise advanced tumors before the advent of the satisfactory anesthesia and perioperative support systems that exist today. Initial attempts at removing the rectum were generally through the perineal route. Frequently, a diverting iliac colostomy had been performed some weeks before the perineal operation. This multistaged approach would permit abdominal exploration for staging while relieving obstruction and permitting some mechanical preparation of the bowel before rectal excision. The primary technical limitation of the perineal approach was the inability to deal with proximal lymphatic spread of tumor [1–3].

Based on his research on the mode of spread of rectal cancer, Miles [4] proposed that the operation should encompass total excision of the rectum and anus with the anal sphincters, and that the levator muscles and ischiorectal fat bilaterally should also be included with the specimen. He advocated virtual total sigmoid resection with ligation of the inferior mesenteric vessels at their origin. He also promoted the need for excision of the pelvic peritoneum surrounding the rectum. Clearly, this operation required the fashioning of a permanent colostomy.

Despite proven oncologic benefit, acceptance of the Miles [4] abdominoperineal resection was slow, based on an operative mortality of 36.2% in his first 61 patients. The operation he proposed was begun from the abdomen. Upon completion of the abdominal portion, the patient was repositioned on the left side to permit completion of the perineal portion of the excision. One surgeon [2] believed this was an excessive physiologic insult and not only delayed

the application of the procedure but also led to a number of staged procedures in an attempt to decrease morbidity and mortality.

Combined synchronous abdominoperineal excision of the rectum was popularized by Lloyd-Davies [5] when he introduced adjustable leg rests that permitted satisfactory simultaneous exposure of both the abdomen and the perineum. The arguments in favor of the synchronous approach include a decrease in overall operating time, with two teams of surgeons working together. Difficult dissections are facilitated by the simultaneous dissection from above and below.

Objections to the combined synchronous approach include the possibility of inferior exposure for both teams of surgeons; however, with attention to patient positioning and care to prevent neuropraxia of the peroneal nerves from the leg rests, adequate exposure for both surgeons is always obtainable. This has become the technique of choice for the performance of abdominoperineal resection throughout the world.

Selection Factors for Abdominoperineal Resection

The number of abdominoperineal resections carried out has decreased in the last two decades. Our current understanding of the routes of spread of rectal cancer, combined with technical innovations such as the circular stapler, intrarectal ultrasonography and the "ultra-low" anastomotic techniques, have contributed to this decline. Nevertheless, abdominoperineal resection has an important role in the treatment of patients with distal rectal cancer and, for many of them, remains the best option to achieve cure of the disease in addition to adequate local control. A number of factors influence the decision to perform an abdominoperineal resection.

Tumor-Related Factors

Although the distance of the tumor from the anal verge helps to guide surgical therapy, it is not an absolute indication for or against abdominoperineal resection. Some tumors of the distal rectum (those within 0–5 cm of the anal verge) may be mobilized adequately with good margins and permit the performance of a sphincter salvage procedure. Others, such as distal rectal tumors in male patients having a narrow pelvis, may not be able to be mobilized sufficiently to provide adequate margins and require abdominoperineal resection. Such decisions are made intraoperatively, based on the tumor clearance after full rectal mobilization. In all instances, cure of the cancer should be the guiding principle; performing a sphincter salvage procedure should not jeopardize the patient's outcome.

The risk of nodal disease depends directly on the depth of penetration of the cancer through the bowel wall. Lesions beyond the muscularis propria have a significant risk of there being nodal disease. Similarly, involvement of other organs, such as invasion into the vagina, usually require abdominoperineal resection. Invasion of the anal sphincter muscle is probably one of the absolute indications for this procedure.

A variety of tumor characteristics help to determine which patients are good candidates for local therapy. These include tumors of relatively small size (<3 cm), tumors involving less than one-third of the circumference of the bowel wall, tumors that are not fixed, and tumors of polypoid configuration. Finally, those staged as T1 or T2 by a combination of clinical examination and transrectal ultrasonography are best suited for local excision. In contrast, tumors that do not meet these criteria are best suited to resective procedures, such as abdominoperineal resection.

Patient Factors

In patients with significant anal sphincter dysfunction and fecal incontinence, abdominoperineal resection is preferred to restoring bowel continuity with a low rectal anastomosis. Although incontinence may be caused by a large obstructing rectal cancer, sphincter assessment may be performed independently of the tumor as a cause of incontinence. Such patients often have a long history of fecal incontinence, predating the diagnosis of rectal cancer. Patients with severe diarrhea and fecal urgency from other gastrointestinal conditions may likewise be better served with an abdominoperineal resection.

Conversely, a colostomy may be extremely difficult to manage for some patients, such as those who are blind or those with severe arthritis. In these circumstances, a low rectal anastomosis, if it can be carried out both technically and in keeping with sound oncologic principles, should be performed. In institutionalized or bedridden patients, a colostomy is usually easier to care for and is preferred to a low rectal anastomosis.

Intraoperative Considerations

In some patients, the decision concerning whether to perform a sphincter salvage procedure or an abdominoperineal resection is made intraoperatively. Both obesity and male sex adversely affect the ability to perform a sphincter salvage procedure because of intraoperative technical considerations. Thin patients and those with a wide pelvis are more suitable for a low anastomosis from a technical standpoint than obese patients with a narrow pelvis.

Preoperative Preparation

After the decision has been made that abdominoperineal resection is the appropriate operation, the patient is prepared to undergo surgery. Complete preoperative evaluation, with particular emphasis on the thorough investigation of co-morbid conditions, is mandatory. Routine laboratory testing (including blood type and cross-matching), urinalysis and electrocardiography are obtained. Radiography of the chest is performed as part of a metastatic evaluation. Consultations with appropriate specialists to evaluate and treat other medical illnesses should be completed.

Consultation with an enterostomal therapist preoperatively is of critical importance. The enterostomal nurse is responsible for most of the preoperative teaching and postoperative problem solving, establishing a working relationship with the patient that is supportive both before and after discharge. In discussion with the patient, the nurse marks the most acceptable site on the patient's abdomen for the stoma, usually in the left lower quadrant.

Except when a high-grade obstruction is present, patients should undergo complete mechanical and antibiotic bowel preparation. Mechanical cleansing

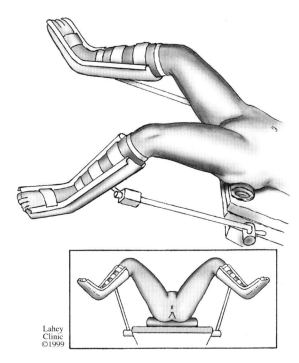

Fig. 7.1. Positioning the patient for combined synchronous abdominoperineal resection (reprinted with permission of the Lahey Clinic, Burlington, MA).

symphysis pubis. If possible, the skin incision should continue to the right of the umbilicus so that it does not interfere with colostomy pouching in the left lower quadrant. Thorough exploration of the abdomen is performed, with particular reference to the liver, the para-aortic nodes, and the parietal peritoneum of the pelvis. Biopsy with frozen-section pathologic analysis should be performed when indicated.

The extent of the abdominoperineal resection is determined by the blood supply of the rectum and sigmoid (Fig. 7.2). Ligation of the main trunk sigmoid vessel preserves the left colic artery off the inferior mesenteric artery and provides a blood supply to the proposed colostomy without sacrificing the oncologic value of the operation. Additional blood supply to the rectum includes the superior rectal artery (the last sigmoid branch) and the middle and inferior rectal arteries. The latter two vessels are divided during mobilization of the rectum.

After the abdominal exploration has been completed, a self-retaining retractor and wound protector are put in place, and the patient is tilted in the mild Trendelenburg position. Congenital adhesions

may be accomplished by several means. Polyethylene glycol lavage or phosphosoda is our preferred method. Oral antibiotics are administered after the preparation has been finished, usually at 7 p.m. and 11 p.m. the night before a scheduled morning operation. Intravenous antibiotics are administered within 1 hour before the skin incision.

On the day of surgery, sequential pneumatic compression stockings are placed on the lower legs before the induction of anesthesia. Once anesthetized, the patient is positioned in the lithotomy Trendelenburg position, with the legs in stirrups that cannot compress the peroneal nerve (Fig. 7.1). A bath blanket is placed under the sacrum to facilitate exposure of the perineum. Foley catheterization is performed under sterile conditions. Routine ureteral catheters are not used; these are saved for the previously operated or radiated pelvis. The anus is occluded with a purse string of heavy suture material to eliminate fecal soiling during rectal mobilization.

Operative Technique

Access to the abdomen is by means of a vertical mid-line incision, the lower end of which is at the

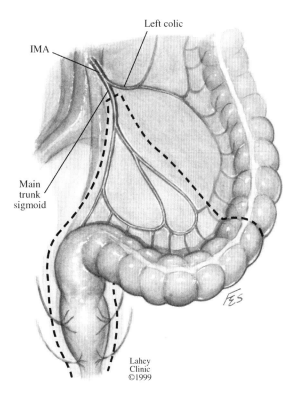

Fig. 7.2. Extent of resection as determined by blood supply (IMA, inferior mesenteric artery) (reprinted with permission of the Lahey Clinic, Burlington, MA).

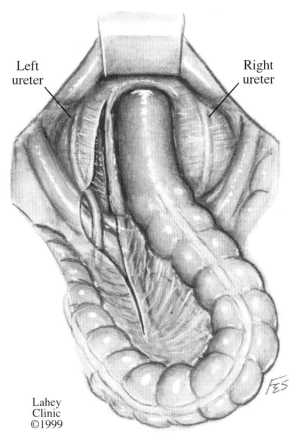

Left
ureter

Right
ureter

Lahey
Clinic
©1999

Fig. 7.3. Peritoneal incisions with identification of the ureters bilaterally (reprinted with permission of the Lahey Clinic, Burlington, MA).

orly. When the blood supply is divided early in the dissection, the viability of the end of the sigmoid will be apparent at the time of construction of the colostomy.

After the colon has been divided, downward traction on the distal sigmoid will facilitate mobilization of the remainder of the mesentery down to the sacral promontory. Autonomic nerves are at risk during this dissection if the plane is not entered properly. The superior hypogastric nerves should not be injured because they are in the retroperitoneum. At the sacral promontory, the loose areolar plane between the mesorecturn and the sacrum is entered sharply, and the posterior and posterolateral dissection can continue to the tip of the coccyx (Fig. 7.4). From this point, all dissection should be performed sharply or with electrocautery under direct vision. Manual extraction is not acceptable because of the higher incidence of bleeding from the presacral veins and disruption of the peritoneal envelope around the mesorecturn, with creation of an inadequate lateral margin.

After the posterior dissection has been completed, the proximal lateral rectal attachments are divided with electrocautery, again under direct vision and without the need for clips or sutures because they are avascular.

At this point, the rectum will be more mobile; upward traction on the rectum will permit com-

of the sigmoid are divided, as is the left lateral peritoneal reflection. In this way, the sigmoid colon is rendered a mid-line structure. Abdominal viscera should be packed only after complete sigmoid mobilization. A steeper Trendelenburg position aids in keeping the small bowel out of the pelvis.

The peritoneum at the base of the rectosigmoid mesentery is incised on both sides of the rectum. These peritoneal incisions are continued to the base of the bladder. In the process, both ureters are identified. The lateral borders of the dissection are the ureters on each side (Fig. 7.3).

Attention is then directed to division of the vasculature. The entire sigmoid mesentery is mobilized off the retroperitoneum, and the "bare area" of the sigmoid mesentery between the left colic and the sigmoid vessels is entered. In this plane, the main trunk sigmoid vessel is easily isolated at its origin, clamped, divided and ligated. The sigmoid colon can then be divided in its mid-portion with a linear cutting stapler. The proximal colon is packed superi-

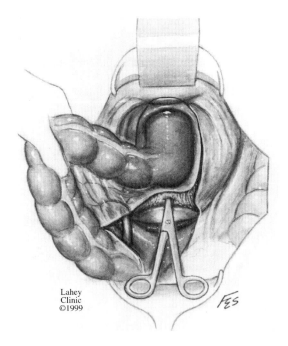

Lahey
Clinic
©1999

Fig. 7.4. Sharp entry into the retrorectal space at the sacral promontory (reprinted with permission of the Lahey Clinic, Burlington, MA).

pletion of the peritoneal incisions anteriorly to it. Continuation of sharp dissection in this plane will expose the back of the bladder and seminal vesicles in the male patient, and the cervix and posterior vagina in females. In males, Denonvillier's fascia must be opened deliberately to permit separation of the prostate and bladder neck from the anterior rectum. The anterior limit of the dissection is below the prostate in males and below the symphysis pubis in female patients.

The lateral and anterolateral dissections are performed under direct vision, using electrocautery with an extender that enables the surgeon to work deep in the pelvis. The lateral ligaments cannot be divided until after the anterior dissection has been completed. Because the lateral ligaments may contain a branch of the middle rectal artery, care must be taken to cauterize this tissue well. It is during this dissection that injury to the pelvic autonomic nerve plexus is most likely to occur (Fig. 7.5). Exposure is facilitated by anterior retraction of the pelvic viscera with either a malleable retractor or a St Mark's retractor.

The completion of rectal mobilization is performed posteriorly, again reflecting the rectum anteriorly to permit visualization of the remainder of the mesorectum. This dissection can continue directly to the levator hiatus. After the rectum has

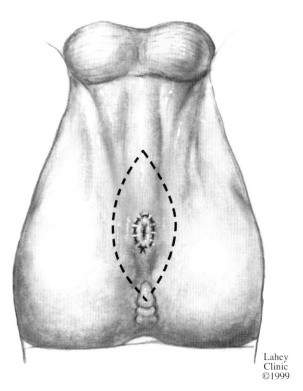

Fig. 7.6. Planned perineal incision (reprinted with permission of the Lahey Clinic, Burlington, MA).

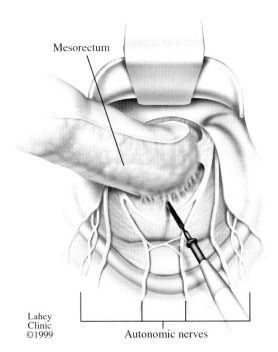

Fig. 7.5. Sharp dissection of the anterolateral rectal attachments, preserving autonomic nerves if possible (reprinted with permission of the Lahey Clinic, Burlington, MA).

been completely mobilized, the top of the levator muscle can be seen in its entirety.

In the combined synchronous approach, during mobilization of the rectum, a second team of surgeons prepares the perineum again with antiseptic solution and makes an elliptical incision, the anterior extent of which is over the perineal body and the posterior extent of which is at the tip of the coccyx. The lateral incisions should extend to the ischial tuberosities to permit excision of the ischiorectal fat on either side of the rectum (Fig. 7.6).

With the use of electrocautery, the lateral incisions are deepened into the ischiorectal fossa bilaterally. Both the anterior and posterior branches of the inferior rectal artery on each side are divided and ligated. After this step has been accomplished, the lateral dissection can easily be completed to the levators. At this point, a self-retaining retractor is put in place and the anterior dissection is completed with electrocautery to the level of the deep transverse perineal muscle. It is only at this point that the anococcygeal ligament is sharply divided (Fig. 7.7). This will provide access to the presacral space. Downward displacement of Waldeyer's fascia by the abdominal surgeon will facilitate the perineal

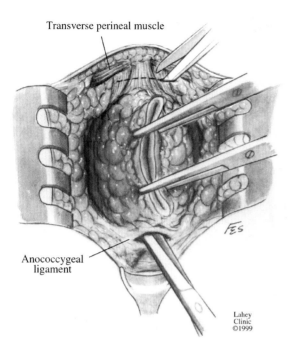

Transverse perineal muscle

Anococcygeal ligament

Lahey
Clinic
©1999

Fig. 7.7. Complete perineal mobilization of the rectum up to the levatores; division of the anococcygeal ligament (reprinted with permission of the Lahey Clinic, Burlington, MA).

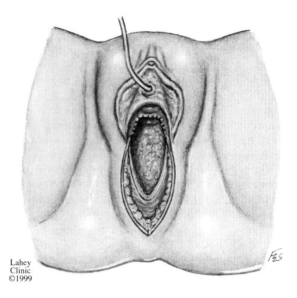

Lahey
Clinic
©1999

Fig. 7.8. Defect after en bloc posterior vaginectomy (reprinted with permission of the Lahey Clinic, Burlington, MA).

surgeon's entry into the appropriate plane. Care should be taken to direct the incision anteriorly to prevent entry into the presacral space, with the attendant risk of bleeding.

After the pelvis has been entered posteriorly, the perineal operator can insert an index finger on the superior aspect of both levator muscles, displacing them into the operative field. Electrocautery is used to divide the levator muscles as close to the lateral pelvic side wall as possible on each side. After the anterolateral portion of the levator muscles has been divided, the remaining attachments are in an anterior position. Care must be taken to keep this dissection out of the urethra in the male patient and the vagina in females. In some instances, passing the specimen out of the perineal wound will facilitate the anterior dissection.

Anterior distal rectal cancer in a female patient may require en bloc partial posterior vaginectomy (Fig. 7.8). Depending on the size of the vaginal defect, the wound may be repaired by freeing the posterolateral vaginal wall on each side and closing with a running synthetic absorbable suture. If this step is not technically feasible, the vaginal wound can be left open to heal by secondary intent.

The perineal wound is irrigated with normal saline solution, hemostasis is ensured, and the wound is closed in layers using synthetic absorbable

sutures to eliminate as much dead space as possible. Skin closure with a running subcuticular absorbable suture eliminates the need for the potentially uncomfortable removal of sutures at a later date.

While the perineal wound is being closed, the abdominal operators irrigate the pelvis and achieve hemostasis. The aperture for the colostomy is created by excising skin and subcutaneous tissue at the site marked preoperatively, within the rectus muscle. The muscle is split in the direction of its fibers and the posterior sheath and peritoneum are incised. The defect is enlarged to two to three fingers breadth. The divided end of the colostomy is brought out for later maturation, which is accomplished after the abdomen has been closed. Care should be taken to be certain that there is no tension on the proposed colostomy, which may require additional mobilization of the descending colon.

Closed suction drains are placed in the pelvis through separate stab wounds in the right lower quadrant. This maneuver avoids the placement of drains through the perineal wound or buttocks, which is uncomfortable for the patient and may contribute to delayed healing of the wound. Placement on the right side avoids potential interference with pouching of the new stoma.

Before closure, it is appropriate to consider the possibility that postoperative radiotherapy may be required. The prevention of migration of the small bowel into the pelvis can be accomplished in most individuals by the creation of an omental pedicle. Dissection of the gastrocolic omentum off the right transverse colon and division of the greater omentum, leaving the left gastroepiploic vessel intact, will permit the omental pedicle to be brought down the left gutter and sutured over the drains into the pelvic inlet. When the omentum is insufficient, an absorbable mesh can be sutured above the pelvic inlet and, with running sutures, circumferentially fixed to the inside of the abdominal wall. With the increasing use of preoperative adjuvant radiotherapy, these maneuvers are less often a consideration.

Maturation of the colostomy is accomplished last by excising the previous staple line. Brisk arterial bleeding is required to ensure viability of the stoma. Protrusion of one-fourth to one-half of an inch is preferred because the patient will be able to use tactile and visual feedback to achieve and maintain independence in care of the stoma. A clear plastic appliance should be put in place at the time of operation for continuous monitoring of the health of the stoma.

Intraoperative and Postoperative Complications

Substantial improvements in both morbidity and mortality have been made since Miles [4] reported a 36.2% mortality rate for his first 61 abdominoperineal resections in 1908. Operative mortality ranges from zero to 6% [6–17], with the majority of operative deaths occurring from cardiorespiratory complications. Despite improvements, the morbidity associated with abdominoperineal resection remains high and may be considered as intraoperative or postoperative complications.

Bleeding

Significant intraoperative bleeding may occur in approximately 4% of resections for rectal cancer [18]. The two most common types of bleeding are pelvic and that from splenic injury. The latter may occur during mobilization of the splenic flexure and is usually the result of a capsular injury. Excessive traction on the splenic flexure during mobilization should be avoided to prevent tearing adhesions to the capsule of the spleen. Most capsular injuries are managed conservatively without the need for splenectomy.

Pelvic bleeding can be massive and life threatening. It can originate from several potential sites. Bleeding from the internal iliac vein or artery occurs in a small percentage of operations. Rothenberger and Wong [13] reported one internal iliac vein injury in a series of 155 patients undergoing abdomino-

perineal resection, and Rosen et al. [14] reported one injury in 230 patients.

Other pelvic bleeding may occur along the anterior surface of the sacrum from the presacral venous plexus of the basivertebral veins. An elegant description of the presacral venous plexus and the basivertebral veins has been given by Wang et al. [19]. Such bleeding is usually precipitated by blunt dissection. Entering the presacral space sharply and continuing in the correct plane avoids such bleeding. Bleeding from the presacral venous plexus is usually controlled by suture ligation or electrocautery. Massive bleeding can occur from stripping the fascia off the sacrum and avulsing the basivertebral veins on their entrance into the sacral foramina. Bleeding from basivertebral veins can be controlled by thumbtacks [20] or titanium tacks [21]. The placement of a tissue expander into the presacral space has also been described [22]. If all of these methods fail to stop the bleeding, consideration should be given to pelvic packing and a second laparotomy performed 24–72 hours later to complete the operation and remove the packs [23].

Unhealed Perineal Wound

The perineal wound has been a major source of potential morbidity after abdominoperineal resection. Unhealed perineal wounds are defined as wounds that have not healed after 6 months. Such wounds may continue to drain foul material and cause significant patient disability. Delayed healing occurs in 14–23% of patients after abdominoperineal resection; ultimately, 25% require further surgery [13,18].

Not surprisingly, the management of the perineal wound has undergone a major evolution since the initial description by Miles [4] in which a perineal anorectal excision was performed and the resultant wound left open and packed. The wound was left open because of concern for postoperative hemorrhage and sepsis or abscess formation if the perineum were closed. However, an open perineal wound caused prolonged hospitalization and the need for regular care of the wound itself to ensure proper and adequate healing.

Subsequent reports of successful primary healing after closure of the perineal wound led to the routine performance of primary closure. In 1974, Altemeier et al. [24] reported 129 patients who underwent primary closure of the perineal wound after abdominoperineal resection, with successful primary healing in 118 (91%).

Wounds that drain persistently or show evidence of slow healing should be treated aggressively with daily wound care, including baths and dressing changes. Curettage and debridement of the wound may be necessary in the operating room in patients with a long thin track or so-called persistent perineal sinus. If healing does not occur or if a wound reopens after healing, consideration should be given to a retained foreign body, a fistula or recurrent cancer.

Despite aggressive wound care, a small percentage will remain unhealed. The bony pelvis tends to be a rigid, non-collapsible space. In such circumstances, the wound is excised and the defect filled with a well-vascularized muscle or myocutaneous flap, such as gracilis, rectus or gluteus muscle.

Inadvertent Perforation of the Rectum

Inadvertent perforation of the rectum during the performance of an abdominoperineal resection has been reported to occur in 14–26% of operations [25–28]. A study [26] of 178 resections for rectal cancer found that, by multivariate analysis, inadvertent perforation of the rectum was associated with an increased risk of death by a factor of 3.4 and a local recurrence rate of >4. This complication may be underestimated because perforation of the rectum is associated with a poor prognosis. Perforation should always be reported in operative and pathology reports [26].

Perineal Hernia

Perineal hernia has been reported to occur in 1% of patients after abdominoperineal resection [13,29,30]. Because only a a small amount of perineal tissue is available for support after abdominoperineal resection, it is perhaps surprising that this complication does not occur more often. Complications of perineal hernia include skin ulceration, evisceration of the bowel, incarceration of the bowel, and perineal enterocutaneous hernia. The repair of a perineal hernia is a major surgical undertaking. Preoperatively, recurrent cancer should be excluded. A combined abdominal and perineal approach is favored. Adequate exposure and full mobilization of the bowel out of the pelvis is necessary. If a substantial amount of omentum is present, this can be mobilized and placed in the pelvis to perform the repair. If the omentum is not present, gracilis and gluteus flaps may be used [29,30].

Urogenital Complications

Bladder Dysfunction
Bladder dysfunction may occur in 7–68% of patients after abdominoperineal dissection, although the incidence is generally quoted at about 30% [13,31]. Dysfunction may include incomplete emptying, urgency, overflow or stress incontinence, loss of bladder sensation, and chronic urinary tract infections. The majority of voiding difficulties have been shown to be neurogenic in origin as a result of parasympathetic denervation. Although a neurogenic bladder may occur in as many as 50% of men after abdominoperineal resection, voiding difficulties resolve in the majority within 3–6 months after surgery [32]. Bladder neck angulation and the presence of benign prostatic hypertrophy may also contribute to these difficulties.

Urinary tract infections, which occur in 6–16% of patients, result from an indwelling Foley catheter, which is usually left in place for 5–7 days postoperatively [33,34]. Strict attention to sterile technique in addition to removing the catheter as soon as possible should minimize this complication.

Sexual Dysfunction
Although the incidence of sexual dysfunction in men (as defined by erectile dysfunction or retrograde ejaculation) has been reported to be as high as 25–100% [35,36] after rectal resection for cancer, more recently the incidence has decreased with the use of autonomic nerve preserving techniques. The incidence of sexual dysfunction after abdominoperineal resection increases with age. Havenga and colleagues [32] and Enker [37] found that 86–96% of men retain their sexual function after rectal resection autonomic nerve preservation.

The incidence of sexual dysfunction in women after abdominoperineal resection of the rectum is less well defined. The most common complaint postoperatively is dyspareunia, although one series found little change when preoperative complaints were compared with postoperative complaints [38]. As in men, advanced age correlates with a higher incidence of sexual dysfunction. Oliveira and coworkers [31] reported a 15% incidence of sexual and urinary dysfunction after pelvic dissection in women. In some women who have undergone a posterior vaginectomy in addition to an abdominoperineal dissection, sexual intercourse may be impossible because of a stenotic vaginal introitus.

Ureteral Injury
The ureters are vulnerable to injury in any pelvic operation. During the performance of abdominoperineal resection, the ureters, particularly the left one, are prone to injury during ligation of the superior rectal artery, during transection of the lateral ligaments, and during the perineal phase of the operation. Prevention of this complication is paramount. In all abdominoperineal resections, care

should be taken to identify the ureters. For patients who are undergoing this procedure for recurrent cancer, those with large tumors, and patients who have undergone prior radiation therapy, consideration should be given to the placement of ureteral stents. These do not prevent injury but may facilitate identification of the ureters and, if injury occurs, may help to identify the injury intraoperatively. Prompt identification of ureteral damage is important because major morbidity can result from an unrecognized injury that presents as a fistula. The reported incidence of this complication is <1%. Rosen et al. [14] noted one ureteral injury in 230 patients undergoing abdominoperineal resection; one of 155 patients at the University of Minnesota [13] had this complication. The treatment of ureteral injury depends on the time of diagnosis, the severity of the damage, and the level of the injury. Every effort should be made to confirm the diagnosis intraoperatively. Although 5–10 ml of indigo carmine or methylene blue dye may be injected intravenously to identify any injury, most often direct exploration of the ureter is necessary. Partial transection of the ureter may be treated by primary closure and the placement of a stent. For injuries below the pelvic brim, ureteroneocystostomy is the procedure of choice.

Urethral Injury

Posterior urethral injuries, particularly in men, may occur during the perineal phase of the operation. The result may be urethral stricture or fistula. The incidence of urethral injuries is small, occurring in one of 230 patients reported by Rosen and colleagues [14].

Colostomy Complications

A large number of potential stoma complications, including ischemia and necrosis, retraction, stenosis, prolapse and parastomal herniation, may occur in patients undergoing abdominoperineal resection. Meticulous operative technique combined with careful site selection and preoperative marking of the stoma site will reduce the incidence of complications substantially. A well-vascularized segment of colon should be brought out through the rectus muscle via an aperture that admits two fingers. Excessive tension should be avoided, as should sutures at the fascial level.

Other Complications

As with any abdominal operation, a number of other complications may occur after abdominoperineal resection, including wound infection, small bowel obstruction, pelvic abscess, cardiorespiratory complications, deep venous thrombosis, and pulmonary embolism. Recent studies have shown that outcome after rectal cancer resection is improved by surgeons undergoing colorectal surgical subspecialty training and carrying out rectal cancer surgery more frequently [39].

Concluding Remarks

Abdominoperineal resection remains an essential procedure in the management of many histologic types of rectal malignancy. The inability to restore gastrointestinal tract continuity should not be perceived by the patient or the patient's family as a failure because the result may be a permanent cure of the underlying cancer. Intraoperative technical challenges, which can be minimized by meticulous attention to technical detail, include massive pelvic bleeding associated with faulty dissection of the mesorectum, autonomic denervation resulting in bladder and sexual dysfunction, and stomal problems associated with inadequate colostomy creation. Postoperatively, perineal wound problems include infection and non-healed perineal wounds; stoma problems such as prolapse, retraction and parastomal hernia may also occur over time. Nevertheless, in appropriately selected individuals, the abdominoperineal resection provides excellent oncologic results; often the functional results are superior to those obtained after a restorative procedure, which may result in a poor quality of life due to substantial alterations in bowel function. Although technical advances in surgical technique and adjuvant therapies continue to decrease the overall role of this operation in the treatment of rectal cancer, there will always be a need to perform total surgical excision of the rectum in some patients.

References

1. Gabriel WB. Perineo-abdominal excision of the rectum in one stage. Lancet 1934;ii:69–74.
2. Goligher JC. Surgery of the anus, rectum and colon. 5th ed. London: Bailliére Tindall, 1984:590–779.
3. Lockhart-Mummery JP. Two hundred cases of cancer of the rectum treated by perineal excision. Br J Surg 1926;14:110–24.
4. Miles WE. A method of performing abdominoperineal excision for carcinoma of the rectum and the terminal portion of the pelvic colon. Lancet 1908;ii:1812–13.
5. Lloyd-Davies OV. Lithotomy–Trendelenburg position for resection of the rectum and lower pelvic colon. Lancet 1939;ii:74–76.

6. Bokey EL, Chapuis PH, Fung C, et al. Postoperative morbidity and mortality following resection of the colon and rectum for cancer. Dis Colon Rectum 1995;38:480–87.

7. Cunsolo A, Bragaglia RB, Petrucci C, Poggioli G, Gozzefti G. Survival and complications after radical surgery for carcinoma of the rectum. J Surg Oncol 1989;41:27–32.

8. Gillen P, Peel AL. Comparison of the mortality, morbidity and incidence of local recurrence in patients with rectal cancer treated by either stapled anterior resection or abdominoperineal resection. Br J Surg 1986;73:339–41.

9. Halpern NB, Cox CB, Aldrete JS. Abdominoperineal resection for rectal carcinoma: perioperative risk factors. South Med J 1989;82:1492–96.

10. Hughes ES, McDermott FT, Masterton JP, Cunningham IG, Polglase AL. Operative mortality following excision of the rectum. Br J Surg 1980;67:49–51.

11. Patel SC, Tovee EB, Langer B. Twenty-five years of experience with radical surgical treatment of carcinoma of the extraperitoneal rectum. Surgery 1977;82:460–65.

12. Theile DE, Cohen JR, Holt J, Davis NC. Mortality and complications of large-bowel resection for carcinoma. Aust N Z J Surg 1979;49:62–66.

13. Rothenberger DA, Wong WD. Abdominoperineal resection for adenocarcinoma of the low rectum. World J Surg 1992;16:478–85.

14. Rosen L, Veidenheimer MC, Coller JA, Corman ML. Mortality, morbidity, and patterns of recurrence after abdominoperineal resection for cancer of the rectum. Dis Colon Rectum 1982;25:202–208.

15. Holm T, Rutqvist LE, Johansson H, Cedermark B. Abdominoperineal resection and anterior resection in the treatment of rectal cancer: results in relation to adjuvant preoperative radiotherapy. Br J Surg 1995;82:1213–16.

16. Michelassi F, Block GE, Vannucci L, Montag A, Chappell R. A 5- to 21-year follow-up and analysis of 250 patients with rectal adenocarcinoma. Ann Surg 1988;208:379–89.

17. Dixon AR, Maxwell WA, Holmes JT. Carcinoma of the rectum: a 10-year experience. Br J Surg 1991;78:308–11.

18. Pollard CW, Nivatvongs S, Rojanasakul A, Ilstrup DM. Carcinoma of the rectum: profiles of intraoperative and early postoperative complications. Dis Colon Rectum 1994;37:866–74.

19. Wang QY, Shi WJ, Zhao YR, Zhao WQ, He ZR. New concepts in severe presacral hemorrhage during proctectomy. Arch Surg 1985;120:1013–20.

20. Nivatvongs S, Fang DT. The use of thumbtacks to stop massive presacral hemorrhage. Dis Colon Rectum 1986;29:589–90.

21. Stolfi VM, Milsom JW, Lavery IC, Oakley JR, Church JM, Fazio VW. Newly designed occluder pin for presacral hemorrhage. Dis Colon Rectum 1992;35:166–69.

22. Cosman BC, Lackides GA, Fisher DP, Eskenazi LB. Use of tissue expander for tamponade of presacral hemorrhage: report of a case. Dis Colon Rectum 1994;37:723–26.

23. Zama N, Fazio VW, Jagelman DG, Lavery IC, Weakley FL, Church JM. Efficacy of pelvic packing in maintaining hemostasis after rectal excision for cancer. Dis Colon Rectum 1988;31:923–28.

24. Altemeier WA, Culbertston WR, Alexander JW, Sutorius D, Bossert J. Primary closure and healing of the perineal wound in abdominoperineal resection of the rectum for carcinoma. Am J Surg 1974;127:215–19.

25. Ranbarger KR, Johnston WD, Chang JC. Prognostic significance of surgical perforation of the rectum during abdominoperineal resection for rectal carcinoma. Am J Surg 1982;143:186–88.

26. Porter GA, O'Keefe GE, Yakimets WW. Inadvertent perforation of the rectum during abdominoperineal resection. Am J Surg 1996;172:324–27.

27. Slanetz CA Jr. The effect of inadvertent intraoperative perforation on survival and recurrence in colorectal cancer. Dis Colon Rectum 1984;27:792–97.

28. Zirngibl H, Husemann B, Hermanek P. Intraoperative spillage of tumor cells in surgery for rectal cancer. Dis Colon Rectum 1990;33:610–14.

29. Beck DE, Fazio VW, Jagelman DG, Lavery IC, McGonagle BA. Postoperative perineal hernia. Dis Colon Rectum 1987;30:21–24.

30. Brotschi E, Noe JM, Silen W. Perineal hernias after proctectomy: a new approach to repair. Am J Surg 1985;149:301–305.

31. Oliveira L, Weiss E, Amarnath B, Nogueras J, Wexler S. Sexual and urinary impairment after low pelvic dissection in colorectal surgery [abstract]. Dis Colon Rectum 1997;40:A43.

32. Havenga K, Enker WE, McDermott K, Cohen AM, Minsky BD, Guillem J. Male and female sexual and urinary function after total mesorectal excision with autonomic nerve preservation for carcinoma of the rectum. J Am Coll Surg 1996;182:495–502.

33. Billingham RP. Conservative treatment of rectal cancer. Extending the indications. Cancer 1992;70(5 Suppl): 1355–63.

34. Cawthorn SJ, Parums DV, Gibbs NM, et al. Extent of mesorectal spread and involvement of lateral resection margin as prognostic factors after surgery for rectal cancer. Lancet 1990;335:1055–59.

35. Yeager ES, Van Heerden JA. Sexual dysfunction following proctocolectomy and abdominoperineal resection. Ann Surg 1980;191:169–70.

36. Weinstein M, Roberts M. Sexual potency following surgery for rectal carcinoma: a follow-up of 44 patients. Ann Surg 1977;185:295–300.

37. Enker WE. Potency, cure, and local control in the operative treatment of rectal cancer. Arch Surg 1992;127:1396–402.

38. van Driel MF, Weymar Schultz WC, van de Wiel HB, Hahn DE, Mensink HJ. Female sexual functioning after radical surgical treatment of rectal and bladder cancer. Eur J Surg Oncol 1993;19:183–87.

39. Porter GA, Soskolne CL, Yakimets WW, Newman SC. Surgeon-related factors and outcome in rectal cancer. Ann Surg 1998;227:157–67.

8. Total Mesorectal Excision with Autonomic Nerve Preservation: "Optimized Surgery"

N.J. Kafka and W.E. Enker

Introduction

The management of rectal cancer has changed markedly since the late 1970s, with both the introduction of novel forms of adjuvant therapy and continued improvements in operative technique. The goals of treatment remain constant. These are:

1. Cure of disease, including the en bloc resection of the primary cancer and prevention of metastatic spread
2. Local control with avoidance of pelvic recurrence
3. Sphincter preservation, involving the restoration of continuity and preservation of normal or near-normal anorectal function
4. Preservation of sexual and urinary function, which entails maintaining the integrity of the autonomic nervous system.

Historically, using traditional operative technique without adjuvant therapy, outcome was poor and carried with it significant morbidity. Local recurrence rates consistently exceeded 20% and were sometimes reported to be much higher [1]. Furthermore, 5-year survival ranged from 27% to 42% [2–5]. The most important advance in operative technique to date has been the advent of total mesorectal excision (TME), which continues to gain acceptance globally and is now used in the management of mid-rectal tumors by 82% of colorectal surgeons affiliated with colorectal surgery training programs [6]. Concurrent autonomic nerve preservation is vital to optimize sexual and urinary function.

This chapter will discuss the anatomic and pathophysiologic bases of TME and autonomic nerve preservation. The operative techniques involved will be described. Their morbidity and mortality, including sexual and urinary function, will be reviewed. The oncologic results, including recurrence and survival will be detailed. Finally, the utility of lateral extended lymphadenectomy, the use of the colonic J-pouch, and the role of TME in proximal rectal cancers will be discussed.

Rationale of Total Mesorectal Excision and its Relationship to the Anatomy of Spread of Rectal Cancer

Most patients (65–80%) presenting with rectal cancer have either full-thickness penetration into the perirectal fat (T3NanyM0) or involvement of regional mesorectal lymph nodes situated along the route of the rectal blood supply to the rectum (TanyN1–2M0) [7,8]. This regional spread is virtually all confined within the mesorectum, which comprises fat, vessels and lymphatics contained within the visceral pelvic fascia [9] (Fig. 8.1).

Recently, pathological evaluation of resected specimens has been undertaken to evaluate the importance of the mesorectum as an anatomical unit in the dissemination of rectal cancer. Mesorectal spread has been identified in a significant percentage of patients. Morikawa et al. [10] evaluated specimens from resections of 171 cancers (38 rectosigmoid, 68 upper rectal, and 65 lower rectal) by lymph node clearing. The rate of lymph node metastases was 57.3%, with 33.3% of T1 rectal cancers having involved lymph nodes. Mesorectal lymphatic spread extended up to 4 cm distal and 10 cm proximal to the primary tumor. Scott et al. [11] evaluated specimens from 20 curative resections of tumors within 18 cm of the anal verge. Distal cancer

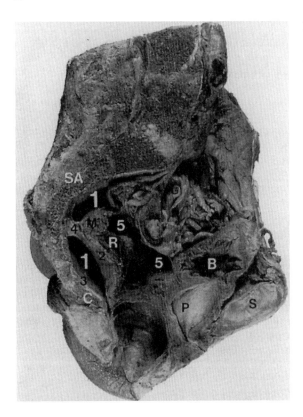

Fig. 8.1. Mid-sagittal hemisection of a male pelvis: 1, retrorectal space; 2, visceral fascia; 3, parietal fascia; 4, rectosacral fascia; 5, peritoneal cavity; R, rectum; M, mesorectum; B, bladder; P, prostate; S, symphysis pubis; SA, sacrum; C, coccyx. (Reproduced with permission from [19] Havenga K, DeRuiter MC, Enker WE, Welvaart K. Anatomical basis of autonomic nerve-preserving total mesorectal excision for rectal cancer. Br J Surg 1996;83:384–88.)

lymph node metastases in association with 12/23 (52%) Dukes' C lesions. In 12 patients (24%), the mesorectum distal to the tumor was involved with cancer. The maximum distance from the primary carcinoma to a metastatic lesion was >2 cm in five of these 12 individuals and was 5 cm in one patient.

Conventional rectal surgery for cancer often employs a blunt technique along undefinable tissue planes. This has been thought to affect lateral clearance of the tumor. Since 1983, several clinicopathologic studies have been undertaken to determine the incidence and effects of positive lateral margins of resection. The first published report was by Quirke et al. [14] in 1986. They evaluated 52 patients using transverse section whole mounts, with a follow-up of 2 years. Unsuspected instances of spread to the lateral resection margin were identified in 27% of the specimens. Eighty-five percent of the patients with positive margins developed local recurrence. Of those patients undergoing "curative" resections, five of 39 (12.8%) had involved lateral margins. There were no local recurrences in those with negative lateral margins, compared with 4/5 (80%) of those with involved margins. Ng et al. [15] reported on 80 patients undergoing proctectomy for cancer, of whom 50 underwent curative resections. The median follow-up was 26.6 months. The lateral resection margins were positive in 20% of cases, with a strong inverse correlation with Dukes' stage (0 Dukes' A; 6.7% Dukes' B; 24.2% Dukes' C; and 75% Dukes' D). Local recurrence rates correlated strongly with involved lateral margins. Among patients undergoing curative resections the local recurrence rate was 17% in those with uninvolved margins and 60% in those with involved margins ($p < 0.001$).

Adam et al. [16] performed a prospective study on 190 patients with a median follow-up of 5 years. They excluded those who had undergone preoperative radiotherapy because of concerns regarding downstaging of the tumors. They utilized transverse and coronal sections, measuring the closest point at which the tumor approached the lateral margin and defining a margin of <1 mm as a positive margin. Local recurrence and survival were correlated with margin status. Local recurrences were defined as pelvic recurrences, with pathologic or radiologic confirmation. Curative operations were limited to those in which all macroscopic tumor was removed and in which the distal margin was uninvolved. Positive lateral margins were identified in 36% of patients and in 25% of those undergoing curative resection. The local recurrence rates were 64% in patients with involved versus 9% in those with uninvolved margins, overall, and 66% versus 8%, respectively, in those undergoing curative resection. The

spread was seen in five (25%). One specimen exhibited distal intramural spread of malignant cells to 2 cm below the macroscopic main tumor and four (20%) exhibited tumor cell spread in the mesorectum of 1–3 cm with or without mural extension. In these specimens the extramural spread generally exceeded the mural spread. Hida et al. [12] performed a retrospective evaluation of 198 specimens resected over a 10-year period, using lymph node clearing and assessing distal intramural spread. Intramural spread was seen in 10.6% of patients, extending up to 2 cm from proximal rectal cancers and 1 cm from distal rectal tumors; it was not identified for T1 or T2 tumors. Distal mesorectal nodal metastases were identified in 20.2% of the patients. The greatest distance to a lymph node metastasis was 4 cm. Reynolds et al. [13] reported on 50 consecutive resections with TME. They identified mesorectal deposits in association with 5/21 (24%) Dukes' B tumors and mesorectal deposits and/or statistical significance of the differences in outcome persisted in multivariate analysis. The hazard ratio was 12.23. Survival was similarly affected. The overall 5-year life table survival was 15% in those with involved margins and 66% in those with uninvolved margins (24% versus 74% in curative resections). These results also persisted in multivariate analysis. Penetration of the muscularis propria was not a significant factor in the multivariate analysis.

These studies suggest that the critical factor in outcome is an inadequate resection, defined as the involvement of the lateral margins of resection. Thus, the primary goal of surgery must be the complete excision of all mesorectal disease, contained within an intact layer of visceral fascia, with negative lateral margins.

Technique of Total Mesorectal Excision with Autonomic Nerve Preservation

The technique of TME utilizes precise, sharp dissection in the areolar tissue between the visceral and parietal layers of the pelvic fascia (Fig. 8.2). When correctly performed, there is a characteristic smooth, bilobed appearance posteriorly and distally, with encapsulation by the visceral fascia [18]

(Fig. 8.3). Anteriorly, the dissection is in the plane between the seminal vesicles and Denonvillier's fascia (Fig. 8.4). This procedure is more difficult but is no more radical than blunt dissection. Indeed, the

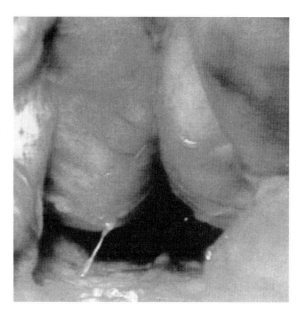

Fig. 8.3. Posterior aspect of mesorectum during surgery, showing the characteristic bilobed appearance. (Modified with permission from [18] MacFarlane JK, Ryall RDH, Heald RJ. Mesorectal excision for rectal cancer. Lancet 1993;341:457–60; © by *The Lancet* Ltd.)

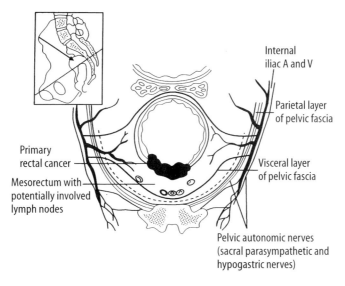

Fig. 8.2. Pelvic anatomy, demonstrating the visceral and parietal pelvic fascial layers, between which is the plane of dissection in total mesorectal excision with autonomic nerve preservation. The parietal pelvic fascia covers the sacrum, the musculoskeletal boundaries of the pelvic side walls, the vessels and the autonomic nerves, protecting them from injury while all regional disease is removed. (Reproduced with permission from [17] Enker WE. Total mesorectal excision – the new golden standard of surgery for rectal cancer. Ann Med 1997;29:127–33; modified from [7] with permission of PRR, Inc., Melville, NY.)

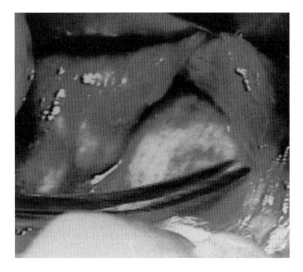

Fig. 8.4. Anterior aspect of the mesorectum during dissection, with the seminal vesicles in front and Denonvillier's fascia behind, of characteristically white appearance. (Modified with permission from [18] MacFarlane JK, Ryall RDH, Heald RJ. Mesorectal excision for rectal cancer. Lancet 1993;341:457–60; © (by *The Lancet* Ltd.)

precise dissection, under direct vision, which leaves the gonadal vessels, ureters, iliac vessels, sacral veins, pelvic autonomic nerves and pelvic wall musculature beneath the parietal fascia, minimizes the risk of damage to these structures. An understanding of the regional anatomy is vital to a correct dissection. Due to the risk of anastomotic leakage at a low rectal or anal anastomosis, routine temporary fecal diversion is recommended. This is usually accomplished by the creation of a loop ileostomy but it can also be effected by the construction of a loop colostomy. The latter may be more technically challenging and runs the risk of injury to the blood supply of the anastomosis, which is often the marginal artery.

Although most surgeons are aware of the visceral and vascular anatomy of the pelvis, the neuroanatomy is less well understood and its importance

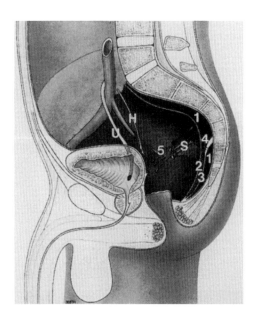

Fig. 8.5. Schematic drawing of the relationship between the pelvic autonomic nerves and pelvic fasciae: 1, retrorectal space; 2, anterior leaf of the visceral fascia; 3, posterior leaf of the visceral fascia; 4, rectosacral fascia; 5, middle rectal artery; S, sacral splanchnic nerves; H, hypogastric nerve; U, ureter. (Reproduced with permission from [19] Havenga K, DeRuiter MC, Enker WE, Welvaart K. Anatomical basis of autonomic nerve-preserving total mesorectal excision for rectal cancer. Br J Surg 1996;83:384–88.)

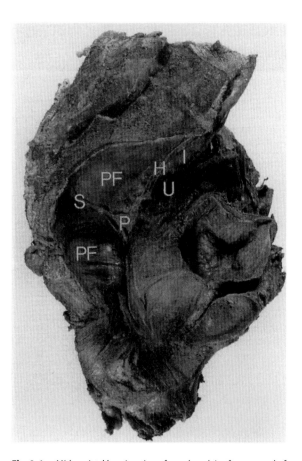

Fig. 8.6. Mid-sagittal hemisection of a male pelvis after removal of the rectum and mesorectum: H, hypogastric nerve; S, sacral splanchnic nerves; P, pelvic autonomic nerve plexus; PF, parietal fascia; I, internal iliac artery; U, ureter. (Reproduced with permission from [19] Havenga K, DeRuiter MC, Enker WE, Welvaart K. Anatomical basis of autonomic nerve-preserving total mesorectal excision for rectal cancer. Br J Surg 1996;83:384–88.)

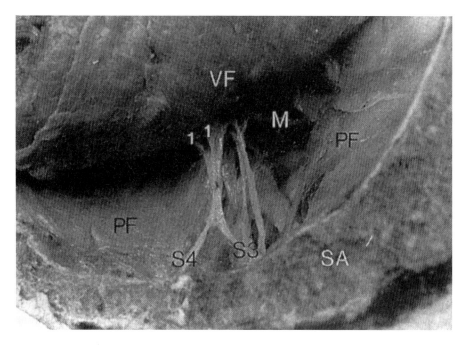

Fig. 8.7. Detail of the third splanchnic nerve, dissected from the parietal fascia: S3, third sacral splanchnic nerve; 1, medial splanchnic branches (to rectum); M, middle rectal vein; VF, visceral fascia; PF, parietal fascia; SA, sacrum. (Reproduced with permission from [19] Havenga K, DeRuiter MC, Enker WE, Welvaart K. Anatomical basis of autonomic nerve-preserving total mesorectal excision for rectal cancer. Br J Surg 1996;83:384–88.)

poorly appreciated. The anatomy of the pelvic sympathetic and parasympathetic nerves has been elegantly described by Havenga et al. [19] (Figs 8.5–8.8). The splanchnic nerves run laterocaudad and anteriorly along the pelvic wall, over the piriformis muscle, then pierce the parietal fascia to enter the visceral space, running between the leaves of the visceral fascia caudal to the rectosacral fascia. They join laterally on the pelvic wall with the hypogastric nerves to produce the pelvic autonomic nervous plexus. Care must be taken not to damage this by excessive lateral dissection of the so-called "lateral ligament" along the pelvic side wall (Fig. 8.9). To reach the lateral pelvic wall, the hypogastric nerves enter the pelvis in the visceral compartment. To spare the hypogastric nerves during dissection, a step in dissection level must be made immediately medial to the nerves where they pass through the visceral compartment. This leaves segments of the visceral fascia attached to the pelvic side walls posterior and lateral to the hypogastric nerves.

Although Heald's group reported prolonged operation times and increased blood loss in their initial experience [18], their more recent reports indicate a mean operative time of 4 hours [20]. Carlsen et al. [21] compared TME directly with "conventional" operations performed previously by the same sur-

geons and found that operative time decreased from 186 to 176 minutes with no difference in blood loss. They additionally noted an increased risk of intra-operative rectal perforation in the "conventional" group (29% versus 16%).

Outcome of Total Mesorectal Excision

Several reports have demonstrated improvements in local recurrence (4–8%) and cancer-specific survival with TME (70–80% at 5 years) (Table 8.1). There have been two single-surgeon series evaluating TME with no or minimal adjuvant therapy. Their reports address local recurrence rate, distant recurrence (metastasis) rate, overall recurrence rate and disease-free and overall survival.

Heald and Karanjia [22], in 1992, presented the initial report of TME, with a local recurrence rate of 2.6% and a 5-year actuarial local recurrence rate of 3.5% in 152 curative anterior resections. These results were updated, with a report in 1998 of 519 rectal cancer resections [20], utilizing a prospectively maintained database. The tumors were located up to 15 cm from the anal verge and the average follow-up was 8.3 years. Nine percent of the patients

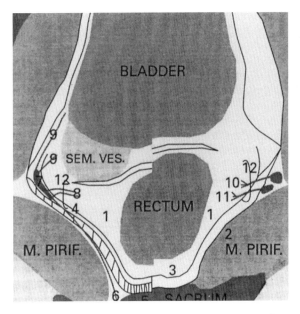

Fig. 8.8. Schematic diagram of an oblique transverse section of the pelvis, posteriorly at the level of S3 and anteriorly at the level of the pubic symphysis. The left half is at a level 2 cm lower than the right half of the figure: M. PIRIF., piriformis muscle; SEM. VES., seminal vesical; 1, mesorectum; 2, parietal fascia; 3, visceral fascia; 4, anterior and posterior leaves of the visceral fascia; 5, rectosacral fascia; 6, sacral splanchnic nerve; 7, pelvic autonomic nerve plexus; 8, mesorectal nerve branches; 9, urogenital nerve branches; 10, middle rectal artery; 11, middle rectal vein; 12, "lateral ligament". (Reproduced with permission from [19] Havenga K, DeRuiter MC, Enker WE, Welvaart K. Anatomical basis of autonomic nerve-preserving total mesorectal excision for rectal cancer. Br J Surg 1996;83:384–88.)

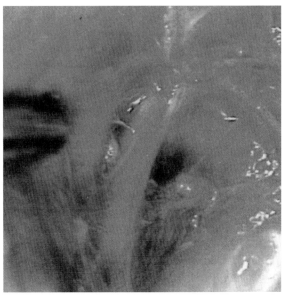

Fig. 8.9. The principal parasympathetic erigent nerve root preserved on the right pelvis side wall. (Modified with permission from [18] MacFarlane JK, Ryall RDH, Heald RJ. Mesorectal excision for rectal cancer. Lancet 1993;341:457–60; © by *The Lancet* Ltd.)

had received preoperative radiation for fixed or inoperable tumors and approximately 6% received chemotherapy postoperatively. The overall local recurrence rate, with or without distant metastasis, was 6% at 5 years and 8% at 10 years. Patients undergoing anterior resections had much better outcomes than those with abdominoperineal resections (5% local recurrence at 5 years and 5% at 10 years versus 17% and 36%, respectively). The local recurrence rate for curative anterior resections was 2% at both 5 and 10 years. These outcomes were unaffected by Dukes' stage, tumor grade, anastomotic leak, the distance of the tumor from the dentate line, and the level of the anastomosis. The actuarial overall recurrence rate at 5 years [18] was 18% for anterior resections (22% when including locally non-curative resections); at 10 years it was 19% for curative anterior resections. The recurrence rates for anterior resections and abdominoperineal resections combined were 19% at 5 years and 22% at 10 years. The 5- and 10-year cancer-specific survivals were 68% and 66% respectively, and 80% and

78% for those undergoing curative resections. Outcome was affected by Dukes' stage and extramural vascular invasion but not by grade, anastomotic leak, the distance from the tumor to the anal verge, or the level of the anastomosis.

MacFarlane et al. [18] reported on a subset of "high-risk" patients from Heald's original series. This group comprised 135 patients with T3 or T4 lesions and/or lymph node metastases but no distant metastases. All had tumors with distal margins located 12 cm or less from the anal verge. All underwent curative resections. The median follow-up was 7.7 years. The local recurrence rate (calculated by life table analysis) was 5% at 5 years. Among those patients with pelvic recurrence, 4/7 had isolated local recurrence and 3/7 developed combined local and distant recurrences. The overall recurrence rate at 5 years was 22%; 32% were in the Dukes' C subgroup. This rate was affected by stage of disease, extramural large vein invasion, and tumor differentiation. The recurrence-free cancer-specific 5-year survival was calculated to be 78%.

Enker et al. [8], in 1995, reported on 246 patients with tumors at 0–12 cm from the anal verge that had been resected for cure between 1979 and 1993. All the tumors were Dukes' stages B or C (T3N0M0 or TanyN1–2M0) lesions, making this group of patients comparable with the high-risk groups of the North Central Cancer Treatment Group adjuvant trial [23] and MacFarlane et al. [18]. Data were collected

Table 8.1. Total mesorectal excision outcomes

Reference	Stage	Year	No. Patients	% Local recurrence (5-year or actuarial 5-year)	overall % recurrence	% 5-Year survival
Heald and Karanjia [22]	All	1992	152	2.6 (3.5)	NR	NR
Heald et al. [20]	All	1998	519	6 (6)	19	68[a] 80 in curative[a]
MacFarlane et al. [18]	T3 or T4, or N1 or N2	1993	135 (curative)	5	22	78[a]
Enker et al. [8]	T3 or T4, or N1 or N2	1995	246 (curative)	7.3 5.7 isolated	30.9	74.2
Enker (unpublished)	T3 or T4, or N1 or N2	1999	545 (curative)	5	NR	74
Arbman et al. [24]	All	1996	230 (curative)	6[b] (vs 14 in controls)	NR	NR
Havenga et al. [25]	Stage II or III	1998	691 (curative)	4–9[c] (vs 32–35 in controls)		62–75[c] 75–80[a,c] (vs 42–44[c], 52[a,c] in controls)
Bjerkeset and Edna [26]	All curative to 25 cm	1996	NR	4	NR	65 85[a]

[a] Cancer specific.
[b] 3 of these 8 did not actually undergo TME.
[c] 95% confidence interval for Kaplan–Meier analysis.
NR, not reported.

prospectively. A total of 28.5% of the patients received perioperative chemotherapy or radiation. The Kaplan–Meier estimate of local recurrence within 5 years was 7.3%. Pelvic recurrences without distant metastatic disease were seen in 5.7%. Recurrence rate was correlated with nodal status and perineural invasion, but not with tumor height, gender, or type of resection (low anterior versus abdominoperineal resection). The rate of distant failure without local recurrence was 23.6%. The overall 5-year survival rate in this group of high-risk patients was 74.2%; it was inversely correlated with stage, nodal status and type of operation (anterior versus abdominoperineal resection). There was no correlation with the sex of the patient or the level of the primary tumor. These results have persisted (W. Enker, unpublished data, presented at the annual meeting of the Society for Surgical Oncology, March, 1998). With a mean follow-up of 5.6 years to December 1998, in 545 patients who had undergone TME, the 5-year survival rate was 74% and the local recurrence-free survival was 95%.

Several regional studies have followed. Arbman et al. [24] studied outcomes in Östergötland, Sweden. They compared 230 patients operated on between 1990 and 1992, the "TME" group, with 211 controls (conventional operations performed between 1984 and 1986). Only one control and three

TME patients underwent radiotherapy and none received chemotherapy. All underwent curative resections. The local recurrence rate in the control group was 14% (12% in cases reported to have been resected with "undoubted radicality") compared with 6% in the TME group, of whom 3/8 actually did not undergo TME. The recurrence rate was 4% in those in the TME group with "undoubted radicality". The difference in recurrence rate was maintained in a 4-year actuarial recurrence model and there was a significant difference in actuarial overall survival. Further confirmation of the importance of TME was demonstrated by a local recurrence rate of 19% in the 21 patients operated on by surgeons who were unfamiliar with the TME technique during the later, "TME", period.

Havenga et al. [25] reported on 691 patients who underwent TME, with or without intrapelvic lymphadenectomy, and 720 patients undergoing conventional surgery by experienced surgeons at three specialized centers. All patients had Stage II or III rectal cancer within 12 cm of the anal verge (meeting the previously discussed high-risk criteria of other operative and adjuvant studies) and all were curatively resected. The study was prospective but not randomized (there were two groups of surgeons, one performing only TME and one conventional surgery). The 95% confidence interval for local recurrence rate by Kaplan–Meier life table analysis was 4–9% in the TME group, compared with 32–35% in the conventional group, a 25% absolute difference in local recurrence rates. The 5-year overall and cancer-specific survival rates in the two groups were 62–75% and 75–80% versus 42–44% and 52%, respectively. These differences persisted in multivariate analysis and for each stage. Also affecting the risk of local recurrence in multivariate analysis were tumor stage and distance from the anal verge. Cancer-specific mortality was affected by tumor stage and type of operation (abdominoperineal resection versus low anterior resection). The differences in death rates were largely but not entirely explained by the differences in local recurrence.

Bjerkeset and Edna [26] reported on the outcome of TME in Norway. They combined all curatively resected patients with tumors at or below 25 cm from the anal verge and reported a local recurrence rate of 4%, an overall 5-year survival rate of 65%, and a 5-year cancer-specific survival rate of 85%. This included five patients who were initially considered to be unresectable and who received neoadjuvant therapy. Dahlberg et al. [27] compared the outcome of rectal resection for adenocarcinoma in Uppsala, where approximately 50% of resections utilized TME, with that in the rest of Sweden, where 0–5% utilized TME and most surgeons performed blunt dissection. The 5-year survival in Uppsala was increased to 61.9% compared with 50.9% elsewhere, with a relative risk of death of 0.61. Köckerling et al. [28] evaluated 1581 curative resections performed in Erlangen, Germany between 1985, when the technique of TME began to be gradually introduced, and 1991. These were compared with historical controls, resected between 1974 and 1984. No patient received adjuvant therapy. The mean follow-up was 13.1 years (minimum 4 years). The local recurrence rate decreased from 39.4% to 9.8% over the study period ($p < 0.0001$) and the 5-year survival increased from 50% to 71% ($p < 0.0001$).

Morbidity of Total Mesorectal Excision

The reported morbidity of TME has been variable. MacFarlane et al. [18] reported an anastomotic leak rate of 17.4% (11% clinical and 6.4% radiological) for anastomoses at 3–6 cm from the anal verge. Long-term anastomotic failure, significant morbidity, and/or a permanent stoma were reported in approximately 5% overall. Enker et al. [8] reported clinical leaks in 2.9% of their patients and 1.8% (all

of whom had had full-course postoperative radiation) had rectal strictures or fistulae resulting in permanent stomas. Arbman et al. [24] found no differences in morbidity or mortality between their TME and conventional groups. Carlsen et al. [21] reported no difference in the number of patients with complications, number of complications per patient, or in-hospital mortality compared with "standard" resection. The most significant complication of TME was anastomotic leak, requiring re-operation; however this was found to be largely avoidable with the use of proximal diversion.

Sexual and Urinary Function After Total Mesorectal Excision

Erectile potency has been reported to be 37–68% after conventional rectal resection [29–34], with significant impairment of urinary function. Havenga et al. [35] evaluated sexual and urinary function after TME was performed with particular attention to autonomic nerve preservation in patients with tumors situated within 12 cm of the anal verge. The ability to engage in intercourse was maintained by 86% of the male patients under 60 years of age and 67% of those aged over 60 or undergoing abdominoperineal resection, with a mean of 80% of preoperative penile rigidity. The ability to achieve orgasm was retained in 87% of men and 91% of women, with arousal and lubrication present in 85% of the women. There was no severe urinary dysfunction.

Masui et al. [36] evaluated sexual function in 134 men who had histologically curative resections with varying degrees of autonomic nerve preservation. All were under 65 years of age and all were sexually active preoperatively; 48.5% had tumors above the peritoneal reflection and 51.5% below. These patients were interviewed at least 1 year after surgery. Erection was maintained in 92.9% of those with complete nerve preservation, 82.3% when there was hemilateral nerve preservation, and 61.1% with only pelvic plexus preservation. The respective proportions with erectile rigidity and duration sufficient for vaginal insertion were 89.9%, 52.9% and 26.3% ($p < 0.01$ between complete preservation and each of the other groups). Ejaculation potencies were 82.5%, 47.1% and 0% (differences between each group were significant at the $p < 0.01$ level). Whereas 96.2% of patients reported orgasm preoperatively, 93.9% of men with complete preservation, 64.7% with hemilateral preservation, and 22.2% with plexus preservation reported orgasm postoperatively (differences between all groups significant at the $p < 0.01$ level). The combining of TME with autonomic nerve preservation is essential to reducing the long-term genitourinary morbidity of rectal cancer resection.

Extended Lateral Lymphadenectomy

One strong adverse factor for outcome appears to be lateral nodal spread, along the middle rectal artery or to lymph nodes within the obturator space. Involved lateral nodes have been reported to be present in 8.8–14.3% of patients with rectal and rectosigmoid cancers [10,37,38] (2.6% rectosigmoid, 8.8% upper rectum, 12.3% lower rectum [10]). Moriya et al. reported lateral spread in 13% of all T2 and more advanced lesions and 27% of Dukes' C patients [39]. Lateral spread may be associated with other adverse histological findings. Yamakoshi et al. [38] identified lateral spread only in patients with T3 and T4 lesions below the peritoneal reflection and with marked lymphatic and extramural venous invasion. Three of the four patients with lateral adenopathy in this study also had tumors with perineural invasion (of seven tumors exhibiting perineural invasion). Local recurrence and 5-year survival rates in one study were 50.0% and 25.1% in patients with involved lateral lymph nodes and 9.1% and 74.3% in those without involved lateral nodes [37].

Extended lateral lymphadenectomy has been reported by several Japanese groups in an attempt to address the poor prognosis associated with lateral lymph node involvement. Unfortunately, reported rates of local control have been variable and there is no improved overall survival when compared with TME. Although subgroups with lateral lymph node involvement may benefit, lateral pelvic lymphadenectomy is associated with consistently high rates of severe urinary and sexual morbidity and no general or definite benefit has been identified [36,37,39,40]. Given the high mortality and local recurrence rates with lateral spread, regardless of the type of operation, patients at high risk of lateral nodal metastases are generally treated with adjuvant chemoradiation in western countries. The overall incidence of lateral lymph node spread is probably too small to define clearly the role of extended lymphadenectomy in a clinical trial. At present, we know that the overall survival of TME is the same as the survival of patients undergoing pelvic lymphadenectomy. Except in the presence of gross, resectable disease, there appears to be no role for routine, elective lymphadenectomy with nerve destruction and its attendant morbidity.

Role of the Colonic J-Pouch

The role of abdominoperineal resection in the management of rectal cancer has been greatly diminished by improvement in the techniques for complete rectal mobilization, the improved ability to perform low anastomoses, and the recognition that these are oncologically equivalent or superior to abdominoperineal resection [41,42]. An important consideration after very low anterior resection with TME is neorecto-anal function. One suggestion to decrease stool frequency and improve continence has been the creation of a colonic J-pouch to serve as a new reservoir proximal to the anastomosis [43–46]. The initial studies showed a significant decrease in mean stool frequency to two or fewer per 24 hours, with one study [46] reporting 96% "satisfactory" continence and another [45] a 23% rate of minor incontinence (versus 40% with straight anastomosis); there was no major incontinence. Similar findings have since been reported from randomized, controlled trials [47–49]. Physiologic evaluation has demonstrated that anal function is no different but that the pouches demonstrate increased maximum volume and compliance with decreased neorectal sensitivity compared with straight anastomosis [50]. Pouch manometry and function are similar to those of the remaining rectum after high anterior resection [51]. The early studies of colonic J-pouches had only brief periods of follow-up. More recently, the relative benefit of a pouch compared with a straight anastomosis has been shown to persist for at least 2 years [52]. Furthermore, pouches, a variant of side-to-end anastomosis, may be associated with a decreased incidence of anastomotic leaks [50], possibly due to improved blood flow at the anastomotic site [53]. Given these findings, the creation of a colonic J-pouch is to be recommended when it is technically feasible. Temporary proximal diversion should be performed with a J-pouch to minimize the risks of anastomotic leak, peritonitis and unscheduled re-operation [54]. A pouch length of 6 cm has been shown to produce equivalent fecal frequency, urgency and continence to larger pouches, with less constipation and fewer difficulties with evacuation on long-term follow-up [55], and is thus to be preferred. Outcome in patients over 75 years of age has been shown to be comparable with that in younger patients in one study [56], although in this report 14–15% in each group were incontinent of feces and 40–46% incontinent of flatus at least weekly, which is a less than ideal functional result.

A colonic "coloplasty"–pouch technique has recently been described for patients in whom the creation of a J-pouch is not possible (C.R. Mantyh and V.W. Fazio, unpublished observations: poster presentation, 1999 annual meeting of The American Society of Colon and Rectal Surgeons). A 10 cm longitudinal colotomy is created at 4 cm proximal to the point of coloric resection and closed transversely in a hand-sewn fashion. In a series of 12 patients, postoperative maximal tolerated volumes and compliances were comparable with those achieved in patients with J-pouches, with good function and improved quality of life scores. There were no pouch-related complications. Although further data and long-term follow-up are needed to evaluate this technique better, it should be considered as an alternative to straight colo-anal anastomosis in patients in whom J-pouch construction is not feasible.

Role of Total Mesorectal Excision in Upper Rectal Cancer

Although TME may be performed for cancers at any level of the rectum and rectosigmoid, the pathological studies that have evaluated the mesorectal spread of cancer [10,11,13] suggest distal spread is limited to 5 cm. Given the differences in vascular supply to the proximal rectum (above 10 cm from the anal verge) and the rectosigmoid compared with the distal rectum, a more limited resection may be undertaken. Although they had initially proposed TME for all rectal cancers, Heald's group has modified their approach to more limited distal resection in the past few years [57,58].

Our goal for cancers of the upper rectum has not included a resection down to the pelvic floor since our own inception of TME. We have practiced complete mobilization of the rectum, with transection of the rectum and the mesorectum at least 5 cm below the lowest edge of palpable tumor. These data are consistent with the pathological findings of Hida et al. [12]. Our circumferential dissection of the rectum in the plane separating the visceral and parietal fasciae is the same, regardless of whether the tumor is above or below the 10 cm level.

A recent report from the Cleveland Clinic [59] supports this management of upper rectal cancers (10–15 cm from the anal verge). They compared the outcome of upper rectal cancer resection with a perpendicular 5 cm margin ($n = 229$) with the outcome of sigmoid colectomy ($n = 225$) and mid- and lower rectal cancers (<10 cm from the anal verge) resected with TME, utilizing en bloc resection of advanced tumors at all levels. The groups were comparable in terms of tumor stage, histology and size. Adjuvant radiation therapy was used in 1.3% of sigmoid, 7.4% of upper rectal, and 23.8% of lower rectal cancers but there was no difference in outcome between the irradiated and non-irradiated patients. Five-year local recurrence, overall recurrence, and cancer death rates in patients with lower rectal cancer (8.6 ± 1.5%, 12.9 ± 1.8%, and 25.6 ± 2.2% respectively) were significantly greater than in the other two groups, whose results were comparable with each other. Furthermore, while mortality was similar in all three groups, there was a trend towards increased morbidity (particularly an increased rate of anastomotic leakage in undiverted patients) in the lower rectal cancer group.

For cancers that are more than 10 cm from the anal verge, complete circumferential excision must still be assured with transection of the mesorectum and rectum at the same level, at 90° to the bowel wall, without total rectal and mesorectal excision to the pelvic floor. The length of rectum and mesorectum resected distal to the tumor must be at least 5 cm.

Summary

The primary determinant of outcome of rectal cancer is operative technique. Local and distant recurrence rates and disease-free and overall survival are markedly improved by TME, with little increase in morbidity, compared with other techniques of resection for rectal cancer. It is therefore vital that all surgeons who are treating rectal cancer should become proficient in the technique. Proximal rectal lesions may be resected with 5 cm of distal rectum and mesorectum. There is currently no good evidence supporting extended lateral lymphadenectomy, which is associated with significant morbidity. Careful anatomic dissection minimizes sexual and urinary dysfunction. The colonic J-pouch improves anorectal function and should be considered when technically feasible. The role of adjuvant therapy has not been studied in conjunction with TME. Neo-adjuvant treatment is indicated in unresectable tumors and when sphincter preservation can be made possible. The results of large prospective studies are required to determine the role of adjuvant therapy in other settings, particularly relating to the local control of disease. Such studies are currently under way.

References

1. Glimelius B, Isacsson U, Jung B, Påhlman L. Radiotherapy in addition to radical surgery in rectal cancer. Acta Oncol. 1995;34:565–70.

2. Fisher B, Wolmark N, Rockette H, et al. Postoperative adjuvant chemotherapy or radiation therapy for rectal cancer: results from NSABP protocol R-01. J Natl Cancer Inst 1988;80:21–29.

3. Gastrointestinal Tumor Study Group. Adjuvant therapy of colon cancer: results of a prospectively randomized trial. N Engl J Med 1984;310:737–43.

4. Gastrointestinal Tumor Study Group. Prolongation of the disease-free interval in surgically treated rectal carcinoma. N Engl J Med 1985;312:1465–72.

5. Minsky BD. The role of adjuvant radiation therapy in the treatment of colorectal cancer. Hematol Oncol Clin North Am 1997;11:679–97.

6. Hool G, Church J, Fazio V. Decision-making in rectal surgery. Dis Colon Rectum 1998;41:147–52.

7. Enker WE. Sphincter-preserving operations for rectal cancer. Oncology 1996;10:1673–89.

8. Enker WE, Thaler HT, Cranor ML, Polyak T. Total mesorectal excision in the operative treatment of carcinoma of the rectum. J Am Coll Surg 1995;181:335–46.

9. Church JM, Raudkivi PJ, Hill GL. The surgical anatomy of the rectum – a review with particular relevance to the hazards of rectal mobilization. Int J Colorect Dis 1987;2:158–66.

10. Morikawa E, Yasutomi M, Shindou K, et al. Distribution of metastatic lymph nodes in colorectal cancer by the modified clearing method. Dis Colon Rectum 1994;37:219–23.

11. Scott N, Jackson P, Al-Jaberi T, et al. Total mesorectal excision and local recurrence: a study of tumour spread in the mesorectum distal to rectal cancer. Br J Surg 1995;82:1031–33.

12. Hida J-I, Yasutomi M, Maruyama T, et al. Lymph node metastases detected in the mesorectum distal to carcinoma of the rectum by the clearing method: justification of total mesorectal excision. J Am Coll Surg 1997;184:584–88.

13. Reynolds J, Joyce W, Dolan L, et al. Pathological evidence in support of total mesorectal excision in the management of rectal cancer. Br J Surg 1996;83:1112–15.

14. Quirke P, Dixon M, Durdey P, Williams N. Local recurrence of rectal adenocarcinoma due to inadequate surgical resection. Lancet 1986;ii:996–99.

15. Ng IOL, Luk ISC, Yuen ST, et al. Surgical lateral clearance in resected rectal carcinomas: a multivariate analysis of clinicopathological features. Cancer 1993;71:1972–76.

16. Adam I, Mohamdee M, Martin I, et al. Role of circumferential margin involvement in the local recurrence of rectal cancer. Lancet 1994;344:707–11.

17. Enker WE. Total mesorectal excision – the new golden standard of surgery for rectal cancer. Ann Med 1997;29:127–33.

18. MacFarlane JK, Ryall RDH, Heald RJ. Mesorectal excision for rectal cancer. Lancet 1993;341:457–60.

19. Havenga K, DeRuiter MC, Enker WE, Welvaart K. Anatomical basis of autonomic nerve-preserving total mesorectal excision for rectal cancer. Br J Surg 1996;83:384–88.

20. Heald RJ, Moran BJ, Ryall RDH, et al. Rectal cancer: the Basingstoke experience of total mesorectal excision, 1978–1997. Arch Surg 1998;133:894–99.

21. Carlsen E, Schlichting E, Guldvog I, et al. Effect of the introduction of total mesorectal excision for the treatment of rectal cancer. Br J Surg 1998;85:526–29.

22. Heald RJ, Karanjia ND. Results of radical surgery for rectal cancer. World J Surg 1992;16:848–57.

23. Krook J, Moertel C, Gunderson LL, et al. Effective surgical adjuvant therapy for high-risk rectal carcinoma. N Engl J Med 1991;324:709–15.

24. Arbman G, Nilsson E, Haalböök O, Sjödahl R. Local recurrence following total mesorectal excision for rectal cancer. Br J Surg 1996;83:375–79.

25. Havenga K, Enker WE, Norstein J, et al. Improved survival and local control after total mesorectal excision or lateral pelvic lymphadenectomy in the treatment of primary rectal cancer: an international meta-analysis comparing surgical outcomes in 1411 patients. Eur J Surg Oncol 1999;25:368–74.

26. Bjerkeset T, Edna T-H. Rectal cancer: the influence of type of operation on local recurrence and survival. Eur J Surg 1996;162:643–47.

27. Dahlberg M, Påhlman L, Bergström R, Glimelius B. Improved survival in patients with rectal cancer: a population-based register study. Br J Surg 1998;85:515–20.

28. Köckerling F, Reymond M, Altendorf-Hofmann A, et al. Influence of surgery on metachronous distant metastases and survival in rectal cancer. J Clin Oncol 1998;16:324–29.

29. Balslev I, Harling H. Sexual dysfunction following operation for carcinoma of the rectum. Dis Colon Rectum 1983;26:785–88.

30. Danzi M, Ferulano G, Abate S, Califano G. Male sexual function after abdominoperineal resection for rectal cancer. Dis Colon Rectum 1983;26:665–68.

31. Fegiz J, Trenti A. Sexual and bladder dysfunction following surgery for rectal carcinoma. Ital J Surg Sci 1986;16:103–106.

32. LaMonica G, Audisio R, Tamburini M, et al. Incidence of sexual dysfunction in male patients treated surgically for rectal malignancy. Dis Colon Rectum 1985;28:937–40.

33. Weinstein M, Roberts M. Sexual potency following surgery for rectal carcinoma: a follow-up of 44 patients. Ann Surg 1977;185:295–300.

34. Yasutomi M, Asao R. Sexual and urinary dysfunction following surgery for rectal carcinoma. Operation 1974;28:571–79.

35. Havenga K, Enker WE, McDermott K, et al. male and female sexual and urinary function after total mesorectal excision with autonomic nerve preservation for carcinoma of the rectum. J Am Coll Surg 1996;182:495–502.

36. Masui H, Ike H, Yamaguchi S, et al. Male sexual function after autonomic nerve-preserving operation for rectal cancer. Dis Colon Rectum 1996;39:1140–45.

37. Hida J-I, Yasutomi M, Fujimoto K, et al. Does lateral lymph node dissection improve survival in rectal carcinoma? Examination of node metastases by the clearing method. J Am Coll Surg 1997;184:475–80.

38. Yamakoshi H, Ike H, Oki S, et al. Metastasis of rectal cancer to lymph nodes and tissues around the autonomic nerves spared for urinary and sexual function. Dis Colon Rectum 1997;40:1079–84.

39. Moriya Y, Sugihara K, Akasu T, Fujita S. Importance of extended lymphadenectomy with lateral node dissection for advanced lower rectal cancer. World J Surg 1997;21:728–32.

40. Sugihara K, Moriya Y, Akasu T, Fujita S. Pelvic autonomic nerve preservation for patients with rectal carcinoma. Cancer 1996;78:1871–80.

41. Heald R, Smedh R, Kald A, et al. Abdominoperineal excision of the rectum – an endangered operation [Norman Nigro Lectureship]. Dis Colon Rectum 1997;40:747–51.

42. Enker W. Designing the optimal surgery for rectal carcinoma. Cancer 1996;78:1847–50.

43. Lazorthes F, Fages P, Chiotasso P, et al. Resection of the rectum with construction of a colonic reservoir and colo-anal anastomosis for carcinoma of the rectum. Br J Surg 1986;73:136–38.

44. Parc R, Tiret E, Frileux P, et al. Resection and colo-anal anastomosis with colonic reservoir for rectal carcinoma. Br J Surg 1986;73:139–41.

45. Nicholls R, Lubowski D, Donaldson D. Comparison of colonic reservoir and straight colo-anal reconstruction after rectal excision. Br J Surg 1988;75:318–20.

46. Berger A, Tiret E, Parc R, et al. Excision of the rectum with colonic J pouch–anal anastomosis for adenocarcinoma of the low and mid rectum. World J Surg 1992;16:470–77.

47. Ho Y, Tan M, Seow-Choen F. Prospective randomized controlled study of clinical function and anorectal physiology after low anterior resection: comparison of straight and colonic J pouch anastomosis. Br J Surg 1996;83:978–80.

48. Kusunoki M, Shoji Y, Yanagi H, et al. Function after ano-abdominal rectal resection and colonic pouch–anal anastomosis. Br J Surg 1991;78:1434–38.

49. Mortensen N, Ramirez J, Takeuchi N, Smilgin Humphreys M. Colonic J pouch–anal anastomosis after rectal excision for carcinoma: functional outcome. Br J Surg 1995;82:611–13.

50. Hallböök O, Nyström P-O, Sjödahl R. Physiologic characteristics of straight and colonic J-pouch anastomoses after rectal excision for cancer. Dis Colon Rectum 1997;40:332–38.

51. Ramirez J, Mortensen N, Takeuchi N, Smilgin Humphreys M. Colonic J-pouch rectal reconstruction – is it really a neorectum? Dis Colon Rectum 1996;39:1286–88.

52. Lazorthes F, Chiotasso P, Gamagami R, et al. Late clinical outcome in a randomized prospective comparison of colonic J pouch and straight coloanal anastomosis. Br J Surg 1997;84:1449–51.

53. Hallböök O, Johansson K, Sjodahl R. Laser-Doppler blood flow measurement in rectal resection for carcinoma – comparison between the straight and colonic J pouch reconstruction. Br J Surg 1996;83:389–92.

54. Dehni N, Sclegel R, Cunningham C, et al. Influence of a defunctioning stoma on leakage rates after low colorectal anastomosis and colonic J pouch–anal anastomosis. Br J Surg 1998;85:1114–17.

55. Lazorthes F, Gamagami R, Chiotasso P, et al. Prospective, randomized study comparing clinical results between small and large colonic J-pouch following coloanal anastomosis. Dis Colon Rectum 1997;40:1409–13.

56. Dehni N, Schlegel R, Tiret E, et al. Effects of aging on the functional outcome of coloanal anastomosis with colonic J-pouch. Am J Surg 1998;175:209–12.

57. Heald R, Ryall R. Recurrence and survival after total mesorectal excision for rectal cancer. Lancet 1986;i:1479–82.

58. Karanjia N, Corder A, Bearn P, Heald R. Leakage from stapled low anastomosis after total mesorectal excision for carcinoma of the rectum. Br J Surg 1994;81:1224–26.

59. Lopez-Kostner F, Lavery I, Hool G, et al. Total mesorectal excision is not necessary for cancers of the upper rectum. Surgery 1998;124:612–18.

9. Laparoscopic Resections for Large Bowel Malignancy: Laparoscopic Colectomy

D. Rosenfeld and R.W. Beart

Laparoscopic Rectal Cancer Surgery

H.J. Cho and J.W. Milsom

Introduction

Since laparoscopy was first introduced as a diagnostic tool for pelvic pathology 15 years ago, this technique has been successfully adopted by general and specialty surgeons as a therapeutic tool for a variety of different diseases [1]. General surgeons initially embraced this new laparoscopic technique for intra-abdominal diseases such a cholecystitis, appendicitis, and inguinal hernias. Within a few years, laparoscopic cholecystectomy and appendectomy became common and standard procedures. Laparoscopic techniques offer the benefits of less perioperative morbidity, a shorter hospital stay, a more rapid return to work, and better cosmesis. Laparoscopic surgery has been a rare event in surgical history in a profound technical revolution. The role of laparoscopic techniques in colon and rectal cancer center around diagnosis and staging, palliative therapy and curative techniques, of which the latter remains the most controversial [2].

This chapter has been divided into two sections, the first focusing on discussion involving laparoscopic resection for benign and malignant disease of the abdominal colon. This will be followed by a second section on laparoscopic proctosigmoidectomy for rectal cancer.

In combination, the current chapter will initially discuss the physiological aspects of laparoscopic surgery as it involves the cardiovascular system, the lungs, the kidneys and the neurohumoral axis, and how minimally invasive techniques affect the patient immunologically. This will be followed by a discussion of colectomy for benign disease, the obvious predecessor to laparoscopic resection for malignant diseases of the colon and rectum, covering indications and techniques for laparoscopic resection of the right colon, the proximal left colon and the sigmoid colon. Laparoscopy for both colon and rectal cancer will then be considered, with discussion of the advantages and disadvantages of a laparoscopic approach to cancer, and also the techniques employed and the oncological results.

Laparoscopic Colectomy

Laparoscopic colectomy is a natural extension of the experience gained in laparoscopic cholecystectomy and inguinal hernia repair. It is a substantially more complex procedure but one that has been shown to be efficacious. First reported in 1990, numerous articles have been published regarding this procedure, and consensus is growing that laparoscopic colorectal surgery is safe, effective, and beneficial for many benign diseases [2–5].

Recently, laparoscopic colectomy has also been applied to malignant diseases. Much discussion has centered on whether laparoscopic surgery is appropriate for the management of potentially curable malignant diseases and whether patients are better served by using minimally invasive techniques that have short-term benefits but unknown long-term effects. The initial results of laparoscopic colon cancer surgery appear to be comparable with those of operations performed in the traditional open manner, but with the additional benefits of this minimally invasive technique. Long-term results are not yet available to assess changes in overall survival and recurrence rates, and many surgeons remain cautiously optimistic.

Physiologic Aspects of Laparoscopic Surgery

Cardiovascular Effects

The general anesthesia, reverse Trendelenburg positioning and carbon dioxide (CO_2) insufflation used in laparoscopic surgery induce a characteristic cardiovascular response. The principal changes in cardiovascular function due to CO_2 insufflation are an immediate decrease in the cardiac index (CI), with an associated increase in the systemic vascular resistance (SVR) and the mean arterial blood pressure. In the subsequent 15–30 minutes, there is a partial recovery of the CI and the SVR, with no change in the blood pressure or heart rate. These changes are the result of the interaction between increased abdominal pressure, neurohormonal responses, and absorbed CO_2 [6]. Although these effects are well tolerated in the healthy patient, those with mild to severe cardiovascular diseases can exhibit more exaggerated cardiovascular changes [7].

Four factors are associated with the basic cardiovascular changes seen in laparoscopic surgery: anesthesia, the position of the patient, increased intra-abdominal pressure, and the neurohormonal effects of CO_2 insufflation. Anesthesia causes depression of the myocardium, vasodilation and a loss of sympathetic tone, which can all contribute to the initial decrease in the CI prior to insufflation. The reverse Trendelenburg position also causes a decrease in the CI, stroke volume and cardiac output prior to insufflation by reducing the blood return to the heart. This lowers the preload, which decreases the contractility or cardiac output as seen on the Starling curve [6].

CO_2 insufflation increases intra-abdominal pressure and serum CO_2 levels. Initially, the increased intra-abdominal pressure constricts the arterial tree and leads to a mobilization of venous blood and an increased venous return. This pressure then serves as a barrier to blood flow by constricting the abdominal vessels and the inferior vena cava [8]. This impedes venous return from the abdomen and lower extremities, thereby increasing systemic vascular resistance and the mean arterial blood

pressure, while decreasing venous return and the CI. The observed depression of the CI is directly related to the insufflation pressure. Prolonged intra-abdominal pressure can also decrease renal, hepatic and jejunal mucosal blood flow, leading to mucosal ischemia, oliguria and concerns for patients with hepatic cirrhosis or renal insufficiency. The increased intra-abdominal pressure also causes a cephalad shift of the diaphragm, leading to pulmonary effects (discussed later). Partial restoration of the CI and SVR is the second part of the biphasic change that involves a neurohumoral response. The pneumoperitoneum induces catecholamine secretion, including antidiuretic hormone, noradrenaline, adrenaline, dopamine, renin and cortisol. This possibly explains the increased CI and SVR observed within 15–30 minutes.

The absorption of CO_2 into the vascular system also has numerous effects, such as an increase in SVR, cardiac output, central venous pressure, and pulmonary artery occlusion pressure. Thus, the alterations in cardiovascular dynamics during laparoscopic surgery are influenced primarily by increased CO_2, either directly via vasodilation or indirectly by stimulating the sympathetic nervous system [9].

Initially it was thought that extensive retroperitoneal dissection during colonic mobilization might result in greater CO_2 absorption and more dramatic physiologic changes. Animal research has not shown substantial differences in cardiovascular physiology with dissection [10].

Pulmonary Effects

Intraoperatively, laparoscopic surgery negatively affects the pulmonary system by increasing intra-abdominal pressure, increasing CO_2 absorption, and causing trauma to the abdominal wall. Insufflation causes a cephalad shift in the diaphragm, reducing lung compliance, thoracic compliance, and functional residual capacity. Atelectasis, which can be worsened in advanced age and obesity, becomes a potential risk. V/Q (ventilation and perfusion) mismatching, another detrimental effect, makes patients with decreased pulmonary compliance at a higher risk for hypoxemia [8,11].

With insufflation there is also a rapid initial increase in the $PaCO_2$ (normally estimated by end-tidal CO_2 ($PaCO_2$)) associated with a decrease in the pH and possible acidosis [12]. This is controlled by an initial increase in the respiratory rate or minute ventilation. In elderly people, the increase in $PaCO_2$ and the drop in pH can be much greater and uncontrollable by minute ventilation, necessitating close monitoring. Increased minute ventilation to control pH can also cause increased airway pressure (due to decreased compliance), with a risk of pneumothorax and lung damage. Owing to lung compression, the $PaCO_2$ is an inaccurate estimate of the $PaCO_2$ in laparoscopic procedures.

Postoperatively, however, the reduction in pulmonary function is much less in laparoscopic than in open procedures. One day postoperatively, open cholecystectomy patients' pulmonary function is generally decreased by 50%, as measured by forced vital capacity, 1-second forced expiratory volume, and 25–75% forced expiratory flow, whereas laparoscopic patients' pulmonary function is decreased by approximately 25%. This can be explained by decreased trauma to the abdominal wall, decreased changes in pulmonary volume, and decreased levels of pain [13].

Renal Effects

Laparoscopic surgery causes acute but reversible renal dysfunction and oliguria. Acute oliguria occurs only during insufflation, after which renal function (blood urea nitrogen and creatinine levels) returns to normal after release of the pneumoperitoneum. Permanent damage is possible but, in the rat model, temporary renal dysfunction has resulted in renal failure only if the intra-abdominal pressure is excessively increased or prolonged. Intra-abdominal pressure should be kept below 15 mmHg.

The acute oliguria is most likely to be a result of the increase in intra-abdominal pressure that compresses the inferior vena cava and the renal vein. This is consistent with the finding of a decreased glomerular filtration rate and an even larger decreased effective renal plasma flow during insufflation. All other metabolic factors (renin, antidiuretic hormone, atrial natriuretic peptide, angiotensin II, aldosterone, fractional excretion, free water clearance) have been shown to be unchanged. Oliguria could be aggravated by decreased cardiac output. Given these findings, patients suffering from renal insufficiency or cardiac disease, or who are taking nephrotoxic agents, should be monitored when undergoing laparoscopic surgery. It should also be noted that the oliguria cannot be overcome with intravenous hydration [14].

Neuroendocrine Effects

Laparoscopic surgery causes less tissue damage and trauma than corresponding open procedures. Recent studies have investigated whether the decreased physical trauma and faster recovery times associated with laparoscopic procedures can be linked to lower levels of stress hormones. Cortisol, adrenocorticotropic hormone, growth hormone, prolactin, norepinephrine, epinephrine and dopamine all increase with laparoscopic and open surgery. These hormones can be grouped as the adrenal (epinephrine, cortisol), sympathetic (dopamine, norepinephrine), and pituitary (adrenocorticotropic hormone, prolactin, growth hormone, cortisol) responses to trauma. There is evidence that with laparoscopic techniques all of these factors have significantly smaller peak levels than with open procedures. Similarly, some studies have shown that glucose, a general indicator of all systems, has a peak increase that is 25% less with laparoscopic techniques [15,16].

Immunologic Effects

Several markers of "trauma" and immunosuppression, including serum cytokines (tumor necrosis factor), interleukins (IL-1, IL-6), endocrine hormones (cortisol, insulin, prolactin), lymphocyte levels and function, and delayed hypersensitivity reactions have been measured after laparoscopic procedures. Comparative studies of open versus laparoscopic procedures have shown the latter to have smaller postoperative increases in the levels of serum IL-1, IL-6, tumor necrosis factor, and granulocytes, indicating less inflammation. There are also smaller postoperative decreases in the number of CD3+ cells and activated lymphocytes, which indicate a smaller acute–phase reaction. The postoperative strength of the delayed hypersensitivity reaction, which is a general estimate of T-cell function, is also increased more after laparoscopic than open procedures. There is also evidence of a greater increase and a longer duration of increase in serum levels of cortisol, glucose, prolactin and C-reactive protein in open procedures. All of these factors indicate less immunosuppression and inflammatory response after laparoscopic procedures [17–24].

Laparoscopic Surgery for Benign Colonic Disease

Laparoscopic colectomy (or laparoscopically assisted colectomy) is a natural extension of the experience gained in laparoscopic cholecystectomy. It is the obvious predecessor to laparoscopic colectomy for malignant disease. Intuitively, laparoscopic management of a benign disease must be mastered prior to its use for resection for malignant disease. In the last 10 years, there has been an increasing volume of information on the use of these minimally invasive techniques in standard colorectal operations. Laparoscopic colorectal procedures are substantially more complex than cholecystectomy, but they have been shown to be safe and efficacious for many colonic diseases, especially segmental colon resection for benign disease.

Laparoscopic colonic resection and diversion were initially attractive because, theoretically, they offered the same benefits as those seen in laparoscopic cholecystectomy, such as decreases in postoperative pain, narcotic requirements, pulmonary complications, and duration of hospital stay. Many of these benefits have been realized, but additional unique difficulties have also been seen.

Advantages and Disadvantages

The touted benefits of laparoscopically assisted surgery in the treatment of benign colonic disease include decreased postoperative pain and ileus, earlier tolerance of feeding, shorter hospital stay, less operative blood loss, improved cosmesis, and less abdominal wall trauma than in corresponding open procedures. Laparoscopy also preserves physiologic function in many situations and incurs no increase in morbidity or mortality relative to open procedures [2–5,25–28].

Some disadvantages of laparoscopy compared with open procedures have included longer operative times, more elaborate and expensive equipment, the requirement for additional surgeons, and the potential for complications associated with CO_2 insufflation as described previously. Laparoscopically assisted procedures may also cause major blood vessel injury, small bowel perforation, and injury to the bladder and surrounding structures, although the occurrence is less than 2% [14]. Laparoscopic procedures have not yielded decreased hospital costs because savings from shorter inpatient stays have been offset by increased operative costs. However, the possible savings from decreases in the time to return to work have not been studied and may ultimately swing the pendulum in favor of laparoscopic procedures.

The Learning Curve

Much of the increased complication rate associated with laparoscopy has been attributed to a steep learning curve. Recent studies have found higher complication rates and longer operating times for surgeons who have performed fewer than 30 procedures. In previous studies on laparoscopic colectomies, operating times and outcomes from these surgeons have been used in the calculation of averages without correcting for the learning curve [29].

Current Indications for Laparoscopic Colectomy

The current indications for laparoscopic colectomy include most benign colonic conditions such as colorectal polyps, rectal prolapse, diverticular disease, intestinal stomas for diversion, cecal or sigmoid volvulus, and symptomatic colonic lipomas. Other colonic conditions such as Crohn's disease and ulcerative colitis have also been treated using laparoscopic techniques; investigators have demonstrated that laparoscopic bowel surgery is safe and effective in selected patients [26,27,30,31].

Preoperative Factors for Laparoscopic Colectomy

Although there are no set criteria for selection, patients who are thin rather than obese and those who have not undergone previous abdominal operations are considered as ideal candidates. Those who suffer from a coagulopathy, liver disease, severe respiratory or cardiac disease, or symptoms suggestive of complex and advanced disease, such as obstruction, contained perforation or diverticulitis-related colovesical fistula, should not be considered for laparoscopically assisted colectomy. Lesions in the right, left or sigmoid colon are generally amenable to laparoscopic resection, whereas lesions of the transverse colon are considerably more difficult to resect because of the omental attachments [32–36].

The operative field must be prepared and draped in the usual fashion. A nasogastric tube and Foley catheter are inserted to decompress the bladder and stomach. Stockings are fitted to minimize the risk of deep vein thrombosis. Intraoperative colonoscopy is notoriously unreliable in localizing the pathology. Therefore, at the time of preoperative colonoscopy, the lesion should be tattooed to assist with intraoperative localization. Alternatively, one may chose simultaneous intraoperative colonoscopy with laparoscopy; light transilluminated through the bowel wall may assist in localization.

Resection of the Right Colon

The patient is positioned supine with both the surgeon and the camera operator situated on his or her left side, and the assistant surgeon, the nurse and monitors on the right. A small right upper quadrant incision is made and a Hassan port is inserted into the abdominal cavity. The abdomen is insufflated with CO_2 to achieve a pneumoperitoneum of 10–12 mmHg. This low pressure helps to minimize the risk of subcutaneous emphysema, which occurs with a retroperitoneal dissection. A 10–12 mm cannula is used to facilitate insertion of the laparoscope into the abdominal cavity. Three additional cannulae are inserted: one in the right middle quadrant, one in the suprapubic area, and one in the left middle quadrant. Each cannula allows the instrument to reach the surgical site.

The camera operator places the laparoscope through the left cannula for mobilization of the cecum. With the table tilted head down and rotated towards the left, the surgeon retracts the cecum cephalad and to the patient's left. As the assistant retracts the peritoneum to the right side, the surgeon begins the dissection along the peritoneum of the ileum. The dissection continues along the ascending colon by incising the peritoneum and retracting the colon medially. The ureter must then be visualized. An inability to visualize the ureter at this point or the presence of dense adhesions from previous surgery may prompt conversion to an open colectomy.

Once the colon is mobilized to the level of the hepatic flexure, the laparoscope is placed in the suprapubic cannula. The table is then tilted head up, still rotated towards the left, and the assistant moves to the surgeon's right. The surgeon then retracts the ascending colon and hepatic flexure inferomedially and dissects the transverse colon from the omentum. Once the hepatic flexure is mobilized, the duodenum and ureter should be visualized.

The mesentery is then also visualized and the superior mesenteric, ileocolic, right colic and middle colic vessels are isolated. Mesenteric windows are created in the avascular planes and the vascular pedicle is ligated with hemoclips or a linear stapler.

A 4–6 cm transverse incision is made at the right cannula, the bowel is exteriorized and resected and a stapled or hand-sewn anastomosis is performed. The mesenteric windows can be sealed or left open, depending on the resection, and the bowel is returned to the peritoneal cavity. The abdominal wound is closed. The abdominal cavity is inspected laparoscopically for hemostasis and irrigated. The cannulae are removed and the sites are closed using single figure-of-eight absorbable sutures in the fascial layer. The skin is closed with subcuticular absorbable sutures and adhesive surgical tape (Steri-strips).

Resection of the Left Colon

Resection of the left colon proceeds in a fashion similar to right hemicolectomy. The patient is again positioned supine, but the surgeon and nurse are on the right (nurse on the surgeon's right) and the camera operator and assistant are on the left. The left upper quadrant trocar is placed, the pneumoperitoneum established, and the laparoscope introduced into the abdominal cavity. Three additional 10–12 mm trocars are used to place three cannulae in the same places as for a right colectomy. The patient is placed head down and rotated right side down.

The descending colon is mobilized by placing the laparoscope in the left upper position. The assistant retracts the peritoneal attachment to the left. The surgeon retracts the descending colon cephalad and to the right and dissects the left lateral peritoneal reflection of the sigmoid and descending colon. Again, the ureter must be identified at this point.

After the colon is mobilized to the splenic flexure, the laparoscope is placed in the lower position and the surgeon and the assistant exchange positions. The table is now positioned head up and tilted to the right. With electrocautery and vascular clips, the omentum is dissected from the splenic flexure as the descending colon and splenic flexure are retracted inferomedially.

The sigmoid and left colic vascular pedicles are exposed and ligated with hemoclips or a linear stapler. A 4–6 cm transverse incision is made at the left cannula and the bowel is exteriorized, resected and anastomosed. The bowel is returned to the abdominal cavity and the fascia is closed as in the right-sided resection. The abdomen is re-insufflated and examined for hemostasis. If an extensive presacral mobilization is carried out, a drain can be placed under direct vision.

Resection of the Sigmoid Colon

Resection of the sigmoid colon uses different operating room organization than the right- and left-sided colectomies. The patient is placed in the lithotomy position and the legs are padded for protection. The surgeon and the scrub nurse are on the patient's right, and the two assistants are on the left. The monitor is placed between the patient's legs. The initial 10 cm trocar is placed in the left upper quadrant and the pneumoperitoneum is achieved. Three additional 10–12 mm trocars are used to place additional cannulae in the right lower quadrant, left lower quadrant and left paramedian space.

The table is positioned head down and tilted to the right. The second assistant operates the laparoscope from the left upper cannula. The first assistant retracts the peritoneal attachments of the sigmoid colon and grasps the descending colon. The surgeon then retracts the sigmoid colon cephalad and to the right while incising the peritoneal attachments with cautery or scissors. The left lateral gutter is entered, and the ureter and pelvic vessels are identified. A colonoscope can also be used to help to identify the lesion; a polyp or a tumor can be located by transillumination. Once the sigmoid colon has been mobilized and the lesion identified, the surgeon continues the dissection caudally. The sigmoid colon is retracted cephalad and to the right, and a left presacral window is opened. The sigmoid is then retracted to the left, and a right presacral window opened. The superior hemorrhoidal and sigmoid vessels are visualized.

The laparoscope is placed in the left lower quadrant for the dissection, which is equivalent to that for the left splenic flexure. The vascular pedicle is ligated and the proximal rectum is divided with a

60 mm linear stapler introduced through a cannula. As in the left and right colectomies, the bowel is exteriorized through a 4–6 mm transverse incision. It is resected, leaving the detachable anvil of the circular stapler (28 mm or larger) in the proximal bowel. The bowel is returned to the abdominal cavity and the pneumoperitoneum is re-established. The stapling device is introduced through the anus, attached to the anvil, and fired, forming an anastomosis.

Technique for Laparoscopic Loop Ileostomy

The loop ileostomy requires only two cannula sites. One is placed in the left abdomen lateral to the rectus muscle and the other on the right over the stoma site. The laparoscope is then placed in the left cannula. The surgeon positions a clamp in the right cannula and grasps the ileum. The bowel is pulled to the port and the stoma is matured. A loop colostomy is created in a similar fashion.

Conversion to Open Colectomy

Several factors may lead to a conversion from a laparoscopic to an open colectomy. As already mentioned, the inability to visualize a ureter and the presence of dense adhesions are two common reasons. Other possible indications include the lack of adequate hemostasis, poor exposure, disorientation, inadequate resection or reconstruction, and the discovery of an enterotomy, stricture, abscess or fistula. Conversion to an open procedure should not be considered as a surgical failure but rather the application of sound surgical judgment [37–39].

Postoperative Care

Postoperatively care is similar to that required after open colectomy, except that the recovery is more rapid. We use epidural anesthesia until patients tolerate oral intake well. We feed the patients on the evening of surgery and advance the diet as tolerated. Patients are discharged when they are eating a regular diet. As already noted, laparoscopic colectomy patients suffer less abdominal wall trauma, smaller decreases in respiratory and immune function, and a more rapid tolerance of food. They are usually discharged from the hospital between the third and sixth postoperative days.

Laparoscopic Surgery for Malignant Colonic Disease

With approximately 135 000 new cases of colorectal cancer in the USA each year, there has been increasing interest in the use of laparoscopy to minimize the short-term morbidity associated with treating malignant diseases. Sufficient research and experience in the laparoscopic treatment of colorectal cancer have shown that these methods are feasible, and many of the benefits associated with the laparoscopic treatment of benign colonic disease, such as decreased trauma and shorter hospital stays, have been seen. The current debate is whether it is appropriate to minimize short-term morbidity through minimally invasive techniques given the possibility of as yet unknown changes in the long-term morbidity and mortality of essentially curable diseases [27,30,40–42].

Questions concerning the efficacy of laparoscopic resections of colon and rectal cancer have centered on the completeness of the bowel resections, the completeness of the lymph node resections, and the lack of long-term survival data for laparoscopically treated patients. Recent studies indicate no differences in proximal and distal margins of resection or adequacy of lymph node dissection when comparing laparoscopic colectomy to open colectomy [2,43,44]. There are also concerns regarding the incidence and pattern of recurrences after laparoscopic treatments, specifically port site and extraction site recurrences.

Thus far, laparoscopic resections have been most successful in right hemicolectomies, sigmoid resections, stoma formation procedures, abdominoperineal resections, and ileal pouch–anal anastomosis. Tumors of the right colon, sigmoid colon and proximal rectum appear to be the most amenable to laparoscopic treatment.

Advantages and Disadvantages

Studies of these procedures have shown the expected benefits of decreased short-term morbidity, decreased abdominal wall trauma, earlier tolerance to food, decreased hospital stay, and reduced pain and narcotic requirements [26,33,43–45]. Furthermore, there have been decreases in surgical blood loss (and the need for transfusion). Increased postoperative cell-mediated immunity and neutrophil function has also been reported. This indicates less immunosuppression after laparoscopic colectomy and therefore a theoretically greater resistance to tumor growth than with laparotomy. As discussed previously, this decrease in immunosuppression appears primarily to follow decreased trauma during surgery.

Studies have also shown comparable short-term outcomes after laparoscopic colectomy. No significant differences in the number of lymph nodes removed or the length of bowel resected have been found between laparoscopic and open colectomies. There is a trend towards resection of a greater length of bowel in laparotomy but no statistically significant difference has been found. Cost differences between the two procedures have also not been identified, given decreased hospital stay but increased operating expenses of these procedures. There are also indications that operating time and therefore cost do decrease with surgical experience.

Particular complications of these procedures have been enterotomy and iliac artery laceration. Reasons for a perioperative conversion to laparotomy have included unclear anatomy, adhesions, abscesses, technical difficulties (in isolating the lesion), enterotomy and bleeding.

Recurrence

Local recurrence from the spillage of malignant cells into the abdominal cavity and the venous blood during surgery is a prominent concern with the surgical treatment of colon and rectal cancers [2,3,14,25,27,28,31,41–43,46–55]. Studies have shown that as many as 67% of patients have malignant cells in the venous blood postoperatively. Other studies have shown that 10–40% of patients have local recurrence from the lymph nodes and primary lesions after surgical treatment. Concerns have been raised about the effect of laparoscopic techniques on recurrence and long-term survival, and on staging patterns, given the increased manipulation and use of CO_2 insufflation. In addition, anecdotal reports of port site and extraction site recurrences have fueled discussion in this area.

Possible mechanisms of port/extraction site metastasis have also been the topic of considerable discussion. Three mechanisms have been proposed: contamination of the wound by tumor cells, increased exfoliation of tumor cells by laparoscopic manipulation, and a pneumoperitoneal effect on tumor cell attachment and growth. In laparoscopic colon cancer surgery, the malignant neoplasm is removed through either a port site or a small incision, or transrectally. There is a theoretical risk of contaminating these sites with tumor. Most reported wound recurrence cases have been at the port or incision sites, where direct contamination could have occurred. It is also possible that malignant serosal cells can be dislodged into the peritoneal cavity after the laparoscopic manipulation of unsuspected malignancy. Some investigators also believe that the pneumoperitoneum may play an important role in wound implantation by generating airborne tumor particles. However, animal studies have so far demonstrated conflicting results on wound recurrence with pneumoperitoneum. They have suggested that tumor recurrence is related to immunosuppression. The increased trauma associated with laparotomy appears to lower the threshold of tumor cell growth, indicating that immunosuppression may play a role in recurrence. One of the more recent studies, by Jacobi et al., however, disputes the immunosuppression theory and suggests the CO_2 infiltration of soft tissues as a vector for port site recurrence [46].

A recent review of a database established by the American Society of Colon and Rectal Surgeons has revealed a wound recurrence rate after laparoscopic colectomy for colon cancer comparable with conventional open colectomy, with the benefits of a minimally invasive procedure [27]. Although anecdotal experiences should be taken seriously, they should not be over- or underinterpreted.

New Developments in Laparoscopic Colectomy

The implantation of malignant cells during surgery was first observed by Gerster in 1885 [47]. Lack, in 1896, discussed the possibility of tumor spread from cancer cell contamination of instruments, sponges and surgeons' hands, with transmission of these cells into the wound [47]. From these observations researchers looked at using tumoricidal agents on sutures and wounds to prevent recurrences. The results were encouraging in vitro, but not in vivo. Furthermore, irrigating the peritoneal cavity with tumoricidal agents may actually increase tumor take within the peritoneal cavity [48]. For these reasons, the irrigation of wounds with tumoricidal agents is not commonly practiced. With the anecdotal reports of port site recurrence after laparoscopic colon resection, a resurgence in the theory that tumoricidal agents may prevent port site recurrence has emerged. Jacobi et al. found that taurolidine combined with heparin decreased tumor cell growth in a rat model [49]. Basha et al., showed in their study that 5% pyrrolidone iodine mixed with chloramine 0.5% killed almost all tumor cells in vitro and prevented their growth in vivo [50]. Beart et al. also found a decrease in tumor cell growth in the laparoscopic ports of mice with the use of Betadine [41]. Placing tumoricidal agents in the wounds or on the trocars to prevent port site recurrences may become standard care if the same results can be obtained in vivo.

The best way to put the port site recurrence question to rest is by a prospective randomized study of laparoscopic colectomy versus open colectomy for colon cancer. In 1995 a multicenter study was initiated to answer this question and others concerning adequacy of safety, staging and 5-year survival rates. The results should be available by 2003. Until this time the opinion is that performing laparoscopic colectomy for cancer should be deferred to those centers involved in the study.

Summary

Laparoscopic treatment for benign colonic disease and as palliative operations for advanced malignant disease have gained widespread acceptance as safe, efficacious and beneficial options. There are also strong indications that laparoscopic treatment for malignant colorectal disease is a viable alternative in selected patients. Further studies with substantial follow-up times to determine the adequacy of resection and the comparability of cure rates are needed to assess any long-term differences in the staging and survival patterns of these treatments.

Laparoscopic Rectal Cancer Surgery

Although the use of laparoscopic techniques in benign colorectal surgery has expanded over the past 10 years, controversy continues to surround the use of laparoscopic resection in patients with rectum or colon carcinoma. For benign diseases, diagnostic laparoscopy, the creation of stomas, and limited resections are all becoming reasonable indications. In cases of malignancy, resection either through a conventional incision or a laparoscope must adhere to the same defined surgical oncologic principles. Current randomized trials comparing open with laparoscopic resection have began to address these concerns [51]. Port site metastasis remains a leading obstacle to the widespread acceptance of laparoscopic resection for colorectal carcinoma, although it may be a rare phenomenon. We will discuss the applications of laparoscopic colorectal surgery for malignant rectal diseases. Further research in this area, combined with advances in laparoscopic technology, will be critical to the future successful application of laparoscopic surgery for colorectal carcinoma.

Laparoscopic Surgery for Rectal Carcinoma

The application of laparoscopic techniques to the radical excision of malignant colorectal disease has progressed since Jacobs et al. first reported its feasibility in 1991 [56]. The current role of laparoscopic surgery in restorative procedures is limited owing to an inability easily to transect the rectum below the tumor. Nonetheless, thorough intraoperative staging is achievable, as is complete mobilization of the rectum, by using laparoscopic methods.

Diagnosis and Staging

Despite recent progress in imaging techniques, these tests may be incapable of permitting as complete an evaluation of a particular lesion as may be necessary preoperatively. Laparoscopy allows inspection of the entire abdominal cavity without a major laparotomy; it additionally permits biopsy of a lesion. In evaluating the liver, intraoperative liver ultrasonography (ILUS) is especially useful for the diagnosis of metastasis from colorectal cancer. ILUS is extremely sensitive in detecting occult metastases, especially small intraparenchymal lesions of the liver that might be missed by the surgeon on palpation [57]. We have made ILUS a standard component of the diagnostic (and the curative) laparoscopic colorectal cancer operation [58]. All components of an abdominal exploration are possible with diagnostic laparoscopy, except for palpation.

Laparoscopic Oncologic Resection

Issues surrounding curative laparoscopic oncologic resection for rectal cancer include the ability to perform an acceptable oncologic resection, the question of morbidity and mortality compared with conventional surgery, and the problem of port site metastases. Whether a resection for colorectal carcinoma is performed at an open operation or laparoscopically, the same principles of oncologic resection must apply. We have defined our oncologic principles for laparoscopic cancer surgery as follows [52]:

1. Wide en bloc resection of the tumor-bearing bowel segment with adjacent soft tissue and mesentery
2. Resection of suitable margins of the normal bowel wall above and below the cancer
3. Excision of draining regional lymph nodes accompanying the major vascular pedicle to the involved bowel
4. Minimal manipulation of the tumor-bearing segment
5. Occlusion of the proximal and distal ends of the tumor
6. Placement of the specimen in an endoscopic impermeable bag before delivery through the abdominal wall
7. Assessment of the peritoneal cavity for metastatic Involvement

To allow for the development of the technical laparoscopic skill necessary to perform an oncologic resection, useful animal [59,60] and cadaver models [61,62] have been employed. In these models we confirmed that a laparoscopic oncologic resection could be performed according to oncologic principles, with proximal vascular ligation of the inferior mesenteric artery (IMA), wide clearance of the pelvic side walls, and complete removal of the mesorectum. Recent studies have also demonstrated the adequacy of laparoscopic resection compared with an open technique [45,53,63–65].

Port site metastasis after laparoscopic colon cancer surgery seems unusual, yet it is uncertain whether this actually represents a truly increased metastasis rate when compared with open surgery. Hughes et al. [66] and Reilly et al. [54] recently reported the incidence of wound recurrence after standard laparotomy for colorectal cancer (0.64–1.0%). Comparing these results with the >4% incidence of port site metastasis postulated by Wexner and Cohen [55] suggests the possibility of a higher recurrence rate after laparoscopic resection. However, as mentioned by Nduka et al. [67], the incidence of cutaneous metastasis at drainage sites after open surgery for malignant disease is more than likely underestimated. After conventional open colectomy, wound recurrences are often asymptomatic and, when reaching an advanced stage, with widespread systemic manifestations, small wound recurrences might easily be overlooked and therefore not recorded [68]. Based on the more recent reports [67,69,70] of larger operative series, the incidence of port site metastasis seems to be only 0–1.1%. This figure approximates to the results of wound metastasis after conventional open surgery.

Whether the true incidence of port site metastasis is greater than 1% or less than 4% awaits the results of the well-designed prospective randomized studies currently under way. The wide variation in the incidence of port site metastasis previously reported may relate to surgical technique. Even in conventional colectomy, the experience of the surgeon performing the operation appears to influence the development of local recurrence and also survival. Franklin et al. [53], who reported no port site recurrences in their series of laparoscopic colorectal cancer surgery in over 100 patients, recommended the following procedures during the laparoscopic operation:

1. Suture all trocars to prevent their dislodgement and sudden desufflation during the pneumoperitoneum
2. Use endoscopic bags for extraction of the specimen
3. Wash trocars with 5% povidone-iodine before removal
4. Remove intra-abdominal fluid before extraction of the trocar to prevent wound contamination

5. Close all trocar sites, including fascia, muscle and peritoneum
6. Avoid direct handling of the tumor
7. Irrigate all skin and subcutaneous sites with povidone-iodine solution before closure

Milsom et al. have conducted a prospective, randomized trial comparing laparoscopic and conventional techniques in 109 patients undergoing bowel resection for colorectal cancers and polyps. According to the preliminary results, laparoscopic techniques were as safe as conventional surgical techniques and offered faster recovery of pulmonary and gastrointestinal function. There were no apparent short-term oncologic disadvantages and no port site metastases (median follow-up 1.5 years) [51].

Laparoscopic Resection of Low Rectal Cancer

Although numerous options are currently available for the treatment of rectal cancer, resection of the rectum and node-bearing mesorectum, with preservation of the autonomic nerves, is rapidly becoming the preferred approach. Laparoscopy may improve the visualization of the operative field within a deep and narrow pelvis. In addition, the magnified view provided by laparoscopic surgery may be more helpful in performing total mesorectal excision and autonomic nerve preservation techniques. Laparoscopic resection of the rectum is technically feasible without the need for a large abdominal incision [61,62]. We have recently assessed the feasibility of the laparoscopic technique for total mesorectal excision in terms of both the resectability of the tumor and preservation of the autonomic nerve system by using a human cadaver model. We achieved very positive results regarding nerve preservation and total mesorectal excision [71]. The availability of an angulating laparoscopic linear stapler, currently under development, will greatly advance our ability to perform total mesorectal excision laparoscopically.

Procedures of Laparoscopic Proctosigmoidectomy

Position and Port Site

Full videoendoscopy facilities are required. The patient is placed in the modified lithotomy position using specialized stirrups (OR Direct Stirrups, Acton, MA). The pneumoperitoneum is created by using a standard technique for insufflation with a Veress needle and maintained at 12–15 mmHg by an automatic CO_2 insufflator. After the initial 10 mm cannula has been placed infraumbilically, two can-

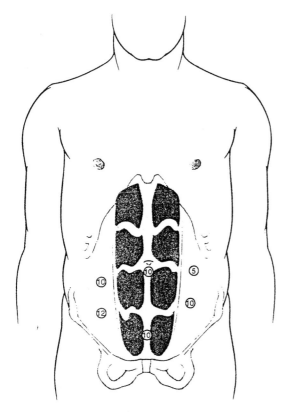

Fig. 9.1. The positions of the cannulae for proctosigmoidectomy.

nulae are positioned in the right and two in the left lateral abdominal wall (Fig. 9.1). For most procedures, because splenic flexure mobilization is necessary, a suprapubic cannula is also placed. For the first phase of the operation (dissection of the mesocolon and pelvic dissection), the surgeon and the second assistant stand on the patient's right side to view a monitor placed near the patient's left knee, while the first assistant stands on the patient's left side to see a monitor placed near the patient's right knee. In the second phase of the operation (mobilization of the splenic flexure), all surgical team members change positions. The monitor at the left knee is moved near the patient's left shoulder when the splenic flexure is being mobilized. The surgeon stands between the patient's legs and both assistants stand on the patient's right side. At this point, the entire team views the monitor at the patient's left shoulder.

Details of the Procedure

Initially, the camera is placed through the umbilical port and the assistant holds the mesosigmoid ventrally and to the left, under tension using a Babcock-like grasper through the left upper cannula and a smaller grasper through the left lower quadrant cannula. The retroperitoneum is incised immediately to the right of the IMA, starting at the sacral promontory. Using blunt dissection, the IMA

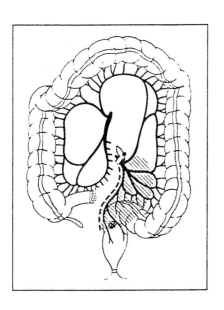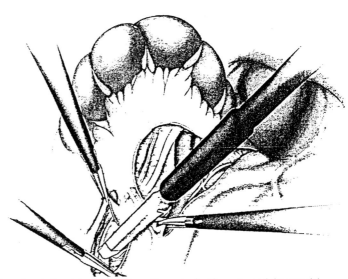

Fig. 9.2. Ligation and division of the inferior mesenteric artery close to its origin using a 30 mm linear stapler. The ureter and the gonadal vessel have been swept clear from the vessels. The inferior mesenteric vein may often be ligated simultaneously.

and vein are swept ventrally and the pre-aortic hypogastric neural plexus is swept dorsally to prevent their injury. Dissection is continued medially beneath the IMA and vein as the left ureter and the gonadal vessels are identified and swept posteriorly.

Once the origin of the IMA is identified, the peritoneum is incised anteriorly over this pedicle and to the left towards the inferior mesenteric vein. This pedicle of the IMA and vein is ligated above or below the left colic artery (according to the surgeon's judgment) using an endoscopic vascular stapler, but only if the left ureter can be clearly identified and retracted to avoid injury (Fig. 9.2).

The lateral attachments of the sigmoid colon are dissected free, and the sigmoid colon is completely mobilized using both sharp and blunt dissection, as in open surgery. The mesosigmoid of the proximal resection line is held by using triangulating tension and then transected. The colon is divided with one or two cartridges of a 30 mm endoscopic stapler. For the second phase, mobilization of the splenic flexure, the surgical team repositions as described above. Once the flexure is dissected from the most

cephalad attachments of the lienocolic ligament, the greater omentum is freed from the transverse colon edge towards the mid-line as far as the surgeon deems necessary to allow the descending colon to reach to the pelvis. To accomplish the third phase of the procedure, that of specimen resection and coloanal anastomosis, members of the surgical team return to their original positions. The rectum is completely mobilized as far distally as required by the tumor location and towards the pelvic floor using the standard open technique, starting with posterior mobilization, and then dissecting postero-laterally to the right and to the left of the rectum. If the proper plane is entered posteriorly, no bleeding will occur, and the connective tissue between the fascia propria of the rectum and the presacral fascia can be separated easily.

Division of the lateral ligaments is readily performed under direct laparoscopic vision and may be better visualized laparoscopically than by open methods. Posteriorly the pelvic nerves are identified and preserved and the mesorectum is completely excised. The close and magnified views of the mesorectum provided by the laparoscope (10–20 ×

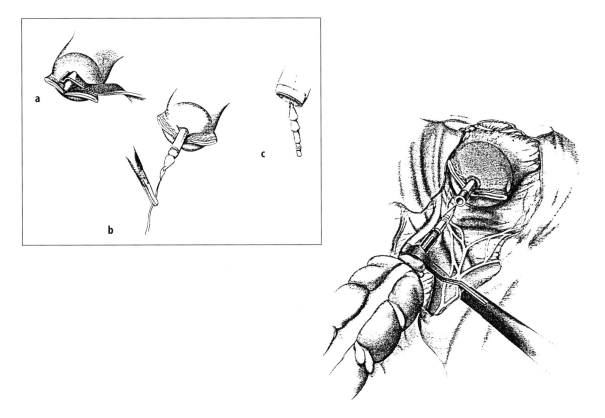

Fig. 9.3. The colorectal anastomosis is created by using an endoscopic Babcock instrument to maneuver the center rod into the center post of the transanally-placed stapler. Inset: **a** Initial protrusion of the plastic trocar of a circular stapler through the rectum, aided by counteraction applied by means of an endoscopic Babcock instrument; **b** The trocar is pushed through the rectum close to the staple line; **c** The trocar is removed through a cannula by pulling on the attached thread.

magnification) ensure identification of the correct planes of dissection and minimal bleeding Once the distal resection line has been freed of the mesorectum, the rectum is transected with two or three applications of the 30 mm endoscopic stapler. This can be difficult in low tumors because currently available staplers cannot successfully transect deep in the pelvis. A bowel bag is brought into the abdominal cavity through the left lower quadrant cannula and the specimen is placed immediately in the bag by using the snare. The left lower quadrant cannula site is widened with a 3–5 cm muscle-splitting incision. The bag containing the specimen is carefully delivered through the incision without exposing the specimen to any abdominal wall tissue.

The mobilized descending colon is then delivered through this same wound using the right upper quadrant grasper to hold it and a purse-string (size 0 polypropylene) suture is placed around the cut edge of the proximal colon after excising the previously placed staples. The anvil of a 28–31 mm circular stapler is placed into the descending colon lumen and the purse-string suture is tied around the center rod in the usual manner. This end of the bowel is carefully returned to the peritoneal cavity without twisting its mesentery. The abdominal wound is closed with size 0 polyglycolic acid figure-of-eight sutures through all layers of the fascia.

The pneumoperitoneum is re-established and the anastomosis is then created. A size 2–0 braided suture is loosely tied to the modified stapler's plastic trocar. The stapler is inserted transanally and, under laparoscopic guidance, passed to the rectal staple line. Next, the plastic tip is protruded through the rectal wall just adjacent to the staple line by turning the wing nut of the stapler counterclockwise. With a grasper in the right upper quadrant cannula, the thread is pulled to dislodge the plastic trocar tip safely from the center rod and to remove it through the cannula. A standard double-stapling technique is used to form the colorectal anastomosis by grasping the groove in the center rod with an endoscopic Babcock instrument through the right lower quadrant cannula and locking the center rod into the center post of the circular stapler. Excellent visualization of the anastomosis before firing the stapler is mandatory (Fig. 9.3). To test the anastomosis for leaks, the pelvis is filled with saline and air insufflation of the rectum is performed with a proctoscope. The tissue donuts created with the circular stapler are checked for completeness and are sent for routine pathologic analysis. At the conclusion of each procedure, after careful irrigation of the pelvis, an atraumatic silicone drain can be placed in the pelvis, using the right lower quadrant cannula site [72–74].

Conclusion

When compared with conventional surgery, the use of laparoscopic techniques offers several advantages to patients requiring rectal resection. Future study will be likely to confirm the reduced postoperative pain, earlier return of gastrointestinal function, and quicker resumption of normal activities seen in previous reports. The most recently reported investigations with a follow-up of up to 2 years have not demonstrated reduced survival. The fear of port site recurrence is the leading concern for the laparoscopic resection of rectal cancer, although more recent studies have documented recurrence rates similar to conventional surgery. Future laboratory and clinical trials will probably confirm the validity of the laparoscopic approach. Advances in instrumentation and surgical techniques will also be likely to demonstrate the feasibility of a laparoscopic oncologic resection of the rectum with autonomic nerve preservation in the majority of patients.

References

1. Semm K. Endoscopic appendectomy. Endoscopy 1983;15:59–64.
2. Milsom JW, Kim SH. Laparoscopic versus open surgery for colorectal cancer. J Surg 1997;21:702–705.
3. Beart RW Jr. Laparoscopic colectomy: status of the art. Dis Colon Rectum 1994;37(Suppl):47–49.
4. Liberman M, Phillips E, Carroll B, Fallas M, Rosenthal R. Laparoscopic colectomy vs traditional colectomy for diverticulitis: outcome and costs. Surg Endosc 1996;10:15–18.
5. Sher M, Agachan F, Bortul M, Nogueras J, Weiss E, Wexner S. Laparoscopic surgery for diverticulitis. Surg Endosc 1997;11:264–67.
6. Reissman P, Salky BA, Pfeifer J, et al. Laparoscopic surgery in the management of inflammatory bowel disease. Am J Surg 1996;171:47–50.
7. Leighton TA, Liu S-Y, Bongard FS. Comparative cardiopulmonary effects of carbon dioxide versus helium pneumoperitoneum. Surgery 1993;113:527–31.
8. Freeman JA, Armstrong IR. Pulmonary function tests before and after laparoscopic cholecystectomy. Anaesthesia 1994;49:579–82.
9. Bongard FS, Pianim NA, Leighton TA, et al. Helium insufflation for laparoscopic operation. Surg Gynecol Obstet 1993;177:140–46.
10. Ho H, Gunther R, Wolfe B. Intraperitoneal carbon dioxide insufflation and cardiopulmonary functions. Arch Surg 1992;127:928–33.
11. Beart RJ. Laparoscopic colorectal surgery [replies]. Dis Colon Rectum 1995;38:1119–20.
12. Coelho JCU, de Araujo RPM, Marchesini JB, et al. Pulmonary function after cholecystectomy performed through Kocher's incision, a mini-incision, and laparoscopy. World J Surg 1993;17:544–46.

13. Wittgen CM, Naunheim KS, Andrus CH, Kaminski DL. Preoperative pulmonary function evaluation for laparoscopic cholecystectomy. Arch Surg 1993;128:880–86.

14. Sackier JM, Slutzki S, Wood C, Halevy A. Concerns about laparoscopic colon cancer surgery [reply]. Dis Colon Rectum 1994;37:625–26.

15. Casey LC, Balk RA, Bone RC. Plasma cytokine and endotoxin levels correlate with survival in patients with the sepsis syndrome. Ann Intern Med 1993;119: 771–854.

16. Wolf JS Jr, Stoller ML. The physiology of laparoscopy: basic principles, complications and other considerations. J Urol 1994;152:294–302.

17. Cioffi WG, Burleson DG, Pruitt BA Jr. Leukocyte responses to injury. Arch Surg 1993;128:1260–67.

18. Colacchio TA, Yeager MP, Hildebrandt LW. Perioperative immunomodulation in cancer surgery. Am J Surg 1994;167: 174–79.

19. Harmon GD, Senagore AJ, Kilbride MJ, Warzynski MJ. Interleukin-6 response to laparoscopic and open colectomy. Dis Colon Rectum 1994;37:754–59.

20. Kloosterman T, Von Blomberg ME, Borgstein P, et al. Unimpaired immune functions after laparoscopic cholecystectomy. Surgery 1994;115:424–28.

21. Lowry SF. Cytokine mediators of immunity and inflammation. Arch Surg 1993;128:1235–41.

22. Patel RT, Deen KI, Youngs D, et al. Interleukin-6 is a prognostic indicator of outcome in severe intra-abdominal sepsis. Br J Surg 1994;81:1306–308.

23. Redmond HP, Watson RWG, Houghton T, et al. Immune function in patients undergoing open vs laparoscopic cholecystectomy. Arch Surg 1994;129:1240–46.

24. Wigmore SJ, Ross JA, Fearon KCH. Modulation of the cytokine and acute–phase response to major surgery by recombinant interleukin 2 [letter]. Br J Surg 1995;82:1289.

25. Falk PM, Beart RW Jr, Wexner SD, et al. Laparoscopic colectomy: a critical appraisal. Dis Colon Rectum 1993;36:28–34.

26. Monson JRT, Hill ADK, Darzi A. Laparoscopic colonic surgery. Br J Surg 1995;82:150–57.

27. Ramos JM, Beart RW Jr, Goes R, et al. Role of laparoscopy in colorectal surgery: a prospective evaluation of 200 cases. Dis Colon Rectum 1995;38:494–501.

28. Ramos JM, Gupta S, Anthone GJ, et al. Laparoscopy and colon cancer: is the port site at risk? A preliminary report. Arch Surg 1994;129:897–99.

29. Benhamou D, Simonneau G, Poynard T, et al. Diaphragm function is not impaired by pneumoperitoneum after laparoscopy. Arch Surg 1993;128:430–32.

30. Cuschieri A. Whither minimal access surgery: tribulations and expectations. Am J Surg 1995;169:9–19.

31. Kmiot WA, Wexner SD. Laparoscopy in colorectal surgery: a call for careful appraisal. Br J Surg 1995;82:25–26.

32. Fernando HC, Alle KM, Chen J, et al. Triage by laparoscopy in a patient with penetrating abdominal trauma. Br J Surg 1994;81:384–85.

33. Houghton AD, Wickham J, McColl I. Preventing complications of laparoscopy [letter]. Br J Surg 1994;81:1546.

34. McDermott JP, Devereaux DA, Caushaj PF. Pitfall of laparoscopic colectomy: an unrecognized synchronous cancer. Dis Colon Rectum 1994;37:602–603.

35. McKittrick LS, Wheelock FC. Carcinoma of the colon. Dis Colon Rectum 1997;40:1494–46

36. Tang E, Stain SC, Tang G, et al. Timing of laparoscopic surgery in gallstone pancreatitis. Arch Surg 1995;130: 496–500.

37. Cadiere GB, Verroken R, Himpens J, et al. Operative strategy in laparoscopic splenectomy. J Am Coll Surg 1994;179: 668–72.

38. Chan ACW, Lee TW, Ng KW, et al. Early results of laparoscopic intraperitoneal onlay mesh repair for inguinal hernia. Br J Surg 1994;81:1761–62.

39. See WA, Cooper CS, Fisher RJ. Predictors of laparoscopic complications after formal training in laparoscopic surgery. JAMA 1993;270:2689–92.

40. Barone JE. Problems with the fourth-year curriculum of students entering surgical residencies. Am J Surg 1995;169:334–37.

41. Beart RW Jr. Wound and port site recurrence [letter]. Surgery 1995;117:719–20.

42. Wexner SD, Cohen SM. Port site metastases after laparoscopic colorectal surgery for cure of malignancy. Br J Surg 1995;82:295–98.

43. Hida J, Yasutomi M, Maruyama T, et al. The extent of lymph node dissection for colon carcinoma: the potential impact on laparoscopic surgery. Cancer 1997;80:188–92.

44. Horvath K, Whelan R, Lier B, et al. A prospective comparison of laparoscopic exposure techniques for rectal mobilization and sigmoid resection. Am Coll Surg 1997;184:506–12.

45. Gray D, Lee H, Schlinkert R, Beart RW Jr. Adequacy of lymphadenectomy in laparoscopic-assisted colectomy for colorectal cancer: a preliminary report. J Surg 1994;57:8.

46. Jacobi C, Ordermann J, Bohm B, et al. The influence of laparotomy and laparoscopy on tumor growth in a rat model. Surg Endosc 1997;11:618–21.

47. McDonald G, Edmondson J, Cole W. Prevention of implantation of cancer cells in the wound by irrigation with anticancer agents. Am J Surg 1961;101:16–19.

48. Docherty JG, McGregor J, Purdie C, Galloway D, O'Dwyer P. Efficacy of tumoricidal agents in vitro and in vivo. Br J Surg 1995;82:1050–52.

49. Jacobi C, Ordemann J, Bohm B, Zieren H. Inhibition of peritoneal tumor cell growth and implantation in laparoscopic surgery in a rat model. Am J Surg 1997;174: 359–63.

50. Basha G, Penninckx F, Geboes K, Yap P. Tumoricidal activity of antiseptics with assessment of cell viability in mice with severe combined immunodeficiency. Tumor Biol 1997;18:213–18.

51. Milsom JW, Böhm B, Hammerhofer KA, Fazio VW, Steiger E, Elson P. A prospective, randomized trial comparing laparoscopic versus conventional techniques in colorectal cancer surgery: a preliminary report. J Am Coll Surg 1998;187:46.

52. Milsom JW, Kim SH. Laparoscopic versus open surgery for colorectal cancer. World J Surg 1997;21:702.

53. Franklin ME Jr, Rosenthal D, Abrego-Medina D, et al. Prospective comparison of open vs laparoscopic colon surgery for carcinoma. Five-year results. Dis Colon Rectum 1996;39:S35.

54. Reilly WT, Nelson H, Schroeder G, Wieand HS, Bolton J, O'Connell MJ. Wound recurrence following conventional treatment of colorectal cancer: a rare but perhaps underestimated problem. Dis Colon Rectum 1996;39:200.

55. Wexner SD, Cohen SM. Port site metastasis after laparoscopic colorectal surgery for cure of malignancy. Br J Surg 1995;82:295.

56. Jacob M, Verdeja JC, Goldstein HS. Minimally invasive colon resection (laparoscopic colectomy). Surg Laparosc Endosc 1991;1:144.

57. John TG, Garden OJ. Laparoscopic ultrasonography: extending the scope of diagnostic laparoscopy. Br J Surg 1994;81:5.

58. Marchesa P, Milsom JW, Hale JC, O'Malley CM, Fazio VW. Intraoperative laparoscopic liver ultrasonography for staging of colorectal cancer. Initial experience. Dis Colon Rectum 1996;39:S73.

59. Böhm B, Milsom JW, Kitago K, Brand M, Fazio VW. Laparoscopic oncologic total abdominal colectomy with intraperitoneal stapled anastomosis in a canine model. J Laparosc Surg 1994;4:23.

60. Böhm B, Milsom JW, Kitago K, Brand M, Stolfi VM, Fazio VW. Use of laparoscopic techniques in oncologic right colectomy in a canine model. Ann Surg Oncol 1995; 2:6.

61. Milsom JW, Böhm B, Decanini C, Fazio VW. Laparoscopic oncologic proctocosigmoidectomy with low colorectal anastomosis in a cadaver model. Surg Endosc 1994;8:1117.

62. Decanini C, Milsom JW, Böhm B, Fazio VW. Laparoscopic oncologic abdominoperineal resection. Dis Colon Rectum 1994;37:552.

63. Monson JRT, Darzi A, Carey PD, Guillou PJ. Prospective evaluation of laparoscopic-assisted colectomy in an unselected group of patients. Lancet 1992;340:831.

64. Phillips EK, Franklin M, Carroll BJ, Fallas MJ, Ramos R, Rosenthal D. Laparoscopic colectomy. Ann Surg 1992; 216:703.

65. Falk PM, Beart RW Jr, Wexner SD, et al. Laparoscopic colectomy: a critical appraisal. Dis Colon Rectum 1993;36:28.

66. Hughes ESR, McDermott FT, Polglase AL, Johnson WR. Tumor recurrence in the abdominal wall scar tissue after large bowel cancer surgery. Dis Colon Rectum 1983; 26:571.

67. Nduka CC, Monson JRT, Menzies-Gow N, Darzi A. Abdominal wall metastases following laparoscopy. Br J Surg 1994;81:648.

68. Hoffman CC, Baker JW, Doxey JB, Hubbard GW, Ruffin WK, Wishner JA. Minimally invasive surgery for colorectal cancer; initial follow-up. Ann Surg 1996;223:790.

69. Fleshman JW, Nelson H, Peter WR, et al. Early results of laparoscopic surgery for colorectal cancer: retrospective analysis of 372 patients treated by Clinical Outcomes of Surgery Therapy (COST) Study Group. Dis Colon Rectum 1996;39:S53.

70. Lord SA, Larach SW, Ferrara A, Williamson PR, Lago CP, Lube MW. Laparoscopic resections for colorectal carcinoma: a three-year experience. Dis Colon Rectum 1996;39:148.

71. Jerby BL, Kessler H, Marcello PW, Gramlich T, Milsom JW. Laparoscopic total mesorectal excision and autonomic nerve preservation in a cadaver model. J Gastrointest Surg (submitted).

72. Milsom JW, Böhm B. Laparoscopic colorectal surgery. New York, NY: Springer-Verlag, 1996.

73. Darzi A, Menzies-Gow N, Guillou PJ, Monson JRT. Laparoscopic abdominoperineal excision of the rectum. Surg Endosc 1995;9:414.

74. Darzi A, Super P, Guillou PJ, Monson JRT. Laparoscopic sigmoid colectomy: total laparoscopic approach. Dis Colon Rectum 1994;37:268.

10. Minimal Access Surgery for Rectal Cancer

V.W. Fazio and F. López-Kostner

Introduction

Abdominoperineal resection of the rectum has been considered to be the preferred treatment for low rectal cancer; however, its cost is a permanent colostomy. From the 1970s to the 1990s, several authors have shown that the chances of cure are not compromised if low anterior resection is used for middle [1–3] and for selected lower rectal cancer [4]. However, 25–60% of patients may experience soiling, increased stool frequency and rectal urgency [5,6]. Significant bladder and sexual dysfunction occurs in 5–70% of patients after low anterior resection and abdominoperineal resection [7–11]. Operative mortality ranges from 1% to 5% and may be markedly higher in elderly patients [12,13].

Local treatment – local excision, contact radiotherapy or electrocoagulation – is a more conservative approach, the main goal of which is to avoid colostomy and major resective surgery without sacrificing local control of the cancer or survival. Most authors report morbidity rates below 10% and no operative mortality; however, there is significant variability in local tumor control rates (0 to 27%). Series with small numbers of patients, different selection criteria or non-use of radiation and short follow-up can explain this discrepancy. The key to success is appropriate patient selection. Patients with small, exophytic, mobile and pathologically favorable tumors (those that are well differentiated and without lymphatic or blood vessel invasion, where there is an absence of colloid histology, and when invasion is to the submucosa only) are ideal candidates for local therapy. Unfortunately, these favorable tumors comprise only 3–5% of all rectal cancers [14,15]. Not all tumors subjected to local therapy have all these features. Some patients who

refuse to have a permanent stoma under any circumstance or who are high-risk candidates for surgery may be treated by local therapy, even though the risk for local recurrence is higher. If the patient develops a local recurrence, there is still a good chance of salvaging the situation with radical resection. More than 50% of patients with locally recurrent rectal cancer can undergo salvage surgery with curative intent.

Preoperative Assessment

Tumor Invasion

The accuracy of digital rectal examination ranges from 44% to 83% for determining the depth of tumor invasion [16–19]. The ability to detect lymph node disease is limited: only about 60% of patients with metastatic lymph nodes were diagnosed accurately by clinical examination [16] in one study. Endorectal ultrasound (ERUS) detects tumor penetration beyond the muscularis propria (T3 disease) with an accuracy of 70–90% in most series [17–23]. However, the ability of ERUS to determine the extent of lesser degrees of invasion is not as good and it is more limited in detecting local lymph node involvement, with accuracy ranging from 50% to 80% [18,20]. ERUS is incapable of detecting microscopic deposits in normal sized lymph nodes, unless ultrasound directed biopsy is done. Computed tomography is useful only for detecting advanced lesions.

The role of rectal endoscopic lymphoscintigraphy in detecting rectal cancer is controversial [24]. Although it seems reasonable to conclude that involved lymph nodes may block the cephalad lymph drainage, particularly in the case of advanced lesions, lymph nodes with partial involvement and non-obstructing lymph flow may be associated with false-negative results on lymphoscintigraphy.

Patient Selection for Local Treatment

Ideally, tumors that are suitable for local treatment are: less than 3 cm in diameter; located within 7 cm of the anal verge; mobile on digital examination; involve less than 25% of the rectal circumference; have no associated palpable perirectal lymph nodes; and have favorable histology (well- or moderately differentiated, no lymphatic or blood vessel invasion, no mucinous component). This corresponds to uT1N0 status according to rectal endosonography. However, patients with less "ideal" characteristics may be eligible for local treatment, depending upon the adequacy of informed consent, fitness (or lack thereof) for major resective surgery, and the use of adjuvant radiation or chemoradiation for T2 lesions.

Size

Most authors exclude patients with tumors >3 cm in diameter for curative local treatment because of the risk of metastases to lymph nodes. However, even small tumors (<3 cm) may have metastatic lymph

nodes. Grigg et al. [25] reported a 17% incidence of lymph node metastasis in tumors <3.0 cm, and Abrams [26] noted 31% of lymph node metastases in tumors ≤3.0 cm. Even though there is a certain association between tumor size and metastatic lymph nodes, this factor is not considered to be an independent variable.

Exophytic Lesions

Polypoid or nodular raised cancers are associated with a better prognosis than ulcerated lesions because these have been reported to have a lower incidence of lymph node metastasis [27]. The main problem is that the definition of polypoid and ulcerative lesions is highly subjective and lacks scientific precision.

Mobile Lesions

Mason [28] pioneered the clinical staging of rectal cancer by digital examination. He argued that the degree of mobility was related to the depth of local invasion. In a prospective study, Nicholls et al. [16] reported that examination by more experienced clinicians achieved an accuracy of 73–80% in lesions confined to the rectal wall. The clinical assessment of negative and positive lymph node status was 65% and 67%, respectively. Characterization of the

Table 10.1. Results with local excision alone

Reference	No. patients	Follow-up (months)	Local failure rates			Overall failure rate	Salvage surgery	Postoperative and chronic complications
			T1	T2	T3			
Lock et al. [29]	89	NS	NS	NS	NS	6/89	3/6	12% wound infection 12% rectovaginal fistula
Stearns et al. [14]	31	>5 years	5/15	2/14	1/2	8/31	5/8	NS
Biggers et al. [30]	141	>5 years	NS	NS	NS	38/141	NS	4% local infection 2% bleeding
Grigg et al. [31]	13	44 (mean)	0/7	0/5	0/1	0/13	–	None
Gerard et al. [32]	14	NS	2/14	–	–	2/14	2/2	None
Balslev et al. [33]	30	27 (mean)	1/24	2/6	–	3/30	1/3	3% temporary fistula
Gall and Hermauck [34]	84	77 (median)	4/54	4/20	3/10	11/84	7/11	NS
Total (%)	402		12/114 (11)	8/45 (17.8)	4/13 (31)	68/402 (17)	18/30 (60)	

NS, not stated.

mobility of the tumor as mobile, tethered or fixed can usually be decided, but quantification – except for extreme ranges of the spectrum – is difficult unless ultrasound is used.

Depth

Modern management of low rectal cancers using local treatment usually requires preoperative endoluminal ultrasonography. As already mentioned, the depth of mural invasion is assessed with a high level of accuracy by using ERUS. This is confirmed by local excision and histological examination.

Assessing the depth of invasion histologically requires careful preparation of the specimen in the operating room. Two important measures are the avoidance of fragmentation of the tumor during excision and pinning the fresh specimen on a cardboard sheet. Despite negative histologic margins, a higher local recurrence rate has been observed for more advanced T stages (Table 10.1 [14,29–34] and Table 10.2 [35–40]). This finding may be explained because of the higher percentage of occult metastatic lymph nodes observed in T2 and T3 tumors (Table 10.3 [41–44]).

Favorable Histology

Simple preoperative biopsy has an error rate of 40% in the assessment of tumor grade owing to the sampling process and inadequacies of biopsy specimens [45] compared with serial histologic examination of the entire excised specimen. Minsky et al. [46] found on univariate analysis that T stage, tumor grade and colloid histology were significant predictors for lymph node metastasis. Logistic regression analysis

Table 10.2. Results after local excision and radiotherapy (with or without chemotherapy)

Reference	No. patients	Follow-up (months)	Local failure rates			Overall failure rate	Postoperative and chronic complications
			T1	T2	T3		
Despretz et al. [35]	25	40.5 (median)	0/7	2/8	3/10	5/25	20% wound dehiscence 4% rectovaginal fistula
Ota et al. [36]	46	36 (median)	0/16	1/15	3/15	4/46	NS
Willet et al. [37]	26	59 (median)	1/10	2/11	1/3	4/26	4% gluteal fissure 4% benign rectal stricture
Minsky et al. [38]	22	37 (median)	0/4	2/12	2/6	4/22	Most patients required lomotil for bowel frequency.
Fortunato et al. [39]	21	56 (median)	1/2	2/15	1/4	4/21	10% proctitis and bleeding
Bleday et al. [40]	48	40.5 (mean)	2/21	0/21	2/5	4/48	20% fecal fistula after transsphincteric or transcoccygeal local excision
Total (%)	188		4/60 (7)	9/82 (11)	12/43 (28)	25/188 (13)	

NS, not stated.

Table 10.3. Percentage of metastatic lymph nodes according to rectal wall involvement

Author	No. patients	Mucosa/submucosa (%)	Muscularis propria (%)	Subserosa (%)
Hojo et al. [41]	423	18	38	46
Hughes et al. [42]	42	6.5	–	–
Hagar et al. [43]	95	8	17	–
Minsky et al. [44]	168	0	28	–

showed that all three factors were independent predictors for metastatic lymph nodes. Brodsky et al.
[47] reviewed 154 patients with pT1 and pT2 rectal
tumors who underwent radical resection. The incidence of lymph node metastases was associated
significantly with T classification (12% for pT1 and
22% for pT2), tumor grade (0 for grade 1, 22% for
grade 2 and 50% for grade 3), and the presence of
lymphatic vessel invasion, blood vessel invasion, or
both (31% for invasive lesions and 17% for non-
invasive lesions). In Morson's series [48], all five T1
tumors with lymph node metastases were poorly
differentiated neoplasms. It is important to stress
that the simple preoperative biopsy can have an
error rate of 40% in the assessment of tumor grade
with respect to biopsy specimens [45] owing to
incomplete sampling.

Margin of Excision

It is useful to think of local excision of rectal cancer
as a (wide) excision biopsy. Given a favorable review
of the lateral and deep margins, histologically and
clinically, as well as the absence of the adverse characteristics mentioned above, this "biopsy" may
prove to: (1) be all that is necessary; (2) require
further non-resective treatment (radiation plus or
minus chemotherapy), for example, for a T2 lesion,
or re-excision, for example, for an involved margin
microscopically: or (3) require a recommendation
for major resective surgery.

The excision is planned to provide a 1 cm or more
radial clearance of the circumference of the tumor.
The depth extends to and includes a layer of perirectal fat. If the circumferential margin is judged to be
incomplete, it is reasonable to re-excise the surgical
bed of the tumor. If the deep margin is involved with
carcinoma and the disc excision has removed the
full depth of rectal wall, then radical excision is indicated as this represents a T3 lesion. Baron et al. [49]
showed better survival when immediate radical
surgery was performed if adverse histologic features
were found in the excision specimen.

Therapeutic Modalities for Local Treatments

Local Excision

Local excision can be performed using endoscopic
[50,51], transanal [31], transsphincteric [52,53], or
transcoccygeal [54,55] approaches. The posterior
transsphincteric approach provides better exposure

but at the risk of fecal fistula and incontinence
due to poor healing of the repair of the divided
sphincters [40].

Transanal Local Excision

In 1977, Morson et al. [53] advocated transanal local
excision (TLE) as definitive treatment in selected
patients. TLE should be considered as an excisional
biopsy. Thereafter, meticulous histologic evaluation
should confirm the curative potential of the excision
and allow for estimation of the risk of lymph node
invasion and, consequently the need for further
treatment. The main advantage of TLE compared
with other local treatment modalities is the ability
to assess the extent of mural involvement by the
tumor.

Surgical Technique   The patient undergoing TLE is
prepared in the same manner as for transabdominal
colonic resection. The prone jack-knife position is
used for lesions in anterior and lateral locations. For
lesions in the posterior rectum the lithotomy position is preferred. A 1.5–2 cm margin around the
tumor is marked with electrocautery (Fig. 10.1). A
personal preference is also to fulgurate the surface
of the neoplasm, in order to render less implantable
any tumor cells shed during excision. The incision
should be full thickness, exposing the extrarectal fat.
The defect in the rectal wall can be left open or
closed with absorbable sutures after fulguration of
the base and irrigation of the bed with a cytotoxic
solution, such as 40% alcohol. The specimen is carefully placed on a piece of cardboard, and the right,
left, caudad, and cephalad aspects are marked. If
adequate resection margins cannot be achieved,
and if the carcinoma is of a high pathologic grade,
rectal resection should be considered in otherwise
good-risk patients.

The morbidity rate after TLE is less than 10%. The
most important complications are bleeding [30],
local infection [29], urinary retention [30], wound
hematoma, and temporary incontinence [15].

Transanal Endoscopic Microsurgery

Transanal endoscopic microsurgery (TEM) was
developed between 1980 and 1983 and began to be
applied clinically in 1983. It was developed to resect
rectal tumors [50]. The ectoscope for TEM has an
outer diameter of 40 mm, with inner tubes of varying length. Four work channels allow the use of
different instruments. A stereoscopic optic system
provides a precise image. Instruments are similar
to those used in laparoscopic surgery. A special
operating rectoscope with a stereo telescope allows
operative manipulation within the distal sigmoid
colon.

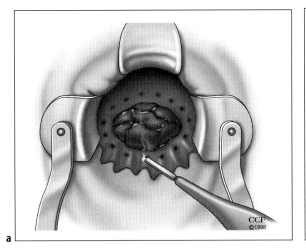

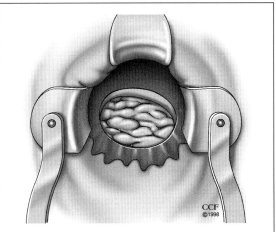

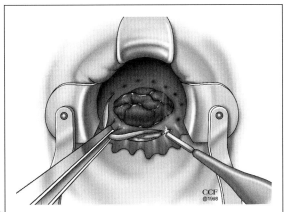

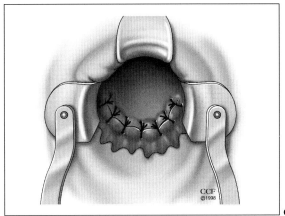

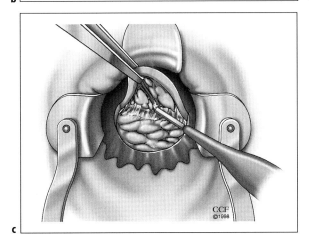

Fig. 10.1. a The margin of planned excision is demarcated with electrocautery 1 cm (plus) from palpable and visible edge of tumor; **b** The lower edge is incised through full thickness bowel wall; **c** The lesion is raised with anterior traction while cautery is used to complete the resection; **d** Excision is complete. The presacral fat is exposed and fulgurated. Alcohol solution (40%) is used to irrigate the exposed fat; **e** Where edges can be approximated, this is done with 20 polyglycolic acid sutures. A proctoscope is then passed to ensure patency of the lumen.

Mentges et al. [57] reported 458 patients undergoing TEM, 113 of them with carcinoma. No patients died from the procedure. The main complications were suture line dehiscence, peritonitis, rectovaginal fistula and bleeding. The complication rate requiring surgical reintervention was 7% (eight of 113). The median follow-up was 29 months, which is too short to draw conclusions about survival. To our knowledge, there has been no prospective randomized study comparing TLE with TEM for low anterior resection and TEM for the treatment of early rectal cancer. Buess et al. [58] reported the results of 74 patients with rectal cancer who were treated by TEM. The complication rate was 5% and mortality was 0.3%. There were 51 T1 lesions, 17 T2 lesions and 6 T3 lesions: 23 of the T2 and T3 lesions were subject to further segmental resection. The 5-year cure rates for patients treated solely by TEM were not fully reported. Recurrence rates can be inordinately high. In one report [59], 10% of patients with T1 cancer developed local recurrence after TEM; 40% of T2 lesions similarly treated recurred. Most recurrences were salvaged by subsequent resection. In a comparative study of TEM versus low anterior resection of the rectum for T1 rectal cancers, Winde and colleagues [60] noted lower morbidity, and similar local recurrence and survival rates favoring TEM. Here, local recurrence rates (4.2%) and 5-year survival rates (96%) did not differ significantly between treatment groups. Saclarides [61], an experienced surgeon and proponent of TEM, has stated, with coworker Brand, that:

> whether or not – TEM can yield lower recurrence rates remains to be seen but this perhaps is not the main reason one should include TEM in one's armamentarium. Rather it is the improved exposure, superior optics, and the opportunity to address lesions in the upper rectum that sets TEM apart from conventional instrumentation.

The limitations to TEM use include:

A substantial learning curve for the surgeon who requires special training

Expensive equipment that can only be justified by adequate patient numbers

Risks of anastomotic disruption, peritonitis, requirement for an ostomy

Possible intraperitoneal dissemination of cancer with full thickness excision of an upper third rectal cancer

The advantages are those listed by Saclarides and Brand. They would seem to be compelling for poor-risk patients with upper rectal cancers that have favorable tumor characteristics. The caveat is that the surgery is carried out by a surgeon experienced with the TEM technique.

Results of Local Excision

The local recurrence rate after local excision varies according to the selection criteria used and the degree of tumor invasion. Local excision of selected rectal adenocarcinomas appears to provide a degree of locoregional control similar to that obtained by radical resection for Stage I tumors. We have reviewed seven published series of patients undergoing local excision (Table 10.1). Of the 402 patients who underwent local excision alone, 68 (17%) ex-

perienced local recurrence. Coco et al. [62] reported a 3% local recurrence rate for T1 and T2 tumors after local treatment, compared with 6% after radical surgery, with both groups followed for at least 5 years. Willet et al. [37] reported similar data, although patients with poor prognostic factors had better local control after radical surgery (89% versus 68%).

In a further review of six series in which the role of radiotherapy as an adjuvant treatment for local excision was assessed, 188 patients were treated with local excision and adjuvant radiotherapy (Table 10.2). Twenty-five experienced local recurrence (13%). Local recurrence rates were 7%, 11% and 28% for T1, T2 and T3 lesions respectively. Although the numbers are too small to draw any conclusions, marked morbidity was observed after radiotherapy.

Attention must be paid to tumor location. Several authors have reported that lesions in the inferior third of the rectum have a higher risk of local recurrence, which is independent of TNM stage [63,64]. In a review of published series in which local excision was used as definitive treatment for patients with invasive rectal carcinoma located within 6 cm of the anal verge, and a minimum postoperative follow-up time of 5 years, Graham et al. [65] found a 66% absolute survival rate, an 89% cancer-specific survival rate, and a 24% local recurrence rate. At present, radiotherapy is used for patients who have microscopic margin involvement of the excised specimen in T1 lesions, in whom re-excision is not feasible or desirable, and in patients with T2 or T3 lesions in whom radical resection is excessively risky or the patient refuses resection, even if the margins are clear.

Contact Radiotherapy

The first application of endocavitary contact irradiation was described by LaMarque in Montpellier in 1946 [66]. It was Jean Papillon in Lyon who established this method by reporting the long-term outcome of treatment. Contact radiotherapy is a non-surgical alternative to local excision. The radiation treatment can be performed in the outpatient setting under local anesthesia. It consists of four endorectal applications (20–30 Gy) over a 6-week period. Each application lasts 2–3 minutes. At a depth of 1 cm, 35% of the dose is delivered and, at 2 cm, another 14% is delivered. This prevents detrimental effects on surrounding tissue. The criteria for patient selection are the same as for TLE. Objective response is provided by the regression of the exophytic component after an average of two fractions and by ERUS. Some authors advise interstitial implants of about 20–30 Gy over 2–3 days when a residual infiltration of the rectal wall is still present [67]. Side effects have been reported after contact radiotherapy but they are uncommon; they are tenesmus, diarrhea, ulceration and bleeding [68]. Follow-up usually reveals atrophy of the mucosa and occasional bleeding from telangiectasia. Based on the greater chance for metastasis to lymph nodes with more advanced T stages and the impossibility of assessing histologically the full extent of tumor wall invasion (no specimen obtained), contact radiation is best used in well-selected patients with a high surgical risk. If the patient cannot tolerate a surgical procedure, contact radiation can also be used to treat tumors of the mid- and sometimes the upper third of the rectum, which are areas that are difficult to treat by local excision. TLE offers a better staging option.

Technique

A proctological tilt table is used. Occasionally, patients with a tumor in the posterior rectal wall are treated in the lithotomy position. Lidocaine gel is used to lubricate the anus. A perineal block using 1% lidocaine is occasionally necessary. The distal end of the applicator is 3 cm in diameter. The radiation source used is a Philips Contact RT50. The maximum dose is delivered to the superficial portion of the tumor, while, as already noted, the dose at 1 cm depth is 35% of the given dose, and at 2 cm it is 14%. The usual treatment schedule is a total dose of 120 Gy in three or four treatments at intervals of 2–3 weeks. For large lesions (e.g. 4–5 cm), where palliation is the goal, overlapping fields can be used.

Results of Contact Radiation

Papillon and Berard [69] reported a series of 312 patients over a period of more than 5 years, with none lost to follow-up. All patients had invasive, sessile, well-differentiated or moderately differentiated adenocarcinoma, polypoid in 209 cases and ulcerative in 103. The 5-year disease-free survival was 74%. Of the 26 patients who experienced pelvic failure (8.3%), seven did not undergo salvage surgery because of their poor general condition; seven others were saved by surgery. Some authors have reported local recurrence rates of between 18% and 30% [70,71]. Most of these patients were selected by clinical and histological features because ERUS was not available. Differences in patient selection, radiotherapy technique and additional treatment with iridium implants can explain these results. Gerard et al. [68] reported on 101 patients treated using Papillon's technique. Local recurrence was observed in 14 patients (14%). Of 36 patients

assessed with ERUS, none with uT1N0 tumors experienced local recurrence.

The Cleveland Clinic Experience with Local Treatment of Rectal Cancer

The long-term outcome was assessed in 111 patients undergoing local treatment for rectal cancer between 1980 and 1989 [72]. These data were compared with those of 59 patients undergoing abdominoperineal resection for Stage I rectal cancer over a similar period (1978–1988). Recurrence was seen in 12 of 66 patients (18.2%) receiving contact radiation and in 12 of 45 patients (26.7%) who underwent local excision. After recurrence, curative resection was possible in five of 12 in the contact radiation group and in eight of 12 in local excision group. The crude 5-year survival rate was 85% and 78% for contact radiation and local excision respectively. There was no difference in survival between these groups and no difference when compared with the abdominoperineal resection group. A multivariate analysis showed the only prognostic factors to be tumor size and distance of the lesion from the anal verge.

Over time, our group has become more selective with the application of local treatment, ideally reserving this for uT1 lesions and selectively for T2 lesions. The latter applies particularly when comorbidity or surgical risk factors are significant, or if the patient refuses major resection. Even so, because of the 20–25% risk of occult nodal metastases with T2 lesions, we advise adjuvant radiation. Additionally, there has been greater use of local excision at the expense of contact radiation over time because the advantages of documenting the pathologic level of mural invasion as well as obtaining a complete histologic examination probably outweigh the advantages of contact radiation. This is so with the single exception of lesions situated in the mid- and upper rectum, where access to the lesion is much easier with contact radiation techniques.

Electrocoagulation

Although the use of electrocautery for treating carcinoma dates back to the nineteenth century, electrocoagulation for treating cancer of the rectum was first described by Strauss et al. in 1935 [73]. Initially, electrocoagulation was used as a palliative measure for patients with disseminated cancer or high surgical risk. However, after the surprising success of this technique in achieving local control, early and potentially curable tumors were also selected for this treatment.

The criteria for patient selection are similar to other local treatments. Because of the potential risk of injury to the prostate or vagina (from transmural thermal injury), special attention must be paid to tumors on the anterior rectal wall, especially if there is evidence of deep infiltration.

Electrocoagulation is performed under general or regional, but not local, anesthesia. The entire surface of the tumor is coagulated, as well as an additional 1–2 cm halo of normal mucosa. The eschar is debrided with a curette. The tumor is repeatedly burned until it is completely destroyed. Electrocoagulation is tedious and requires a methodical approach, with operating time averaging 60 minutes. Most patients may be discharged within 24–72 hours and are followed monthly for evidence of persistent or recurrent tumor.

Crile and Turnbull [27] reported on 62 patients treated with electrocoagulation. No postoperative deaths occurred, and the 5-year survival rate was 60%. Compared with ulcerating tumors, patients with exophytic lesions had a better outcome (82% versus 46%). Madden and Kandalaft [74] reported one of the largest studies of electrocoagulation. Of 204 patients, 156 were treated with curative intent; 97 of these patients (62%) had no evidence of metastatic or recurrent disease for at least 5 years. Postoperative complications occurred in 48 patients (23.5%). Eisentat and Oliver [75] reported on 114 patients treated with electrocoagulation for tumors of the distal rectum. Of these, 81 were treated with curative intent and followed up for at least 5 years. The operative mortality and morbidity rates were 2.4% and 21%, respectively. The most important postoperative complications were bleeding and stricture. Because local control was not achieved, an abdominoperineal resection was required in 31 patients (38%). The 5-year survival rate in the remaining 50 patients was 58%.

Electrocoagulation has the same limitation as that of contact radiotherapy in that no specimen is obtained, so the depth of the tumor wall invasion is unknown. Although no prospective randomized study comparing electrocoagulation and contact radiotherapy has been reported, morbidity and long-term outcome appear to be worse after electrocoagulation.

Adjuvant Therapy after Local Treatment

Theoretically, the use of radiation therapy with local treatment may reduce the risk of local recurrence and also control subclinical disease in the regional lymph nodes. For T1 tumors, most authors report a local control rate above 90%. For T2 tumors, the local control rate is closer to 80%, and, for T3 lesions, this rate is below 70% (Table 10.2). Local control rates in these series appear to depend on the depth of tumor invasion, resection margin status, radiation dose and histologic features, especially blood vessel or lymphatic vessel invasion.

Analyzing the real effect of radiation therapy is difficult because of bias in patient selection. On the other hand it is important to be aware of the treatment-related complications, the most important of which are severe proctitis, stricture and fistula.

The main advantage of local treatments (low morbidity) can be lost with the use of radiation. The optimal radiation dose is not well defined. Willet et al. [37] reported no local failures among six patients with positive microscopic resection margins who received total doses of 60–65 Gy. However, the risk of complications increases when the radiation dose is over 55 Gy. The number of patients in this series is too small to draw any conclusion about optimal radiation dose. Birnbaum and colleagues [76] published their outcomes of treating rectal cancer by adding external beam radiotherapy to the index procedure of contact radiation. In an invited commentary on this article, Stocchi and Nelson [77] agreed that this technique was appropriate for patients at high surgical risk. As observed in an earlier section, the rates of lymph node metastasis are fairly constant with T staging (i.e. T1 approximately 10%; T2 approximately 20–30%; and T3 approximately 50–60%). The rates of pelvic failure in this St Louis series, as well as in most other series, parallel the T stage and rates of occult nodal metastases. This suggested that excessive pelvic recurrence rates are associated with non-resective treatments and are probably due to persistent malignancy in lymph nodes. Stocchi and Nelson further commented that, as Birnbaum et al., others had examined their local recurrence outcomes according to defining the terms "ideal" and "non-ideal" lesions. That is, the selection of an early (very early ?) T stage and lesions without adverse prognostic indicators is the best way to achieve excellent results. Willett et al. [37] had reported recurrence-free survival and local control for favorable lesions to be approximately 90% for both local excision (with or without external radiation) and abdominoperineal resection. When non-ideal lesions were similarly treated (e.g. poor differentiation, venous and lymphatic invasion), local excision provided lower (worse) recurrence-free survival (57%) and local control (68%) compared with abdominoperineal resection, 79% and 89% respectively. This implied that resectional surgery is indicated for any T2 lesion (and probably also for T1 lesions) with adverse histological features.

The addition of chemotherapy to radiotherapy appears to decrease local failure in certain subgroups. A prospective study [78] enrolled 20 patients suffering from cancer in the lower third of the rectum. Those with T1 tumors received postoperative radiotherapy only, whereas 15 of 20 patients with T2 and T3 lesions received postoperative radiotherapy plus 5-fluorouracil. There were no local failures at a median follow-up of 47 months. In another prospective series [79] ten of 13 patients with T2 tumors and a single patient with a T3 tumor received 5-fluorouracil concurrently with radiation. All patients had maintained local control at a median follow-up of 25 months.

Salvage Treatment

After local therapy, most failure recurrences are local or perirectal [80]. Because the recurrence site can be examined digitally, patients must be followed every 3–4 months, especially within the first 3 years. Follow-up studies should include digital, endoscopic and endosonographic examination. If local recurrence is confirmed, radical surgery must be performed.

The salvage surgery rate after TLE ranges between 0% and 100%. This high variability can be explained by the fact that most series are small, retrospective and use different criteria for follow-up. Series with follow-up rates longer than 5 years have a mean rate of 42% [65].

Salvage surgery does not mean definitive cure. In fact, about 50% of these patients will experience further recurrence and will die from cancer [49,81,82]. Although no scientific evidence has been reported, we believe that more accurate and frequent follow-up may further improve the outcome of local therapy.

Palliative Local Surgery

Certain patients may present with obstructing rectal cancers. These may be total (rare) or near total in obstructing the rectal lumen; they are often advanced, fixed tumors. Radiation therapy is usually indicated e.g. 45–60 Gy but, when this is administered, the tumor may completely obstruct. The alternatives, therefore, are several. First, such patients may undergo a loop sigmoid colostomy followed by external beam radiation, with later definitive curative or palliative surgery. Secondly, local treatment

has been used to reduce the obstructive mass so that the irradiation is less likely to produce the degree of edema necessary to obstruct the bowel. The alternatives described in this situation include electrocoagulation, laser beam creation of a channel by tumor vaporization, and even the use of the (prostatic) resectoscope. These modalities may also be utilized as the sole therapy for local palliation of advanced rectal cancer, especially when life expectancy is limited.

A further method used in recent years has been the deployment of an intraluminal metal stent. The value of this mesh-like stent is that good palliation (treatment of obstruction) can be obtained without recourse to a colostomy. Stent use is limited by the ability of the endoscopist to traverse the stricture segment. Thus, very irregular and angulated strictures, especially those that are long, may not allow for stent deployment. Complications may include stent migration into adjacent structures. If this in turn produces serious disability, major surgery may be necessary, which negates much of the benefit.

Summary

The main goal of local therapy is local tumor control, therefore accurate preoperative staging is important to identify lesions suitable for such treatment and to avoid or minimize the risk of leaving untreated involved lymph nodes. At present, clinical, histologic and endosonographic staging for tumor invasion and metastatic lymph nodes has a sensitivity and specificity of between 70% and 80%. There is still a significant risk of leaving subclinical disease behind. Advances in the field of molecular markers may improve the staging system in the future. The risk of local recurrence is clearly associated with the degree of tumor invasion (pT stage), so local excision seems to be the best choice of the local treatment options because it allows complete specimen assessment. Among local excision modalities, TLE is associated with the lowest morbidity. If the surgical risk is too high, contact radiotherapy is a good option because it can be carried out under local anesthesia on an outpatient basis. Electrocoagulation has no advantages over the other two local modalities. TEM, when performed by experts, is another alternative whose place remains to be determined. Even though rigid criteria have been followed, the local recurrence rate after local excision for pT1, pT2 and pT3 tumors is 10%, 20% and 30%, respectively. Chemoradiotherapy as an adjuvant treatment has been associated with a decrease in local recurrence rate, especially for pT1 and pT2 tumors (pT1 = 7%; pT2 = 11%; pT3 = 28%). If one of the main advantages of local therapy is its low morbidity, the use of chemoradiotherapy as an adjuvant treatment is debatable. Chemoradiotherapy may not only increase morbidity rates but can adversely affect anal function and quality of life. Small numbers of patients and short follow-up do not allow conclusions to be drawn about the real place of chemoradiotherapy. Patients with pT3 tumors should not be considered for local therapy if curative intent is the option.

It is hard to answer the question about the oncologic effectiveness of local therapy compared with radical resection. No prospective randomized trials have been done and probably will never be. After radical resection the local recurrence rate for patients with Stage I tumors should be below 10%, which is better than those described after local excision. With "ideal" T1 lesions treated by local excision, comparable rates should apply. One cannot assume that local recurrence after local treatment or excision can allow for routine curative salvage surgery. In fact, only about 50% of patients are suitable to undergo curative salvage surgery and the 5-year survival is variable.

In summary, local therapy is a good alternative for patients with small T1 tumors with exophytic, mobile and pathologically favorable characteristics. Patients with T2 tumors and unfavorable histologic features (poorly differentiated tumor, lymphatic or blood vessel invasion, colloid tissue) are advised to undergo rectal resection. In patients with T2 lesions and favorable histology, local excision followed by radiation is an acceptable option but, as with all patients, careful explanation of the risks and benefits (i.e. *informed* consent) must be given. In patients with T2 lesions and comorbidity or other serious risk factors for tolerating the procedure, or for patients who refuse resectional surgery, local excision or contact radiation is appropriate, providing radiation treatment is added to the particular local index therapy.

References

1. Slanetz CA, Herter FP, Grinell RS. Anterior resection versus abdominoperineal resection for cancer of the rectum and rectosigmoid. Am J Surg 1972;123:110–15.
2. Nicholls RJ, Ritchie JK, Wasworth J, Parks AG. Total excision or restorative resection for carcinoma of the middle third of the rectum. Br J Surg 1979;66:625–27.
3. Williams NS, Johnston D. Survival and recurrence after sphincter saving resection and abdominoperineal resection for carcinoma of the middle third of the rectum. Br J Surg 1984;71:278–82.
4. Lavery IC, Lopez-Kostner F, Fazio V, Fernandez-Martin M, Milsom J, Church J. Chances of cure are not compromised with sphincter-saving procedures for cancer of the lower third of the rectum. Surgery 1997;122:779–85.
5. Karanjia ND, Schache DJ, Heald RJ. Function of the distal rectum after low anterior resection for carcinoma. Br J Surg 1992;79:114–16.
6. Otto IC, Katsuki I, Chunlin Y, et al. Causes of rectal incontinence after sphincter-preserving operations for rectal cancer. Dis Colon Rectum 1996;39:1423–27.
7. William NS, Johnston D. The quality of life after rectal excision for low rectal cancer. Br J Surg 1995;70:90–95.
8. Balsev I, Harling H. Sexual dysfunction following operation for carcinoma of the rectum. Dis Colon Rectum 1983;26:785–88.
9. Fazio VW, Fletcher J, Montague D. Prospective study of the effect of resection of the rectum on male sexual function. World J Surg 1980;4:149–52.
10. Kontturi M, Larmi TK, Tuononen S. Bladder dysfunction and its manifestations following abdominoperineal extirpation of the rectum. Ann Surg 1974;179:179–82.
11. Havenga K, Enker WE, Mc Dermott K, Cohen AM, Minsky BD, Guillem J. Male and female sexual urinary function after total mesorectal excision with autonomic nerve preservation for carcinoma of the rectum. J Am Coll Surg 1996;182:495–502.
12. Hughes ESR, McDermott FT, Masterton JP, Cunningham IGE, Polglase AL. Operative mortality following excision of the rectum. Br J Surg 1980;67:49–51.
13. Payne JE, Chapuis PH, Pheils MT. Surgery for large bowel cancer in people aged 75 years and older. Dis Colon Rectum 1986;29:733–37.
14. Stearns MW, Sternberg SS, DeCosse JJ. Treatment alternatives: localized rectal cancer. Cancer 1984;54:2691–94.
15. Horn A, Halvorsen JF, Morild I. Transanal extirpation for early rectal cancer. Dis Colon Rectum 1989;32:769–72.
16. Nicholls RJ, York-Mason AM, Morson BC, Dixon AK, Kelsey-Fry I. The clinical staging of rectal cancer. Br J Surg 1982;69:404–407.
17. Beynon J, Mortensen NJ, Channer JL, Virjee J, Goddard P. Pre-operative assessment of local invasion in rectal cancer: digital examination, endoluminal sonography or computed tomography? Br J Surg 1986;73:1015–17.
18. Waizer A, Zitron S, Ben-Baruch D, Baniel J, Wolloch Y, Dintsman M. Comparative study for preoperative staging of rectal cancer. Dis Colon Rectum 1989;32:53–56.
19. Anderson BO, Hann LE, Enker WE, Dershaw DD, Guillem JG, Cohen AM. Transrectal ultrasonography and operative selection for early carcinoma of the rectum. J Am Coll Surg 1994;179:513–17.
20. Solomon MJ, McLeod RS. Endoluminal transrectal ultrasonography: accuracy, reliability, and validity. Dis Colon Rectum 1993;36:638–42.
21. Hulsmans FJ, Tio TL, Fockens P, Bosna A, Tygat GN. Assessment of tumor infiltration depth in rectal cancer with transrectal sonography: caution is necessary. Radiology 1994;190:715–20.
22. Derksen EJ, Cuesta MA, Meijer S. Intraluminal ultrasound of rectal tumors: a prerequisite in decision making. Surg Oncol 1992;1:193–98.
23. Milsom JW, Lavery IC, Stolfi VM, et al. The expanding utility of endoluminal ultrasonography in the management of rectal cancer. Surgery 1992;112:832–41.
24. Arnaud JP, Bergamaschl R, Schloegel M, et al. Progress in the assessment of lymphatic spread in rectal cancer: rectal endoscopic lymphoscintigraphy. Dis Colon Rectum 1990;33:389–401.
25. Grigg M, McDermott FT, Pihl EA, Hughes ESR. Curative local excision in the treatment of carcinoma of the rectum. Dis Colon Rectum 1984;27:81–83.

26. Abrams JS. Clinical staging of rectal cancer. Am J Surg 1980;139:539–43.

27. Crile G Jr, Turnbull RB Jr. The role of electrocoagulation in the treatment of carcinoma of the rectum. Surg Gynecol Obstet 1972;135:391–96.

28. Mason AY. Rectal cancer: the spectrum of selective surgery [President's address]. Proc R Soc Med 1976;69:237–44.

29. Lock MR, Cairns DW, Ritchie JK, Lockhart-Mummery HE. The treatment of early colorectal cancer by local excision. Br J Surg 1978;65:346–49.

30. Biggers OR, Beart RW, Ilstrup DM. Local excision of rectal cancer. Dis Colon Rectum 1986;29:374–77.

31. Grigg M, McDermott FT, Pihl EA, Hughes ES. Curative local excision in the treatment of carcinoma of the rectum. Dis Colon Rectum 1984;27:81–83.

32. Gerard A, Pector JC, Ferreira J. Local excision as conservative treatment for small rectal cancer. Eur J Surg Oncol 1989;15:544–46.

33. Balslev I, Pedersen M, Teglbjaerg PS, et al. Major or local surgery for cure in early rectal and sigmoid carcinoma. Eur J Surg Oncol 1986;12:373–77.

34. Gall FP, Hermanek P. Update of the German experience with local excision of rectal cancer. Surg Oncol Clin North Am 1992;1:99–109.

35. Despretz J, Otmezguine Y, Grimard L, Calitchi E, Julien M. Conservative management of tumors of the rectum by radiotherapy and local excision. Dis Colon Rectum 1990;33:113–16.

36. Ota DM, Skibber J, Rich TA. MD Anderson Cancer Center experience with local excision and multimodality therapy for rectal cancer. Surg Oncol Clin North Am 1992;1:147–52.

37. Willet CG, Compton CC, Shellito PC, Efird JT. Selection factors for local excision or abdominoperineal resection for early stage rectal cancer. Cancer 1994;73:2716–20.

38. Minsky BD, Enker WE, Cohen AM, Lauwers G. Local excision and postoperative radiation therapy for rectal cancer. Am J Clin Oncol 1994;38:411–16.

39. Fortunato L, Ahmad NR, Yeung RS, et al. Long-term follow-up of local excision and radiation therapy for invasive rectal cancer. Dis Colon Rectum 1995;38:1193–99.

40. Bleday R, Breen E, Jessup JM, Burgess A, Sentovich SM, Steele G. Prospective evaluation of local excision for small rectal cancers. Dis Colon Rectum 1997;40:388–92.

41. Hojo K, Koyama Y, Moriya Y. Lymphatic spread and its prognostic value in patients with rectal cancer. Am J Surg 1982;144:350–54.

42. Hughes TG, Jenevin EP, Poulos E. Intramural spread of colon carcinoma. Am J Surg 1983;146:697–99.

43. Hager T, Gall FP, Hermaneck P. Local excision of cancer of the rectum. Dis Colon Rectum 1983;26:149–51.

44. Minsky BD, Mies C, Recht A, Rich TA, Chaffey JT. Resectable adenocarcinoma of the rectosigmoid and rectum: I. Patterns of failure and survival. Cancer 1988;61:1408–16.

45. Madsen PM, Braenstrup O. Carcinoma recti: the predictive value of diagnostic biopsies for histologic grading. Dis Colon Rectum 1985;28:676–77.

46. Minsky BD, Rich T, Recht A, Harvey W, Mies C. Selection-criteria for local excision with or without adjuvant radiation therapy for rectal cancer. Cancer 1989;63:1421–29.

47. Brodsky J, Richard G, Cohen A, Minsky B. Variables correlated with the risk of lymph node metastasis in early rectal cancer. Cancer 1992;69:322–26.

48. Morson BC. Factors influencing the prognosis of early cancer of the rectum. Proc R Soc Med 1966;59:607–608.

49. Baron PL, Enker WE, Zakowski MF, Urmacher C. Immediate vs. salvage resection after local treatment for early rectal cancer. Dis Colon Rectum 1995;38:177–81.

50. Buess G, Hutterer F, Theiss R, Boebel M, Isselhard W, Pichlmaier H. Das system fur die transanale endoskopische Rektumoperation (German). Chirurg 1984;55:677–80.

51. Said S, Huber P, Pichlmaier H. Technique and clinic results of endorectal surgery. Surgery 1993;113:65–75.

52. Bergman L, Solhaug JH. Posterior trans-sphincteric resection for small tumours of the lower rectum. Acta Chir Scand 1986;152:313–16.

53. Madsen HT, Kronborg O. Posterior transsphincteric rectotomy. Dis Colon Rectum 1987;30:939–41.

54. Sweeney WB, Deshmukh N. Modified Kraske approach for disease of mid-rectum. Am J Gastroenterol 1991;86:75–78.

55. Huber AK, Koella C. The Swiss experience with the parasacral-transsphincteric approach to rectal cancer. Surg Oncol Clin North Am 1992;1:87–97.

56. Morson BC, Bussey HJ, Samoorian S. Policy of local excision for early cancer of the colorectum. Gut 1977;18:1045–50.

57. Mentges B, Buess G, Effinger G, Manncke K, Becker HD. Indications and results of local treatment of rectal cancer. Br J Surg 1997;84:348–51.

58. Buess G, Mentges B, Manncke K, Starlinger M, Becker HD. Minimal invasive surgery in the local treatment of rectal cancer. Int J Colorectal Dis 1991;6:77–81.

59. Smith LE, Ko ST, Saclarides T, Caushaj P, Orkin BA, Khanduja KS. Transanal endoscopic microsurgery. Initial registry results. Dis Colon Rectum 1996;39:S79–S84.

60. Winde G, Nottberg H, Keller R, Schmid KW, Bunte H. Surgical cure for early rectal carcinomas (T1). Transanal endoscopic microsurgery vs. anterior resection. Dis Colon Rectum 1996;39:969–76.

61. Saclarides TJ, Brand MI. Evolving trends in the treatment of anorectal diseases. Dis Colon Rectum 1999;42:1245–52.

62. Coco C, Magistrelli P, Granone P, Roncolini G, Picciocchi A. Conservative surgery for early cancer of the distal rectum. Dis Colon Rectum 1992;35:131–36.

63. Bentzen SM, Balslev I, Pedersen M, et al. Time to loco-regional recurrence after resection of Dukes' B and C colorectal cancer with or without adjuvant postoperative radiotherapy. A multivariate analysis. Br J Cancer 1992;65:102–107.

64. Takahashi T, Kato T, Kodaira S, et al. Prognostic factors of colorectal cancer. Results of multivariate analysis of curative resection cases with or without adjuvant chemotherapy. Am J Clin Oncol 1996;19:408–15.

65. Graham RA, Garnsey L, Jessup JM. Local excision of rectal carcinoma. Am J Surg 1990;160:306–12.

66. LaMarque PL, Gros CG. La radiotherapie de contact des cancers du rectum. J Radiol Electrol 1946;27:333–48.

67. Horiot JC. Local curative treatment of rectal cancer by radiotherapy alone. Int J Colorect Dis 1991;6:89–90.

68. Gerard JP, Ayzac L, Coquard R, Romestaing P, Ardiet JM, Rocher FP. Endocavitary irradiation for early rectal carcinomas T1 (T2). A series of 101 patients treated with Papillon's technique. Int J Radiat Oncol Biol Phys 1996;34:775–83.

69. Papillon J, Berard P. Endocavitary irradiation in the conservative treatment of adenocarcinoma of the low rectum. World J Surg 1992;16:451–57.

70. Hull TL, Lavery IC, Saxton JP. Endocavitary irradiation. An option in selected patients with rectal cancer. Dis Colon Rectum 1994;37:1266–70.

71. Myerson RJ, Walz BJ, Kodner IJ, Fry R. Endocavitary radiation for early rectal carcinoma: the experience at Washington University [abstract]. Int J Radiat Oncol Biol Phys 1987;13:194.

72. Bohm B, Fazio FW, Lavery IC, Milsom JW, Oakley JR, Hull TL. Local curative treatment of low rectal cancer. Int J Surg Sci 1994;11:26–32.

73. Strauss AA, Strauss SF, Crawford RA, Strauss HA. Surgical diathermy of carcinoma of the rectum: its clinical end results. JAMA 1935;104:1480–84.

74. Madden JL, Kandalaft SI. Electrocoagulation as a primary curative method in the treatment of carcinoma of the rectum. Surg Gynecol Obstet 1983;157:347–52.

75. Eisentat TE, Oliver GC. Electrocoagulation for adeno-carcinoma of the low rectum. World J Surg 1992;16:458–62.

76. Birnbaum EH, Ogunbiyi DA, Gagliardi G, et al. Selection criteria for treatment of rectal cancer with combined external and endocavity radiation. Dis Colon Rectum 1999;42:727–33.

77. Stocchi L, Nelson H. Selection criteria for treatment of rectal cancer with combined external and endocavitary radiation [editorial]. Dis Colon Rectum 1999;42:733–35.

78. Wood WC, Willet CG. Update of the Massachusetts General Hospital experience of combined local excision and radio-therapy for rectal cancer. Surg Oncol Clin North Am 1992;1:131–36.

79. Jessup JM, Bothe A, Stone MD, et al. Preservation of sphincter function in rectal carcinoma by a multimodality treatment approach. Surg Oncol Clin North Am 1992;1:137–45.

80. Faivre J, Chaume JC, Pigot F, Trojani M, Bonichon F. Transanal electroresection of small rectal cancer: a sole treatment. Dis Colon Rectum 1996;39:270–78.

81. Bailey HR, Huval W, Max E, Smith KW, Butts DR, Zamora LF. Local excision of carcinoma of the rectum for cure. Surgery 1992;111:555–61.

82. Killingback MJ. Indications for local excision of rectal adenocarcinoma. Br J Surg 1985;72:S54–S56.

11. Postoperative Adjuvant Combined Modality Therapy

B.D. Minsky, C.H. Kohne and C. Greco

Introduction

Significant advances have been made in the adjuvant management of resectable rectal cancer during the 1990s. In patients with clinically resectable disease, pelvic radiation therapy decreases local recurrence. The addition of systemic chemotherapy further decreases local recurrence and improves survival.

This chapter will examine the results and selected controversies concerning patients with clinically resectable rectal cancer treated in the postoperative adjuvant setting. This will include a discussion of the development and results of ongoing and recently completed randomized trials, as well as the design of innovative Phase I/II programs. The role of adjuvant therapy in patients with locally advanced/unresectable disease, as well as after less radical surgery such as a local excision, has been previously reviewed and will not be discussed [1,2]. The role of neoadjuvant (preoperative) combined modality therapy has been discussed in Ch. 5.

Postoperative Therapy

Rationale of Postoperative Combined Modality Therapy

The majority of patients in the USA undergo surgery and, if needed, receive postoperative adjuvant therapy. The most compelling advantage of this approach is pathologic staging. Although advances in preoperative imaging techniques allow more accurate patient selection, it still remains the most common approach. The primary disadvantages include an increased amount of small bowel in the radiation field [3], a potentially hypoxic post-surgical bed, and, if the patient has undergone an abdominoperineal resection, the radiation field must be extended to include the perineal scar.

Results of Postoperative Therapy

In patients who have received conventional doses of radiation (45–55 Gy), non-randomized data reveal a decrease in local recurrence to 4–31% in patients with stage T3–4N0M0 disease and 8–53% in those with stage T3–4N1–2M0 disease [4–6]. Five randomized trials have examined the use of adjuvant postoperative radiation therapy alone in stages T3 and/or N1–2 rectal cancer [7–13]. None has shown an improvement in overall survival. Two revealed a decrease in local failure (National Surgical Adjuvant Breast and Bowel Project (NSABP) RO-1: 16% versus 25%; $p = 0.06$ [7]; and the Medical Research Council: 21% versus 34%; $p = 0.001$ [12]). Of the five trials, the NSABP is the only one in which the radiation was delivered with standard doses and modern techniques.

After publication of the randomized trials from the Gastrointestinal Tumor Study Group (GITSG) [14] and the Mayo Clinic/North Central Cancer Treatment Group (NCCTG) 79-47-51 [15], which revealed a significant improvement in local control (Mayo/NCCTG) and survival (GITSG and Mayo/NCCTG) with postoperative radiation plus bolus 5-fluorouracil/methylchloroethylcyclohexyl-nitrosourea (5-FU/MeCCNU), the National Cancer Institute (NCI) Consensus Conference concluded in 1990 that combined modality therapy was the standard postoperative adjuvant treatment for patients with T3 and/or N1–2 disease [16].

The majority of combined modality therapy regimens include six cycles of 5-FU-based chemotherapy plus concurrent pelvic radiation. Six cycles of chemotherapy are thought to be necessary to treat systemic disease. In contrast, in a trial from Norway, 144 patients were randomized to postoperative radiation plus bolus 5-FU (500–750 mg/m^2 limited to days 1 and 2 of weeks 1, 2 and 3 of radiation therapy) versus surgery alone [17]. Despite the fact that 5-FU was delivered as a radiosensitizer rather than as systemic therapy, this combined modality therapy regimen significantly decreased local recurrence (12% versus 30%; $p = 0.01$) and improved 5-year survival (64% versus 50%; $p = 0.05$). Although these results with limited dose 5-FU are encouraging, additional experience with this approach is needed before modifying the standard recommendation of six cycles of systemic chemotherapy.

Since the 1990 NCI Consensus Conference, the focus of the Intergroup postoperative trials has been the identification of the optimal chemotherapeutic agents and their method of administration. In the follow-up trial to the 79-47-51 trial, the Mayo/NCCTG designed a four-arm trial (86-47-51) to determine if MeCCNU was necessary, as well as to compare the relative effectiveness of 5-FU when delivered as a bolus versus a continuous infusion. MeCCNU did not improve either local control or survival; it is therefore no longer recommended for use in the adjuvant treatment of rectal cancer [18].

When compared with bolus 5-FU (with or without MeCCNU), patients who received continuous infusion 5-FU had a significant decrease in the overall rate of tumor relapse (37% versus 47%; $p = 0.01$), distant metastasis (31% versus 40%; $p = 0.03$), as well as an improvement in 4-year survival (70% versus 60%; $p = 0.005$). These data suggest that when 5-FU is used as a single agent with radiation therapy, it is more effective as a continuous infusion compared with a bolus.

There were also differences in the individual acute toxicities of continuous infusion and bolus 5-FU

INTERGROUP RECTAL TRIAL 0144

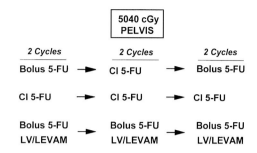

Fig. 11.1. Intergroup 0144 randomized trial of postoperative combined modality therapy. (5-FU, 5-fluorouracil; CI, continuous infusion; LV, leukovorin; LEVAM, levamisole)

regimens. For example, during the combined modality segment, patients who received continuous infusion 5-FU had a significant increase in grade 3+ diarrhea (24% versus 14%; $p < 0.01$), whereas they had a significant decrease in grade 3+ leukopenia (2% versus 11%; $p < 0.01$) compared with bolus 5-FU.

Building on the positive results of continuous infusion 5-FU reported in the Mayo/NCCTG 86-47-51 trial, the replacement postoperative Intergroup trial INT 0144 was designed. The primary endpoint of this trial was to determine whether there is a benefit from continuous infusion 5-FU throughout the entire chemotherapy course (six cycles) when compared with continuous infusion during the combined modality segment only (two cycles) and bolus 5-FU during the remaining four cycles. The control arm is arm 4 (bolus 5-FU/leucovorin (LV)/levamisole) of INT 0114 (Fig. 11.1). The trial opened to accrual in 1993 and completed in 2000.

Table 11.1. Acute toxicity, local control, and survival results of INT 0114

	5-FU	5-FU/LV	5-FU/LEVAM	5-FU/LV/LEVAM
Grade 3+ toxicity (%)				
White blood cells	33	23	23	24
Platelets	49	37	39	38
Diarrhea	19	28	20	35
Maximum toxicity	76	72	70	75
Local failure and survival (%)				
3-y disease-free survival	62	68	62	63
3-y survival	78	80	79	79
Local failure (component)	12	9	13	9

5-FU, 5-fluorouracil; LV, leukovorin; LEVAM, levamisole.

The NSABP RO-1 three-arm trial of postoperative methotrexate, Oncovin and 5-FU (MOF) versus radiation therapy versus surgery alone revealed a significant improvement in 5-year disease-free survival (42% versus 30%; $p = 0.006$) and overall survival (53% versus 43%; $p = 0.05$) with postoperative MOF chemotherapy compared with surgery [7]. The advantage in overall survival of the chemotherapy arm was most evident in males (60% versus 37%) and males less than 65 years of age (44% versus 26%). In contrast, females who received chemotherapy experienced a lower survival (37% versus 54%). It should be emphasized that the trial was not stratified by gender.

As a follow-up to the R-01 trial, the NSABP designed a four-arm trial (R0-2) in which patients were randomized, depending on gender, to either MOF with or without radiation or 5-FU/LV, with or without radiation. A preliminary analysis revealed a significant decrease in local recurrence in the two combined modality therapy arms compared with the two that included chemotherapy alone (7% versus 11%; $p = 0.045$) [19]. However, this did not result in an increase in median survival. Other results are pending.

The most recent Intergroup postoperative trial to report results was INT 0114 [20]. This was a four-arm trial in which all patients received six cycles of postoperative bolus chemotherapy plus concurrent radiation therapy during cycles 3 and 4. The goal of this trial was to determine if combinations of 5-FU-based chemotherapy (5-FU/low-dose LV) versus 5-FU/levamasole versus 5-FU/LV/levamisole) were superior to single-agent 5-FU.

As seen in Table 11.1, with a median follow-up of 4 years, there were no significant differences in local control or survival between the four arms. Although the total incidence of acute grade 3+ toxicity was similar for all four arms, there were differences between the regimens. For example, the 5-FU alone arm had a higher incidence of hematological toxicity, whereas the 5-FU/levamisole arm had a higher incidence of diarrhea [20]. A subset analysis revealed that, in all four arms, women had a significantly greater incidence of acute grade 3+ toxicity compared with men. The reason for this gender difference in toxicity is unclear.

The choice of which postoperative adjuvant regimen to recommend in the non-protocol setting remains controversial. Given that the Mayo/NCCTG 86-47-51 trial revealed that continuous infusion 5-FU is more effective that bolus 5-FU and, since modulation with LV, levamisole, or both, did not improve the results of bolus 5-FU alone in the INT 0114 trial, one could argue that continuous infusion 5-FU is the regimen of choice. INT 0144 directly compares continuous infusion 5-FU with bolus 5-FU/LV/levamisole; however, the results are not yet available. Therefore, for patients not enrolled in a clinical trial, acceptable regimens at this time include either continuous infusion 5-FU or bolus 5-FU plus modulation with LV. These regimens probably have equal efficacy and the choice of a regimen should be based on factors such as their acute toxicity profiles and patient compliance.

Functional Results with Postoperative Therapy

The effect on sphincter function is most likely related to the cumulative impact of all three components of therapy (surgery, radiation and chemotherapy). Not only is there a lack of prospective, randomized data examining functional results but most series use subjective assessment tools such as telephone and mail surveys.

Kollmorgen et al. from the Mayo Clinic examined the impact of postoperative combined modality therapy on bowel function and compared it with a matched group of patients who underwent surgery alone [21]. They used a non-randomized, non-blinded, retrospective telephone survey. Patients who received combined modality therapy had a significant increase in the number of bowel movements, clustering of bowel movements, night-time bowel movements, occasional incontinence, urgency, and wore pads more often compared with those who had undergone surgery alone. Retrospective survey data from the Memorial Sloan-Kettering Cancer Center also suggest that postoperative radiation therapy (with or without chemotherapy) can have a negative impact on sphincter function (increased stool frequency and difficulty with evacuation) in patients who undergo a coloanal anastomosis [22].

In summary, the limited data suggest that postoperative combined modality therapy may affect sphincter function adversely. This potential morbidity needs to be weighed against the benefits of a decrease in local recurrence and improvement and survival with adjuvant therapy. Postoperative combined modality therapy is the most commonly used adjuvant therapy for rectal cancer and remains the benchmark against which other approaches need to be compared.

Decreasing the Toxicity of Pelvic Radiation Therapy

As with other cancer therapies, pelvic radiation, especially in the postoperative setting, is associated with acute and long-term toxicity [23]. A recent analysis of patients treated on the Mayo Clinic/ NCCTG 79-47-51 trial reveals that 5-FU-based chemotherapy further increases the diarrhea associated with pelvic radiation [24].

In general, complications of pelvic radiation are a function of the volume of the radiation field, overall treatment time, fraction size, radiation energy, total dose and technique. A number of simple radiotherapeutic techniques are available to decrease radiation-related small bowel toxicity. For example, the use of multiple field techniques (preferably three fields) allow a larger amount of small bowel to be blocked from the pelvis compared with an anteroposterior/posteroanterior (two-field) technique. In the series from Mak and associates, the incidence of small bowel obstruction in patients with rectal cancer who received pelvic radiation was higher with a single field (21%) compared with a multiple field technique (9%) [25]. The small bowel obstruction rate increased to 30% when extended field radiation was used. Placing the patient prone will usually allow the small intestine to be excluded from the lateral fields.

The treatment should be designed with the use of computed radiation dosimetry and be delivered by high-energy linear accelerators, which, by nature of their depth dose characteristics, deliver a higher dose to the tumor volume while sparing the surrounding normal structures. The treatment of all fields each day results in a lower integral dose and a more homogeneous dose distribution. Sigman and colleagues reported that patients with endometrial or rectal cancer who receive pelvic radiation by a continuous course compared with a planned split course have fewer chronic bowel complications [26]. The use of lateral fields for the boost as well as positioning the patient in the prone position further decreases the volume of small bowel in the lateral radiation fields.

In a number of series, small bowel-related complications are directly proportional to the volume of small bowel in the radiation field [27,28]. In patients who receive conventional doses by standard techniques of preoperative combined modality therapy [29], the small bowel may be the dose-limiting organ [30], restricting the ability to escalate the dose of 5-FU [3]. Small bowel contrast is essential to determine its position during simulation; therefore it should be used routinely during the radiation simulation. Herbert et al. reported that patients with endometrial or rectal cancer who had small bowel contrast used at the time of radiation simulation commonly had a change in the treatment field as well as a lower incidence of overall and chronic complications [31].

In addition to positioning the patient in the prone position and using lateral radiation fields, various physical maneuvers are available to help to exclude the small bowel from the pelvis. These include bladder distension [32], Trendelenburg or inclined procubitis positions [33], and the use of a belly board [34]. However, these measures may be associated with patient discomfort, thereby leading to increased patient movement and daily set-up errors. Therefore, physical maneuvers may not be beneficial in all patients and their use should be individually tailored.

In summary, the toxicities of pelvic radiation need to be examined in perspective. As previously discussed, the primary benefit of postoperative pelvic radiation is to decrease local recurrence. This is all the more reason to pay careful attention to routinely available techniques that help to decrease acute and delayed toxicities.

Is Adjuvant Therapy Necessary after Total Mesorectal Excision?

Some physicians contend that, if patients undergo more extensive surgery, postoperative adjuvant therapy is not necessary. In one series, total mesorectal excision, which involves sharp dissection around the integral mesentery of the hind gut, decreased the local recurrence rate to 5% [35]. However, these data must be interpreted with caution because: these are personal series, they include highly selected patients, and the procedure allows the identification and exclusion of patients with more advanced disease compared with those treated in the adjuvant trials in which total mesorectal excision was not usually performed [36,37]. Likewise, some patients received adjuvant radiation therapy with or without chemotherapy (i.e. 28% in the series from Enker et al. [38] and 18% in the series by Haas-Kock et al. [39]). Furthermore, total mesorectal excision may also be associated with higher complication rates. In the Basingstoke Hospital experience of 219 patients who underwent total mesorectal resection, 16% had anastomotic leaks [40]. In the series from Aitken, operative deaths were excluded from the analysis [41].

On a positive note, advocates of total mesorectal excision have increased the awareness of the importance of careful surgical techniques, which are central to the successful management of rectal cancer. However, they should be considered as a valuable component of therapy, not in competitition with adjuvant therapy. The relative benefits and risks of total mesorectal excision (focusing on endpoints such as local control, survival, sphincter preservation and function, surgical morbidity and mortality, and quality of life) need to be more carefully documented.

Investigational Approaches

Although there have been advances in adjuvant therapy, the development of innovative treatment techniques needs to continue. Selected approaches include radiation fractionation schemas and new chemotherapeutic agents. Some of these modalities have been developed in patients with advanced disease and have not yet been used in the adjuvant setting.

Altered Radiation Fractionation Schemes

Various fractionation programs have evolved with the goal of enhancing tumor cell damage by radiation without increasing normal tissue injury [42]. The repair of subcellular injury, regeneration, cell cycle redistribution, and reoxygenation are all factors at the cellular level that contribute to differences in how various normal tissues and tumors respond to fractionated radiation. The use of hyperfractionation and accelerated fractionation schemes take advantage of some of these factors. A Phase I trial from Lausanne of postoperative accelerated hyperfractionation (1.6 Gy b.i.d. to 48 Gy) reported acceptable acute toxicity [43]. A follow-up report from this group suggests that twice daily radiation is better tolerated when delivered preoperatively compared with postoperatively [44]. Although the late effects should be the same as or, more likely, less than conventional fractionation schemes, the major limitation of accelerated hyperfractionation is acute normal tissue toxicity.

In a randomized trial of patients receiving radiation therapy for pelvic malignancies, three-dimensional conformal radiation therapy decreased the volume of normal tissue in the radiation field; however, it did not decrease acute toxicity [45]. Other techniques such as neutron beam radiation [46], hyperthermia [47,48], radiosensitizers [49], radioprotectors [50,51], altered radiation fractionation schemes [43,44], and proton and three-dimensional treatment planning [52,53], are encouraging but they remain experimental.

New Chemotherapeutic Agents

Selected new chemotherapeutic agents with activity in colorectal cancer, which are in either in development or have been approved, include CPT-11, tomudex, trimetrexate, oxaliplatin, and a combination of uracil and ftorafur (UFT) [54–57]. Clinical trials examining the combination of some of these agents with pelvic radiation are under way [58,59]. In patients with unresectable disease, Marsh and associates have combined chronobiologically-shaped 5-FU infusions with preoperative radiation therapy [60].

Summary

For patients with T3 and/or N1–2 disease, the standard adjuvant postoperative management is combined modality therapy. This includes six cycles of 5-FU-based chemotherapy and concurrent pelvic irradiation during cycles 3 and 4. Ongoing trials will help to determine the ideal chemotherapeutic agents and methods of administration.

References

1. Minsky BD. Management of locally advanced/unresectable rectal cancer. Radiat Oncol Invest 1995;3:97–107.
2. Minsky BD. Results of local excision followed by postoperative radiation therapy for rectal cancer. Radiat Oncol Invest 1997;5:246–251.
3. Minsky BD, Conti JA, Huang Y, Knopf K. The relationship of acute gastrointestinal toxicity and the volume of irradiated small bowel in patients receiving combined modality therapy for rectal cancer. J Clin Oncol 1995;13:1409–16.
4. Willett CG, Tepper JE, Kaufman DS, et al. Adjuvant postoperative radiation therapy for rectal adenocarcinoma. Am J Clin Oncol 1992;15:371–75.
5. Romsdahl MM, Withers HR. Radiotherapy combined with curative surgery: its use as therapy for carcinomas of the sigmoid colon and rectum. Arch Surg 1978;113:446–53.
6. Vigliotti A, Rich TA, Romsdahl MM, Withers HR, Oswald MJ. Postoperative adjuvant radiotherapy for adenocarcinoma of the rectum and rectosigmoid. Int J Radiat Oncol Biol Phys 1987;13:999–1006.
7. Fisher B, Wolmark N, Rockette H, et al. Postoperative adjuvant chemotherapy or radiation therapy for rectal cancer: results from NSABP protocol R-01. J Natl Cancer Inst 1988;80:21–29.
8. Balslev I, Pedersen M, Teglbjaerg PS, et al. Postoperative radiotherapy in Dukes' B and C carcinoma of the rectum and rectosigmoid: a randomized multicenter study. Cancer 1986;58:22–28.
9. Gastrointestinal Tumor Study Group. Prolongation of the disease-free interval in surgically treated rectal carcinoma. N Engl J Med 1985;312:1465–72.
10. Gastrointestinal Tumor Study Group. Adjuvant therapy of colon cancer: results of a prospectively randomized trial. N Engl J Med 1984;310:737–43.
11. Arnaud JP, Nordlinger B, Bosset JF, et al. Radical surgery and postoperative radiotherapy as combined treatment in rectal cancer. Final results of a Phase III study of the European Organization for Research and Treatment of Cancer. Br J Surg 1997;84:352–57.

12. Medical Research Council Rectal Cancer Working Party. Randomized trial of surgery alone versus surgery followed by post-operative radiotherapy for mobile cancer of the rectum. Lancet 1996;348:1610–15.

13. Medical Research Council Rectal Cancer Working Party. Randomized trial of surgery alone versus radiotherapy followed by surgery for potentially operable, locally advanced rectal cancer. Lancet 1996;348:1605–609.

14. Douglass HO, Moertel CG, Mayer RJ, et al. Survival after postoperative combination treatment of rectal cancer. N Engl J Med 1986;315:1294–95.

15. Krook JE, Moertel CG, Gunderson LL, et al. Effective surgical adjuvant therapy for high-risk rectal carcinoma. N Engl J Med 1991;324:709–15.

16. National Institutes of Health Consensus Conference. Adjuvant therapy for patients with colon and rectal cancer. JAMA 1990;264:1444–50.

17. Tveit KM, Guldvog I, Hagen S, et al. Randomized controlled trial of post-operative radiotherapy and short-term time-scheduled 5-fluorouracil against surgery alone in the treatment of Dukes' B and C rectal cancer. Br J Surg 1997;84:1130–35.

18. O'Connell MJ, Martenson JA, Weiand HS, et al. Improving adjuvant therapy for rectal cancer by combining protracted infusion fluorouracil with radiation therapy after curative surgery. N Engl J Med 1994;331:502–507.

19. Rockette H, Deutsch M, Petrelli N, et al. Effect of post-operative radiation therapy (RTX) when used with adjuvant chemotherapy in Dukes' B and C rectal cancer: results from NSABP-RO2 [abstract]. Proc ASCO 1994;13:193.

20. Tepper JE, O'Connell MJ, Petroni GR, et al. Adjuvant post-operative fluorouracil-modulated chemotherapy combined with pelvic radiation therapy for rectal cancer: initial results of Intergroup 0114. J Clin Oncol 1997;15:2030–39.

21. Kollmorgen CF, Meagher AP, Pemberton JH, Martenson JA, Ilstrup DM. The long term effect of adjuvant postoperative chemoradiotherapy for rectal cancer on bowel function. Ann Surg 1994;220:676–82.

22. Paty PB, Enker WE, Cohen AM, Minsky BD, Friedlander-Klar H. Long-term functional results of coloanal anastomosis for rectal cancer. Am J Surg 1994;167:90–95.

23. Coia L, Myerson R, Tepper JE. Late effects of radiation therapy on the gastrointestinal tract. Int J Radiat Oncol Biol Phys 1995;31:1213–36.

24. Miller RC, Martenson JA, Sargent DJ, Kahn MJ, Krook JE. Acute diarrhea during rectal adjuvant postoperative pelvic radiation therapy (RT) with or without 5-fluorouracil: a detailed analysis of toxicity from a randomized North Central Cancer Treatment Group study [abstract]. Proc ASCO 1998;17:279a.

25. Mak AC, Rich TA, Schultheiss TE, Kavanagh B, Ota DA, Romsdahl MM. Late complications of postoperative radiation therapy for cancer of the rectum and rectosigmoid. Int J Radiat Oncol Biol Phys 1994;28:597–603.

26. Sigman WR, Randall ME, Olds WE, McCunniff AJ, St.Clair WH, Craven TE. Increased chronic bowel complications with split-course pelvic irradiation. Int J Radiat Oncol Biol Phys 1993;28:349–53.

27. Mameghan H, Fisher R, Mameghan J, Watt WH, Tynan A. Bowel complications after radiotherapy for carcinoma of the prostate: the volume effect. Int J Radiat Oncol Biol Phys 1990;18:315–20.

28. Gunderson LL, Russell AH, Llewellyn HJ, Doppke KP, Tepper JE. Treatment planning for colorectal cancer: radiation and surgical techniques and value of small-bowel films. Int J Radiat Oncol Biol Phys 1985;11:1379–93.

29. Minsky BD, Cohen AM, Enker WE, et al. Combined modality therapy of rectal cancer: decreased acute toxicity with the pre-operative approach. J Clin Oncol 1992;10:1218–24.

30. Frykholm GJ, Isacsson U, Nygard K, et al. Preoperative radiotherapy in rectal carcinoma – aspects of acute adverse effects and radiation technique. Int J Radiat Oncol Biol Phys 1996;35:1039–48.

31. Herbert SH, Curran WJ, Solin LJ, Stafford PM, Lanciano RM, Hanks GE. Decreasing gastrointestinal morbidity with the use of small bowel contrast during treatment planning for pelvic radiation. Int J Radiat Oncol Biol Phys 1991;20:835–42.

32. Gallagher MJ, Brereton HD, Rostock RA, et al. A prospective study of treatment techniques to minimize the volume of pelvic small bowel with reduction of acute and late effects associated with pelvic irradiation. Int J Radiat Oncol Biol Phys 1986;12:1565–73.

33. Caspers RJL, Hop WCJ. Irradiation of true pelvis for bladder and prostatic carcinoma in supine, prone, or Trendelenburg position. Int J Radiat Oncol Biol Phys 1983;9:589–93.

34. Das IJ, Lanciano RM, Movsas B, Kagawa K, Barnes SJ. Efficacy of a belly board device with CT-simulation in reducing small bowel volume within pelvic irradiation fields. Int J Radiat Oncol Biol Phys 1997;39:67–76.

35. MacFarlane JK, Ryall RD, Heald RJ. Mesorectal excision for rectal cancer. Lancet 1993;341:457–60.

36. Hida JH, Yasutomi M, Maruyama T. Lymph node metastasis detected in the mesorectum distal to carcinoma of the rectum by the clearing method: justification of total mesorectal excision. J Am Coll Surg 1997;184:584–80.

37. Arenas RB, Fichera A, Mhoon D, Michelassi F. Total mesenteric excision in the surgical treatment of rectal cancer. A prospective study. Arch Surg 1998;133:608–12.

38. Enker WE, Thaler HT, Cranor ML, Polyak T. Total mesorectal excision in the operative treatment of carcinoma of the rectum. J Am Coll Surg 1995;181:335–45.

39. Haas-Kock DFM, Baeten CGMI, Jager JJ, et al. Prognostic significance of radial margins of clearance in rectal cancer. Br J Surg 1996;83:781–85.

40. Carlsen E, Schlichting E, Guldvog I, Johnson E, Heald RJ. Effect of the introduction of total mesorectal excision for the treatment of rectal cancer. Br J Surg 1998;85:526–29.

41. Aitken RJ. Mesorectal excision for rectal cancer. Br J Surg 1996;83:214–16.

42. Withers HR. Biological basis for altered fractionation schemes. Cancer 1985;55:2086–95.

43. Coucke PA, Cuttat JF, Mirimanoff RO. Adjuvant post-operative accelerated hyperfractionated radiotherapy in rectal cancer: a feasibility study. Int J Radiat Oncol Biol Phys 1993;27:885–89.

44. Coucke PA, Sartorelli B, Cuttat JF, Jeanneret W, Gillet M, Mirimanoff RO. The rationale to switch from postoperative hyperfractionated accelerated radiotherapy to preoperative hyperfractionated accelerated radiotherapy in rectal cancer. Int J Radiat Oncol Biol Phys 1995;32:181–88.

45. Tait DM, Nahum AE, Meyer LC, et al. Acute toxicity in pelvic radiotherapy; a randomised trial of conformal versus conventional treatment. Radiother Oncol 1997;42:121–36.

46. Duncan W, Arnott SJ, Jack WJL, Orr JA, Kerr GR, Williams JR. Results of two randomized trials of neutron therapy in rectal adenocarcinoma. Radiother Oncol 1987;8:191–98.

47. Ichikawa D, Yamaguchi T, Yoshioka Y, Sawai K, Takahashi T. Prognostic evaluation of preoperative combined treatment for advanced cancer in the lower rectum with radiation, intraluminal hyperthermia, and 5-fluorouracil suppository. Am J Surg 1996;171:346–50.

48. Ohno S, Tomoda M, Tomisaki S, et al. Improved surgical results after combining preoperative hyperthermia with chemotherapy and radiotherapy for patients with carcinoma of the rectum. Dis Colon Rectum 1997;40:401–406.

49. Liu T, Liu Y, He S, Zhang Z, Kligerman MM. Use of radiation with or without WR-2721 in advanced rectal cancer. Cancer 1992;69:2820–25.

50. Stelzer KJ, Koh WJ, Kurtz H, Greer BE, Griffin TW. Caffeine consumption is associated with decreased severe late toxicity after radiation to the pelvis. Int J Radiat Oncol Biol Phys 1994;30:411–17.

51. Rhomberg W, Eiter H, Hergan K, Schneider B. Inoperable recurrent rectal cancer: results of a prospective trial with radiation therapy and razoxane. Int J Radiat Oncol Biol Phys 1994;30:419–25.

52. Tatsuzaki H, Urie MM, Willett CG. 3-D comparative study of proton vs X-ray radiation therapy for rectal cancer. Int J Radiat Oncol Biol Phys 1991;22:369–74.

53. Isacsson U, Montelius A, Jung B, Glimelius B. Comparative treatment planning between proton and X-ray therapy in locally advanced rectal cancer. Radiother Oncol 1997;41:263–72.

54. Pitot HC, Wender DB, O'Connell MJ, et al. Phase II trial of irinotecan in patients with metastatic colorectal carcinoma. J Clin Oncol 1997;15:2910–19.

55. Cunningham D, Zalcberg JR, Rath U, et al. Final results of a randomised trial comparing "Tomudex" (raltitrexed) with 5-fluorouracil plus leucovorin in advanced colorectal cancer. Ann Oncol 1996;961:961–65.

56. Saltz LB, Leichman CG, Young CW, et al. A fixed-ratio combination of uracil and ftorafur (UFT) with low dose leucovorin. Cancer 1995;75:782–85.

57. Gorlick R, Metzger R, Danenberg K, et al. Higher levels of thymidylate synthase gene expression are observed in pulmonary as compared with hepatic metastases of colorectal adenocarcinoma. J Clin Oncol 1998;16:1465–69.

58. Botwood N, James R, Vernon C, Price P. A Phase I study of "Tomudex" (raltitrexed) with radiotherapy (RT) as adjuvant treatment in patients (pt) with operable rectal cancer [abstract]. Proc ASCO 1998;17:277a.

59. Rich TA, Kirichenko AV. Camptothecin radiation sensitization: mechanisms, schedules, and timing. Oncology 1998;12:114–19.

60. Marsh RW, Chu NM, Vauthey JN, et al. Preoperative treatment of patients with locally advanced unresectable rectal adenocarcinoma utilizing continuous chronobiologically shaped 5-fluorouracil infusion and radiation therapy. Cancer 1996;78:217–25.

12. Follow-up After Potentially Curative Therapy for Rectal Cancer

D.E. Nadig, K.S. Virgo, W.E. Longo and F.E. Johnson

Introduction

Colorectal cancer is a relatively common malignancy, particularly in developed countries in the western world. In the USA approximately 130 200 new cases were identified and approximately 56 300 died of their disease in 2000 [1]. In approximately 70% of patients, colorectal cancer is surgically treatable for cure. However, 30–50% eventually develop recurrence and die of their disease [2,3]. Today, physicians have at their disposal a variety of biochemical and imaging modalities to aid their efforts in detecting these recurrences while they are still potentially curable. It remains a real dilemma, both practically and economically, whether any specific test or combination of tests offers the best results. Furthermore, the optimal interval between tests is based primarily on anecdotal evidence.

As the treatment of cancer began to reach levels of sophistication and reproducibility, it became apparent early on that treatment failures were common, and often fatal. In 1951 Wangensteen et al. recognized the unfortunate consequences of recurrence and the high mortality rates for treatment failures of colorectal cancer. They proposed second-look laparotomy as a method to enhance the cure rate in asymptomatic patients who were judged to be at high risk for developing recurrent disease [4]. This was based on the premonition that the discovery of early recurrent disease would permit potentially curative resection, which is the cornerstone of salvage treatment. After a 13-year experience, Wangensteen [5] and Gilbertsen and Wangensteen [6] reported that the morbidity and mortality of this approach outweighed its benefits. Despite this, the belief persisted that earlier detection of recurrence would lead to greater patient benefit.

Modern imaging techniques have led to improved detection of recurrent disease, especially in asymptomatic patients. A number of reports have now documented clear benefit in terms of survival duration and cure rates in highly selected patients after resection of recurrent colorectal disease. These reports provide a rationale for postoperative follow-up, but the assumption that high intensity postoperative surveillance is more beneficial than low intensity surveillance is controversial. To date no study has definitively shown that aggressive postoperative follow-up leads to prolonged disease-free survival or cure. Indeed, several studies have brought into question the usefulness of any follow-up regimen [7–11].

When discussing follow-up after potentially curative treatment for rectal cancer, most pre-existing data center around patients with both colon and rectal cancer. However, there are certain follow-up issues that are unique to rectal cancer: first, the fact that the pelvis represents the most common site for recurrence; and secondly, that local full-thickness excision represents a unique way to treat rectal cancer but not colon cancer. This chapter will discuss: the background of detecting recurrent disease; the utility of the various methods of detecting recurrent disease, such as history and physical examination; laboratory findings, including tumor markers; the role of endoscopic follow-up; and the utility of various imaging modalities such as computed tomographic (CT) scanning, magnetic resonance imaging (MRI), and immunoscintigraphy. Finally, evidence-based recommendations regarding suggested follow-up will be provided. The ultimate goal is the development of a follow-up plan that will be simple, effective and economic. The authors have been fortunate enough at the time of writing this chapter to be able to incorporate the recommendations for colorectal cancer surveillance published by the American Society of Clinical Oncology (ASCO) [12].

Background

Serious interest in the follow-up of patients with colon and rectal cancer began in the late 1980s and lasted into the early 1990s. Steele remarked in 1993 that there is no evidence that earlier diagnosis of asymptomatic, or even symptomatic, colon and rectal cancer recurrences will lead to any greater chance of cure [13]. He added that, with the exception of a subset of patients found to have isolated regional failure, the early diagnosis of asymptomatic recurrent colorectal cancer does not lead to any reasonable probability of curative therapy.

A 1993 survey of the members of the American Society of Colon and Rectal Surgeons examined patterns of surveillance in patients whose colon cancer had been treated with potentially curative surgery [14]. This survey assessed the use of nine follow-up measures, including office visits, complete blood counts, liver function tests, serum carcinoembryonic antigen (CEA) levels, chest radiography, bone scanning, CT, colonoscopy and flexible sigmoidoscopy. Among the responding members of this organization of colorectal cancer experts, wide variation in practice was found and no clear consensus patterns could be identified. In a similar study of the Society of Surgical Oncology there was also wide variability in test ordering patterns among respondents. The practices of members of the Society of Surgical Oncology differed moderately from those of the previously surveyed members of the American Society of Colon and Rectal Surgeons. It is interesting that the charge differential between high- and low-intensity follow-up regimens for each patient cohort was about $800 million per year [15]. Other studies have demonstrated how geographic variation, surgeon's age and tumor stage affect follow-up [16–18]. Charges vary extensively between follow-up strategies, with no indication that higher-cost strategies increase survival or quality of life [19]. It can be presumed that the results of these studies and the similar lack of consensus would also pertain to rectal cancer.

The main aims of follow-up programs include: (1) to measure the efficacy of the original therapy; (2) to detect metachronous or new malignancies; and (3) to detect potentially curable recurrence [20]. Estimating the curative potential of treatment does not require sophisticated tests because recurrent disease eventually declares itself in most patients [21]. Some argue that, at this time, the only

irrefutable benefit of postoperative follow-up is in the identification of metachronous disease (i.e. adenomatous polyps, new colorectal malignancies, and new primaries in other organ systems). The final aim and the focus of much debate is the identification of recurrent disease that is amenable to resection. Still others reasons for postoperative follow-up are listed below:

- Early detection of recurrence, leading to early treatment
- Detection of a second primary, leading to early treatment
- Detection of complications of initial therapy, leading to remedial efforts
- Audit of results of initial therapy
- Rehabilitation
- Psychological support
- Risk counseling for patient and family
- Avoidance of medical malpractice risks
- Maintaining rapport with patients and referring physicians
- Routine health care maintenance to improve overall quality of life

In devising a plan for patient follow-up, it is important to recognize the anatomic and temporal patterns of recurrence as well as their relationship to the initial tumor staging. The recurrence of colorectal cancer is for the most part a time-limited phenomenon. In all, 60–80% of recurrences become apparent within the first 2 years after initial resection and 90% within the first 4 years [21–23]. Pihl et al. showed that the risk of recurrence is related to the stage of the primary cancer [24]. In their study of 1315 patients, 801 had rectal cancer and the 5-year disease-free survival rate after rectal cancer surgery was 86% for Dukes' stage A, 77% for stage B, 60% for stage C, and 4% for stage D. The overall recurrence rate for rectal cancer was 42% at 5 years. Those with rectal cancer had a 12% incidence of local recurrence. In this group, systemic recurrence occurred in the absence of local disease in 18%. Systemic disease occurred in the liver (12%), lung (3%), bone (0.9%), brain (0.7%), lymph nodes (4%) and peritoneum (2%). Rectal cancer, when compared with colon cancer, was associated with a higher recurrence rate as well as a shorter overall survival duration.

Although no strong evidence supports a single follow-up strategy, there is little argument that some patients with recurrent colorectal disease do benefit from the resection of recurrences. In fact, surgery represents the only reasonable chance for cure in these patients. Carcinoma of the rectum typically spreads laterally within the pelvis and metastasizes by lymphatic and/or hematogenous routes [25]. Patients with local recurrence, hepatic metastases and pulmonary metastases can sometimes be cured with repeat resection. Local recurrence is thought to be related to the anatomic confines of the pelvis, which make the initial wide resection difficult. Some authors report that pelvic recurrence is incurable [26], others that cure is likely only when the disease is localized to the suture line [27,28].

At least 20% of people with a history of colorectal carcinoma will develop hepatic metastases. Of these, around 15–20% will have disease confined to a localized volume within the liver that is amenable to cure [29]. Following successful resection of an isolated hepatic metastasis, 5-year survival rates in large multi-institutional studies range from 20% to 30%, with operative mortality rates of less than 5% [30,31]. The mean survival duration with untreated hepatic metastases from colorectal carcinoma is approximately 6 months [32].

Pihl et al., in 1987, reported a review of 1578 patients over 32 years who underwent resection of colorectal carcinoma [33]. They stated that 11.5% of those with primary rectal carcinoma developed pulmonary metastasis. Sixteen patients underwent surgery for isolated lung metastases and four patients remained alive at 2, 6 and 15 years. The conditional probability of survival for the 16 patients was $38 \pm 13\%$ at 5 years. Goldberg et al. reported a 27% 5-year survival rate for individuals who underwent curative resection of solitary pulmonary colorectal metastases [32].

Although there is little proof that the identification of recurrent disease in follow-up programs increases the likelihood of resectability, cure or prolonged survival, many physicians have witnessed the successful treatment of recurrent colorectal cancer. These anecdotal experiences, the unproven belief that follow-up is beneficial, and traditions imparted during training, are among the likely motivating factors for most physicians caring for colorectal cancer patients.

Methods of Recurrence Detection

History and Physical Examination

Beart et al. reported on 168 colorectal cancer patients who were followed prospectively after primary resection [34,35]. Each patient was seen for follow-up at a minimum of every 4 months. Diagnostic studies used to complement the history and physical examination included chest radiographs, liver function tests, complete blood counts, CEA serum levels, barium enema, flexible sigmoidoscopy, and colonoscopy. Of the 168 patients followed, 48 developed recurrence. Of these, 41 had symptoms prior to confirmation of recurrence on physical examination, serologic testing or radiologic examination. These symptoms included coughing, abdominal or pelvic pain, changes in bowel habits, rectal bleeding and malaise. Physical examination was less sensitive than patient history, suggesting that the reporting of symptoms may lead to an earlier diagnosis of recurrence than frequent physical examinations. Those with positive findings had either symptoms or elevated CEA levels. It is generally believed, but not proven, that recurrent disease that is symptomatic or can be detected on physical examination is more likely to be advanced and incurable. Cochran et al. reported that only one of 71 patients whose history and physical examination led to the diagnosis of recurrence was later cured surgically [36]. Small anastomotic recurrences after low anterior resection, which might be evident on physical examination, may still be amenable to cure. In the follow-up of rectal cancer patients, digital rectal examination, palpation of groin nodes, and bimanual pelvic examination in women can be useful.

Laboratory Investigations

Fecal Occult Blood

The detection of fecal occult blood is a useful and cost-effective tool in screening for primary and metachronous colorectal malignancy [37]. It is of little value, however, in the detection of recurrent disease because most recurrences are extraluminal and do not interrupt the mucosa. Beart et al. reported that only six of 48 patients with recurrent disease had positive fecal occult blood tests [34,35]. Crowson et al. showed that 7.2% of patients with anastomotic recurrence had positive tests [38].

Liver Function Tests

The liver is the most common site of metastasis from colorectal carcinoma, representing approximately 50% of all recurrences [39]. Measurement of the serum alkaline phosphatase level was described in 1940 to be the best non-invasive means of testing for hepatic metastases [40]. In a study of 327 patients with a history of colorectal cancer, 43 of the 56 patients subsequently found to have liver metastases also had elevated levels of alkaline phosphatase, giving a sensitivity of 77% [41]. There were, however, 110 patients without metastases who also had elevated levels, a false-positive rate of 34%. Thirteen patients with metastatic disease had normal levels, giving a false-negative rate of 4%. Given its low specificity to predict hepatic metastases, as well as the development of a more sensitive and specific serological marker (CEA), the serum alkaline phosphatase level has fallen out of favor as a screening tool.

Carcinoembryonic Antigen

CEA was first identified in colorectal cancer tissue in 1965 by Gold and Freedman [42]. CEA is a glycoprotein oncofetal tumor-associated antigen whose biological function remains unclear. A role in the turnover of digestive epithelium has been suggested but not proven [43]. In general, a serum CEA level of greater than 5 ng/ml is considered abnormal. It was initially hoped that CEA measurement would provide a sensitive and specific marker for the presence of colorectal malignancy, but the sensitivity [44] and specificity [45–47] are low. It is also a relatively expensive test, so it is not useful as a screening tool for any cancer. However, CEA has some value as a tumor marker in patients with known cancer. It has been shown to correlate with tumor volume [48], response to antitumor therapy [49], and the likelihood of persistent tumor remaining after primary resection [50]. After curative resection, an elevated CEA level should fall to normal within 4–8 weeks [44]. If this does not occur, then incomplete resection is likely. Unfortunately, 20–30% of individuals with recurrent disease will have normal CEA levels. The sensitivity and specificity of CEA in detecting recurrent colorectal cancer are approximately 70% and 80%, respectively [51]. The utility of rising CEA levels in predicting recurrent disease has also been confirmed in individuals with normal preoperative levels. In a study of node-positive colorectal cancer patients with normal preoperative CEA levels, 96% (109/114) had tumors that were positive for CEA by immunohistochemistry [52]. From this group, 32 had recurrent disease. Forty-four percent (14/32) demonstrated elevated CEA levels at the time of diagnosis of recurrence. Several studies have reported that CEA monitoring can lead to a diagnosis of recurrent disease before it is revealed by the history and physical examination, with a median lead time of approximately 6 months [51,53–55].

A common question is what CEA level should trigger further work-up for recurrent disease or lead to exploratory surgery. Some use a single value above a certain cut-off point, such as 5 ng/ml. Others require two consecutive elevated results and still others require a specific slope of the rise in CEA levels to indicate likely recurrence [56]. At present

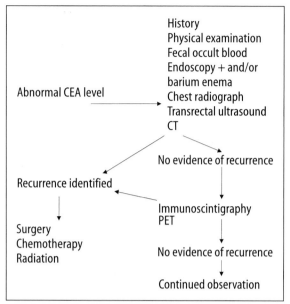

Fig. 12.1.   CEA algorithm.

there is no consensus, although most agree that a single test is less reliable than two or more. Additionally, the ideal frequency of CEA level assessment has not been established. The fundamental utility of CEA monitoring has been questioned by more than one investigator because it has not been shown convincingly that earlier diagnosis using CEA monitoring leads to prolonged survival or increased cure rates [47,57]. Northover et al. randomized patients after undergoing curative surgery to an active intervention group or a control group [58]. CEA was measured in all patients at frequent intervals and, in the active intervention group, a rising CEA prompted further investigation, including second-look laparotomy when appropriate. Preliminary analysis showed no difference in survival between the two groups. Fig. 12.1 depicts an algorithm showing how abnormal CEA levels can be used to identify the presence of recurrence and lead to evaluation and treatment.

Other Tumor Markers

Since the discovery of CEA, other colorectal cancer-associated antigens, including TAG-72 and CA19-9 have been discovered [59–61]. Neither of these has been found to have greater utility than CEA, although TAG-72 has been suggested to complement CEA [60]. The development of a test with high sensitivity and specificity remains a worthwhile goal. Molecular biological approaches hold some promise.

Endoscopy

Colonoscopy is an important part of follow-up for colorectal cancer patients because they are at increased risk for the development of metachronous colorectal neoplasms. Additionally, when possible, these patients should undergo preoperative colonoscopy to the cecum in order to identify synchronous lesions. Three to seven percent of patients about to undergo colorectal cancer resection are found to have a second or synchronous malignancy requiring resection at another location within the colon or rectum [62]. An additional 25% have adenomas that also require removal. Those individuals who present with obstruction or perforation should undergo colonoscopy within 3–6 months after resection. In addition to the detection of synchronous lesions, endoscopy is useful in identifying metachronous lesions as well as anastomotic recurrences. Patients with prior rectal cancer are clearly at high risk for a second colorectal malignancy. Reilly et al. showed that six of 78 patients (8%) undergoing routine endoscopy developed a metachronous neoplasm within an average of 3.7 years after resection of a colorectal cancer [63]. Endoscopy provides added benefit in that potentially troublesome polyps can be removed.

Endoscopy can also be useful in the identification of intraluminal anastomotic recurrences. Anastomotic and local recurrence occurs more frequently with rectal cancers than with colon cancers. Slanetz et al. showed a 13% anastomotic recurrence rate for tumors located 8–13 cm from the anal verge [64]. The reasons given for anastomotic recurrence include lapses in surgical technique, implantation of viable tumor cells, and inadequate distal or lateral margins [65]. The great majority of those presenting with anastomotic recurrence are found to have either extensive local or systemic disease [65,66].

In a retrospective analysis of anastomotic recurrences in 50 patients, Rodriguez-Bigas et al. reported that five patients were alive without disease after 5 years [65]. Eighty-two percent of these anastomotic recurrences were identified on endoscopy. All of these patients were noted to have been asymptomatic at the time of diagnosis and the recurrence was limited to the anastomosis on postoperative microscopic inspection. This study suggests that routine endoscopy, particularly in those with a history of rectal cancer resection (low anterior resection), may lead to potential cure of recurrent disease. The ideal interval between endoscopic examinations has not been determined. The ascertainment of what subset of patients benefit most has not been shown. A prospective trial is needed.

Imaging Modalities

Rectal cancer recurrence can occur in multiple locations. This discussion will therefore be broken down by potential area of recurrence (locoregional, hepatic, pulmonary, brain, bone) and appropriate modalities will then be discussed. As is true for all follow-up modalities to date, no postoperative imaging strategy has been shown unequivocally to improve cure rates or to extend survival time.

Locoregional Metastases

Local recurrence is recurrence at or adjacent to the site of the primary tumor, including the anastomosis, tumor bed and regional lymph nodes. Barium enema has been the most used method of postoperative surveillance. Although not as sensitive as endoscopy (97%), air-contrast barium enema has been shown to detect approximately 90% of intraluminal malignancies [67]. The radiologic features include intraluminal filling defect, eccentric anastomotic narrowing, and local extrinsic mass effect. When the local recurrence does not involve the anastomosis, it is referred to as an extraluminal recurrence. Approximately two-thirds of local recurrences are extraluminal [68].

CT scanning has become the preferred method for evaluating local recurrence. It has a sensitivity of approximately 95% [69]. It is important in rectal cancer recurrences that rectal contrast should be administered. A CT scan can show not only the anastomosis but the tumor bed as well as regional lymph nodes. Any pelvic lymphadenopathy is likely to be secondary to recurrent disease. In the early postoperative period a mass of soft tissue density is not unexpected due to the presence of granulation tissue, hemorrhage, edema and/or fibrosis. Postradiation changes can produce streaky densities, presacral masses, or diffuse thickening of the rectal wall. All of these changes can easily be confused with recurrent disease. A soft tissue mass may persist in the rectal bed for up to 24 months [70]. A CT scan at 3–4 months will frequently show a soft tissue mass, even in patients who have no recurrence. A repeat study at 6–12 months often reveals a decrease in the size of the mass as well as an increase in its definition.

For a time, it was felt that MRI could allow for the differentiation of malignant from benign postoperative pelvic masses based on differences in signal intensity. Subsequently, this has been discounted [71]. Both CT scanning and MRI are sensitive modalities for detecting masses but neither is able reliably to distinguish malignant from benign lesions.

Transrectal ultrasound is sometimes useful to diagnose recurrent rectal cancer. For demonstrating mural involvement as well as local adenopathy, it has been shown to be superior to CT scanning [72]. Ultrasound, like CT, is unable to distinguish malignant from benign masses. Additionally, transrectal ultrasound can only be used after sphincter preserving surgery. Transvaginal ultrasound, however, is a possible alternative in women after abdominoperineal resection.

Another method for the detection of recurrent disease is immunoscintigraphy. Its first reported use in the detection of human colorectal carcinoma was in 1978 when Goldenberg et al. introduced ^{131}I-labeled anti-CEA antibody into 18 patients with advanced colorectal disease and followed this with a whole body scan [73]. A study of 42 patients suspected of having recurrent colorectal carcinoma was performed in order to compare conventional diagnostic methods (barium enema, CT) with immunoscintigraphy [74]. Eighty-three percent of the patients had recurrent disease localized by conventional methods and 57% by immunoscintigraphy, which has subsequently been found to be useful under specific circumstances. One of these is in the localization of recurrent disease when CEA levels are elevated but no lesion can be identified by other means (physical examination, barium enema, CT) and in the characterization of suspicious masses as malignant rather than undetermined. The reported sensitivity has ranged from 18% to 90% and specificity from 76% to 97% in detecting recurrent colorectal malignancy [75–77]. Immunoscintigraphy tends to perform poorly for intrahepatic recurrences. While this modality can be very useful in follow-up, it also has a notable false-negative rate.

Finally, the latest modality introduced and currently gaining great acceptance is positron emission tomography (PET). This is a functional imaging modality that relies on physiological, metabolic changes within tissue to allow for the detection of disease. [18F]fluoro-2-deoxy-D-glucose (FDG) is a radioactive glucose analog. The accumulation of FDG within cells is proportional to the metabolism and transport of glucose by these cells. PET scanning depends on the increased utilization of glucose by malignant cells to allow for detection. PET does not depend on gross morphological abnormalities and for this reason can be helpful in assessing patients with suspicion for recurrence that is based on elevated CEA levels or on physical or radiological findings that are indeterminate. Flanagan et al. studied 22 patients with abnormal CEA levels and normal results of conventional methods of tumor detection [78]. Each patient underwent FDG-PET scanning and the results were compared with patho-logic findings ($n = 9$) and long-term radiologic and clinical follow-up. PET scanning was abnormal in 17 and normal in five patients. Of 17 with abnormal PET scan results: seven underwent resection for cure, eight were later found to have extensive disease, and two were regarded as false positives. The five with negative PET scans were found to have no recurrence. Overall, the positive predictive value of PET scan imaging in these clinically difficult situations was 89% and the negative predictive value was 100%. Multiple similar studies have confirmed the utility of FDG-PET in the follow-up of selected colorectal cancer patients [79]. The relatively high cost and paucity of PET imaging centers have caused this modality to be limited primarily to university medical facilities. More studies are needed to determine if immunoscintigraphy or PET imaging protocols in follow-up programs may affect survival and cure rates.

Hepatic Metastases

Multiple modalities exist for the detection of recurrent disease in the liver, including radionuclide scintigraphy, ultrasonography, CT, MRI, immunoscintigraphy, and PET. Radionuclide scintigraphy was widely used in the 1970s and early 1980s. The agent ^{99m}Tc sulfur colloid accumulates in the Kupffer cells, which are abundant in the liver and absent in metastatic colorectal cancer tumor cells. The tumor, therefore, appears as a photopenic or cold area on the scan. This test lacks spatial resolution, sensitivity and specificity, and has essentially been supplanted by CT and ultrasonography.

Ultrasound is relatively inexpensive, but it is quite operator dependent. It can be greatly influenced by patient-specific factors such as bowel gas overlying the liver and obesity. The sensitivity of ultrasound in detecting metastatic liver disease is low (57%) and, for lesions less than 1 cm in diameter, this falls to around 20% [80]. Intraoperative ultrasound, on the other hand, is very sensitive, and many believe it should be mandatory prior to resection. In a multi-institutional trial evaluating liver metastases from colorectal cancer, more than half of those determined to be resectable based on preoperative evaluation were later found at surgery to be unresectable by ultrasound [81].

Following its introduction, CT soon became the gold standard for detecting hepatic recurrences and remains the primary modality used. Liver metastases from colorectal cancer appear as areas of low attenuation on non-contrast scans. After the administration of a bolus of contrast material, these metastases often show early rim enhancement or hyperdensity, then they go through an isodense period and subsequently a hypodense phase. The appearance of the tumor on a CT scan is therefore dependent on the timing of the intravenous contrast. CT with arterial portography involves repeat scanning 4 hours after the injection of contrast and has been reported to increase further the sensitivity of CT scanning for hepatic recurrence. The sensitivity of CT for metastatic colorectal carcinoma in the liver is high (78–90%) [82,83].

MRI can be used to detect hepatic recurrences but current techniques provide for no better imaging than contrast-enhanced CT and at a greater cost [82]. The sensitivity of both CT and MRI increase with increasing tumor size.

For hepatic recurrence, immunoscintigraphy has been found to be clearly inferior to contrast-enhanced CT, with its reported sensitivity being from 65% to 86% and specificity from 77% to 92% [84]. Nevertheless, some argue that immunoscintigraphy is helpful because it can evaluate the entire body and help to rule out sites of metastasis that might make resection of the hepatic lesion undesirable. Others argue that FDG-PET is superior to immunoscintigraphy and is useful for the same reasons. Vitola et al. studied 24 patients who had been previously treated for colorectal carcinoma and who returned with a suspected hepatic recurrence [85]. All patients underwent either CT of the abdomen ($n = 17$), CT portography ($n = 17$), or both ($n = 11$). The final diagnosis was obtained by tissue pathology ($n = 19$) or through clinical follow-up ($n = 5$). A total of 60 suspicious lesions were identified. Of the 55 hepatic lesions, 39 were malignant and 16 were benign. FDG-PET had an accuracy of 93%, while CT and CT portography both had accuracy rates of 76%. PET imaging also detected unsuspected extrahepatic lesions in four patients. The sensitivity of PET was 90% versus 86% for CT and 97% for CT portography. The specificity of PET was 100% versus 58% and 9% for CT and CT portography, respectively. The excellent sensitivity and specificity of PET imaging in examining hepatic recurrences has also been noted by other researchers [86,87]. As the evidence accumulates, the cost-effectiveness of PET, as well as its influence on survival and cure rates, should be examined carefully.

A difficult and continuing issue concerns the effect of follow-up on survival. A recent study from Edinburgh sought to determine whether frequent liver imaging could detect liver metastases that were suitable for surgical or chemotherapeutic intervention while they were at an asymptomatic stage [88]. Among 157 patients, 21 of 24 who were asymptomatic developed histologically proven liver metastases. Twelve had metastases diagnosed by both ultrasound and CT scanning and the remain-

ing nine by CT alone. Patients with liver metastases detected at an asymptomatic stage had a median survival of 16 months (range 7–41) from the time of diagnosis, while survival in the symptomatic group was less than 4 months.

Pulmonary Metastases

Between 5% and 10% of all patients undergoing operations for colorectal malignancy will develop pulmonary metastases [33]. The results of resection of pulmonary metastases have been encouraging, with 5-year survival rates reportedly being between 15% and 35%. Thus, it seems worthwhile to attempt to uncover these metastatic implants while they are potentially resectable for cure. However, the optimal method and timing for their detection remains unclear. Graffner et al. reported that recurrent disease was found on routine chest radiography in three of 47 patients, all of whom were asymptomatic [62]. Tornqvist et al. identified solitary lung metastases in 13 patients; seven of these underwent resection and four had long-term survival [8]. Plain chest radiography has been the imaging modality primarily described in the literature. If suspicion arises from the radiograph or from clinical findings, chest CT has a higher sensitivity and specificity than plain chest radiography. The ideal interval for postoperative chest radiography has not been determined.

Aggressive follow-up for the detection of pulmonary metastases appears to be worthwhile. In a review of 159 patients who underwent pulmonary resection for metastatic colorectal cancer over a 22-year period, the cumulative survival rates at 5 years and 10 years were 40.5% and 27.7%, respectively [89]. Other investigators have demonstrated similar results [90–97]. In an effort to identify factors predicting improved survival after the resection of isolated pulmonary metastases from colorectal cancer, a retrospective analysis of the records of 86 patients who underwent thoracic surgery with curative intent was performed [98]. Analysis of the data demonstrated that complete resection, less than two pulmonary metastases, and a normal prethoracotomy serum CEA level were predictors of a longer survival duration by univariate analysis, but only complete resection ($p = 0.024$) and preoperative CEA level ($p = 0.001$) were independent prognostic factors by multivariate analysis. The efficacy of resecting solitary metachronous metastases to the liver and then the lung is evolving.

Brain Metastases

Approximately 15–20% of patients dying from cancer will have intracranial metastases at autopsy [99]. In a collective review by Alden et al., which included 19 patients identified from their institution, the authors determined the time interval between treatment of the primary tumor and the diagnosis of metastatic disease, presentation, treatment and outcome [100]. Among their own patients, over 50% had metastatic disease when the colon primary was first diagnosed. Forty-two percent presented within 25 months and 74% within 50 months. The brain was the sole site of metastatic disease in 21%. All patients were symptomatic, with a variety of neurological complaints. The median survival was 2.8 months with no 1-year survivors. Collectively, among five series involving 86 patients with colorectal cancer metastatic to the brain there were no 2-year survivors [101–104]. In the Mayo Clinic series [105], 16% of the 150 patients with brain metastases from colorectal carcinoma survived more than 1 year, of which 92% had single cerebral metastases and 38% had no systemic metastases. In view of the fact that there are very few long-term survivors [106] and that the brain is infrequently the sole site of metastasis, the routine follow-up of asymptomatic patients in an effort to detect brain metastases is not warranted. Nevertheless, certain prognostic variables related to a favorable outcome after the treatment of brain metastases have been identified.

Bone Metastases

Rectal cancer has a greater propensity than colon cancer to metastasize to bone, with the vertebral column, skull, pelvic bones and long bones of the extremity most often affected [107]. Osseous metastases from colorectal cancer are rare. Among 1046 patients with 10 years of follow-up, a 4% incidence of bone metastases was found [108]. It is commonly felt that, in the absence of symptoms, the routine surveillance of the bony skeleton in search of metastases is not warranted. If symptoms do develop, bone scanning is the most sensitive study for the detection of such metastases [19].

Issues Specifically Regarding Rectal Cancer

It is of paramount importance that accurate staging should be performed prior to embarking on treatment of rectal cancer. Accurate staging will direct physicians in determining whether local therapy, radical surgery or adjuvant therapy, either in the preoperative setting or postoperatively, should be employed. These efforts are obviously made to decrease the local recurrence rate and theoretically to impact on the development of distant metastases. Accurate staging can also impact on the functional

result achieved after the appropriate procedure giving the best oncological outcome.

Patterns of recurrence are different in colon cancer than in rectal cancer. For example, follow-up programs after rectal cancer surgery should emphasize the detection of locoregional recurrence in the pelvis and pulmonary metastases as opposed to follow-up after colon cancer surgery where the detection of liver metastases is more pressing. Furthermore, a variety of surgical procedures are available for the treatment of rectal cancer, including local excision, restorative proctosigmoidectomy and abdominoperineal resection. Each of these predisposes the patient to different forms of local recurrence.

After restorative procedures, a change in the caliber of the stools, rectal bleeding or pelvic pain may represent either a luminal recurrence at the previous colorectal or coloanal anastomosis or a recurrence in the pelvis. These symptoms should lead to prompt evaluation. Recurrence after abdominoperineal resection typically causes perineal pain or a perineal mass. In this setting, there is often a delay from the onset of symptoms to CT detection and diagnosis of recurrence.

The reported recurrence rate after local excision ranges between 1% and 50%. Risk factors for local recurrence include transmural tumors, unfavorable histologic characteristics and positive excision margins. Efforts to reduce the local recurrence rates have employed the addition of chemoradiation to local excision. Currently there is no consensus about the most effective way to follow these patients. Often, anecdotal approaches employing digital examination or direct inspection of the rectal mucosa are used.

Endorectal and endovaginal ultrasound has been used to detect asymptomatic local recurrence after rectal surgery. Among 120 patients followed in such a manner after radical restorative procedures, 17/120 (14%) recurrences were detected [109]. There were two false positives. Currently, data are insufficient to support the routine use of intrarectal ultrasound in patients who have undergone radical surgery for rectal cancer.

Recommendations

Given the lack of strong statistical evidence for benefit and the limitations of cost weighed against the numerous reasons for postoperative surveillance, a thorough yet cost-effective and minimally invasive strategy is needed. Until 1995 there were no randomized clinical trials published on follow-up. In 1994, a meta-analysis of seven non-randomized trials involving over 3000 patients comparing routine and intensive follow-up determined that, although more asymptomatic recurrences were detected and resected in the intensive follow-up group, there was no significant difference in survival [110]. When the analysis was restricted to those studies that included CEA measurements, there was an apparent 9% increase in 5-year survival in the intensively investigated group.

In the largest study [111] of the three randomized trials [11,111,112] comparing minimal and intensive follow-up, recurrence rates were similar in both groups, but tumor recurrence in the intensive group was detected an average of 9 months earlier, often at an asymptomatic stage. There was, however, no difference in overall or cancer-related survival rates between the two groups. A similar result was reported by Northover et al. [58], in whose study a rising CEA prompted further investigation.

In 1999, in an effort to determine the most effective, evidence-based, postoperative surveillance strategy for the detection of recurrent colon and rectal cancer, ASCO published their recommendations in the *Journal of Clinical Oncology* [12]. This was based on a complete MEDLINE literature search performed for the previous 20 years. All tests described in the literature for postoperative monitoring were considered and an expert panel recommended a postoperative monitoring schema. The ASCO recommendations are described in Table 12.1 and summarized herein. Postoperative serum CEA testing should be performed every 2–3 months in patients

with Stage II or III disease for ≥ 2 years after diagnosis only, if the patients are medically fit enough to undergo a liver resection. A clinical history and pertinent physical examination should be performed every 3–6 months for the first 3 years and annually thereafter. Colonoscopy should be performed every 3–5 years for patients with previous colon or rectal cancers to detect new cancers or polyps. Patients with rectal cancer, specifically those with Stage II or Stage III disease who did not receive pelvic radiation, should have direct imaging (flexible proctosigmoidoscopy) of the rectum at periodic intervals. Routine complete blood count, liver function tests, chest radiography, CT scanning and other pelvic imaging are not recommended unless directed by symptoms or an elevated serum CEA level.

Conclusion

Many advances have been made in the field of colorectal cancer follow-up since the pioneering efforts of Wangensteen and others with second-look operations in the 1950s. The understanding of the biology and natural history of colorectal malignancy has been advanced. Diagnostic methods for the detection of recurrent disease have also advanced tremendously with CEA monitoring, immunoscintigraphy, CT, MRI and PET imaging. As has been discussed in this chapter, however, no strategy of postoperative follow-up has been shown unequivocally to produce improved survival benefit or cure rate. It is quite possible that benefit will be shown but well-controlled trials will be required. Cost considerations will probably prove to be of importance because the rate of detection of curable disease is likely to be low. Quality of life issues will also be important in such trials. Better treatment and outcome of recurrent disease would provide a strong rationale for vigorous postoperative surveillance.

Table 12.1. Recommended follow-up of patients after curative resection for rectal cancer

	Year				
	1	2	3	4	>4
Office visit (history and physical)	2–4	2–4	2–4	1	1
Serum CEA level[a]	4–6	4–6	As needed in years 3+		
Colonoscopy	1	0	0	Every 3–5 years	
Proctosigmoidoscopy[b]	At periodic intervals				
Pelvic CT[b]	At periodic intervals at least in first 3 years				
Chest radiography	Prompted by abnormal CEA or symptoms of pulmonary metastases				
Abdominal CT/MRI/ Ultrasound	Prompted by abnormal CEA or clinical symptoms				

[a] If Stage II or III tumor and the patient is medically fit enough to undergo liver resection.
[b] For patients who have not undergone pelvic radiation.

References

1. Greenlee RT, Murray T, Bolden S, Wingo PA. Cancer Statistics 2000. CA Cancer J Clin 2000;50:7–33.
2. August D, Ottow R, Sugarbaker P. Clinical perspective of human colorectal cancer metastasis. Cancer Metast Rev 1984;3:303–24.
3. Hughes KS, Simon R, Songhorabodi S, et al. Resection of the liver for colorectal carcinoma metastases: a multi-institutional study of patterns of recurrence. Surgery 1986;100:278–84.
4. Wangensteen OH, Lewis FJ, Tongen TA. The second-look in cancer surgery. Lancet 1951;ii:303–307.
5. Wangensteen OH. Experience with cancer of the stomach and the colon and second look procedure. Minn Med 1968;51:1833–38.

6. Gilbertsen VA, Wangensteen OH. A summary of thirteen years' experience with the second-look program. Surg Gynecol Obstet 1962;114:438–42.

7. Beart RW Jr, Metzger PP, O'Connell MJ, Schutt AJ. Postoperative screening of patients with adenocarcinoma of the colon. Dis Colon Rectum 1981;24:585–88.

8. Tornqvist A, Ekelund G, Leondoer L. The value of intensive follow-up after curative resection for colorectal carcinoma. Br J Surg 1982;69:725–28.

9. Safi F, Link KH, Beger HG. Is follow-up of colorectal cancer patients worthwhile? Dis Colon Rectum 1993;36:636–44.

10. Bohm B, Schwenk W, Hoche HP, Stoch W. Does methodological long-term follow-up affect survival after curative resection of colorectal carcinoma? Dis Colon Rectum 1993;36:280–86.

11. Ohlsson B, Bieland V, Ekberg H, Graffner H, Tranberk KG. Follow-up after curative surgery for colorectal carcinoma: randomized comparison with no follow-up. Dis Colon Rectum 1995;38:619–26.

12. Desch CE, Benson AB, Smith TJ, et al. Recommended colorectal cancer surveillance guidelines by the American Society of Clinical Oncology. J Clin Oncol 1999;17:1312–21.

13. Steele G. Standard postoperative monitoring of patients after primary resection of colon and rectum cancer. Cancer 1993;71:4225–35.

14. Vernava AM, Longo WE, Virgo KS, Coplin MA, Wade TP, Johnson FE. Current follow-up strategies after resection of colon cancer: results of a survey of members of the American Society of Colon and Rectal Surgeons. Dis Colon Rectum 1994;37:573–83.

15. Virgo KS, Wade TP, Longo WE, Coplin MA, Vernava AM, Johnson FEJ. Surveillance after curative colon cancer resection: practice patterns of surgical specialists. Ann Surg Oncol 1995;2:472–82.

16. Cooper GS, Yuan Z, Chak A, Rimm AA. Geographic and patient variation among Medicare beneficiaries in the use of follow-up testing after surgery for non-metastatic colorectal carcinoma. Cancer 1999;85:2124–31.

17. Johnson FE, Longo WE, Wade TP, Coplin MA, Vernava AM, Virgo KS. Practice patterns in cancer patient follow-up are minimally affected by surgeon age. Surg Oncol 1996;5:127–31.

18. Virgo KS, Vernava AM, Longo WE, McKirgan LW, Johnson FE. Cost of patient follow-up after potentially curative colorectal cancer treatment. JAMA 1995;273:1837–41.

19. Johnson FE, Longo WE, Vernava AM, Wade TP, Coplin MA, Virgo KS. How tumor stage affects surgeons' surveillance strategies after colon surgery. Cancer 1995;76:1325–29.

20. Macintosh EL, Rodriguez-Bigas AR, Petrelli NJ. Colorectal carcinoma In: Johnson FE, Virgo KS, editors. Cancer patient followup. St Louis, MO: Mosby; 1997:118–31.

21. Polk H, Spratt JS. Recurrent colorectal carcinoma: detection, treatment, and other considerations. Surgery 1971;69:9–23.

22. Carnovas J, Enriquez JM, Devesa JM, Morales V, Millan I. Value of follow-up in the management of recurrent colorectal cancer. Eur J Surg Oncol 1991;17:530–35.

23. Makela J, Haukipauro K, Laitinen S, Karralvoma MI. Surgical treatment of recurrent colorectal cancer: five-year follow-up. Arch Surg 1989;124:1029–32.

24. Pihl E, Hughes ESR, McDermott FT, Milne BJ, Price AB. Disease-free survival and recurrence after resection of colorectal cancer. J Surg Oncol 1981;16:333–41.

25. Galandiuk S, Moertel CG, Fitzgibbons RJJ. Patterns of recurrence after curative resection of carcinoma of the colon and rectum. Surg Gynecol Obstet 1992;174:27–32.

26. Segall MM, Goldberg SM, Nivatvongs S. Abdominoperineal resection for recurrent cancer following anterior resection. Dis Colon Rectum 1980;23:359–61.

27. Vassilopoulos PP, Yoon JM, Ledesma EJ. Treatment of recurrence of adenocarcinoma of the colon and rectum at the anastomotic site. Surg Gynecol Obstet 1981;152:777–80.

28. Pihl E, Hughes ESR, McDermott FT. Recurrence of carcinoma of the colon and rectum at the anastomotic suture line. Surg Gynecol Obstet 1981;153:495–96.

29. Holm A, Bradley G, Aldrete JS. Hepatic resection of metastases from colorectal carcinoma. Ann Surg 1989;209:428–34.

30. Nordlinger B, Parc R, Delva F. Hepatic resection for colorectal liver metastases: influence on survival of preoperative factors and surgery for recurrence in 80 patients. Ann Surg 1987;205:256–63.

31. Hughes KS, Rosenstein RB, Saghorabodis S. Resection of the liver for colorectal carcinoma metastases. Dis Colon Rectum 1988;31:1–4.

32. Goldberg RM, Fleming TR, Tangen CM, et al. Surgery for recurrent colon cancer: strategies for identifying resectable recurrence and success rates after resection. Ann Intern Med 1998;129:27–35.

33. Pihl E, Hughes ESR, McDermott FT. Lung recurrence after curative surgery for colorectal cancer. Dis Colon Rectum 1987;30:417–19.

34. Beart RW, Metzger PP, O'Connell MJ. Postoperative screening of patients with carcinoma of the colon. Dis Colon Rectum 1981;24:585–89.

35. Beart RW, O'Connell MJ. Postoperative follow-up of patients with carcinoma of the colon. Mayo Clin Proc 1983;58:361–63.

36. Cochran JP, Williams JT, Faber RG, Slack WW. Value of outpatient follow-up after curative surgery for carcinoma of the large bowel. BMJ 1980;280:593–95.

37. Decosse JJ. Early cancer detection: colorectal cancer. Cancer 1988;62:1787–90.

38. Crowson MC, Jewkes AJ, Acheson N. Haemoccult testing as an indicator of recurrent colorectal cancer: a 5-year prospective study. Eur J Oncol 1991;17:281–84.

39. Gilbert JM, Jeffrey I, Evan M. Sites of recurrent tumor after curative colorectal surgery: implications of adjuvant therapy. Br J Surg 1984;71:203–205.

40. Gutman AB, Olson KB, Gutman GB, Flood CA. Effect of disease of the liver and biliary tract upon the phosphatase activity of serum. J Clin Invest 1940;19:129–51.

41. Baden H, Anderson B, Augustenborg G. Diagnostic valve of gamma-glutamyl transpeptidase and alkaline phosphatase in liver metastases. Surg Gynecol Obstet 1971;133:769–73.

42. Gold P, Freedman SO. Demonstration of tumor-specific antigens in colonic carcinomata by immunological tolerance and absorption techniques. J Exp Med 1965;121:439–62.

43. Jessup J, Thomas P. CEA: function in metastasis by human colorectal carcinoma. Cancer Metast Rev 1989;3:263–80.

44. Arnaud JP, Koehl C, Adloff M. Carcinoembryonic antigen (CEA) in the diagnosis and prognosis of colorectal carcinoma. Dis Colon Rectum 1980;23:141–44.

45. Fletcher RH. Carcinoembryonic antigen. Ann Intern Med 1986;104:66–73.

46. Hine KR, Leonard JC, Booth SN, Dykes PW. Carcinoembryonic antigen concentrations in undiagnosed patients. Lancet 1978;ii:1337–40.

47. Moertel CG, Fleming TR, MacDonald JS, Haller DG, Lavine TA, Tangen C. An evaluation of carcinoembryonic antigen (CEA) test for monitoring patients with resected colon cancer. JAMA 1993;270:943–47.

48. Bronstein RR, Steele G, Ensminger W. The use and limitations of serial plasma carcinoembryonic antigen (CEA) levels as a monitor of changing metastatic liver tumor volume in patients receiving chemotherapy. Cancer 1980;46:266–72.

49. Mayer R, Garnick M, Steele G. CEA as a monitor of chemotherapy in disseminated colorectal cancer. Cancer 1978;42:1428–32.
50. Goslin R, Steele G, MacIntyre J. The use of preoperative plasma CEA levels for the stratification of patients after curative resection of colorectal cancers. Ann Surg 1980;192:747–51.
51. Hine FR, Dyke PW. Serum CEA testing in the postoperative surveillance of colorectal carcinoma. Br J Surg 1984;49:689–93.
52. Zeng Z, Cohen AM, Urmacher C. Usefulness of carcinoembryonic antigen monitoring despite normal preoperative valves in node-positive colon cancer patients. Dis Colon Rectum 1993;36:1063–68.
53. Armitage NC, Davidson A, Tsikos D, Wood CB. A study of the reliability of carcinoembryonic antigen blood levels in following the course of colorectal cancer. Clin Oncol 1984;10:141–47.
54. McCall JL, Black RB, Rich CA, et al. The valve of serum carcinoembryonic antigen in predicting recurrent disease following curative resection of colorectal cancer. Dis Colon Rectum 1994;37:875–81.
55. Staab HJ, Anderer FA, Stumpf E, Horning A, Fischer R, Kreninger G. Eighty-four potential second-look operations based on sequential carcinoembryonic antigen determinations and clinical investigations in patients with recurrent gastrointestinal cancer. Am J Surg 1985;149:198–204.
56. Carl J, Bentzen SM, Norgaard-Pedersen B, Kronborg O. Modelling of serial carcinoembryonic antigen changes in colorectal cancer. Scand J Clin Lab Invest 1993;53:751–55.
57. Kievit J, van de Velde CJ. Utility and cost of carcinoembryonic antigen monitoring in colon cancer follow-up evaluation: a Markov analysis. Cancer 1990;65:2580–87.
58. Northover J, Houghton J, Lennon T. CEA to detect recurrence of colon cancer. JAMA 1994;272:31.
59. Iemura K, Moriya Y. A comparative analysis of the serum levels of NCC-ST-439, CEA and CA 19-9 in patients with colorectal carcinoma. Eur J Surg Oncol 1993;19:439–42.
60. Guadagni F, Roselli M, Cosimelli M, et al. Biologic evaluation of tumor-associated glycoprotein-72 and carcinoembryonic antigen expression in colorectal cancer Part I. Dis Colon Rectum 1994;37:S16–S23.
61. Fillela X, Molina R, Pique JM, et al. Use of CA 19-9 in the early detection of recurrences in colorectal cancer: comparison with CEA. Tumour Biol 1994;15:1–6.
62. Graffner H, Holtberg B, Johansson B, Moller T, Petersson BG. Detection of recurrent cancer of the colon and rectum. J Surg Oncol 1985;28:156–59.
63. Reilly JC, Rusin LC, Theverkauf FJ. Colonoscopy: its role in cancer of the colon and rectum. Dis Colon Rectum 1982;25:532–38.
64. Slanetz CA, Herter FP, Grinell RS. Anterior resection vs. abdominal-perineal resection for cancer of the rectum and rectosigmoid. Am J Surg 1972;123:110–17.
65. Rodriguez-Bigas MA, Stulc JP, Davidson B, Petrelli NJ. Prognostic significance of anastomotic recurrence from colorectal adenocarcinoma. Dis Colon Rectum 1992;35:838–42.
66. Cass AW, Million RR, Pfaff WW. Patterns of recurrence following surgery alone for adenocarcinoma of the colon and rectum. Cancer 1976;37:2861–65.
67. Thoeni RF, Menuck C. Comparison of barium enema and colonoscopy in detection of small colonic polyps. Radiology 1977;124:631–35.
68. Barkin J, Cohen M, Flaxman M. Value of routine follow-up endoscopy for the detection of recurrent colorectal carcinoma. Am J Gastroenterol 1988;88:1355–60.
69. Moss AA, Thoeni RF, Schnyder P. Valve of computed tomography in the detection and staging of recurrent rectal carcinomas. J Comput Assist Tomogr 1981;5:870–74.
70. Kelvin FM, Korobkin M, Heaston DK. The pelvis after surgery for rectal carcinoma: serial CT observations with emphasis on non-neoplastic features. AJR Am J Roentgenol 1983;141:959–64.
71. DeLange EE, Fechner RE, Wanebo HJ. Suspected recurrent rectosigmoid carcinoma after abdominoperineal resection: MR imaging and histopathologic findings. Radiology 1989;170:323–28.
72. Rifkin MD, Ehrlich SM, Marks G. Staging of rectal carcinoma: prospective comparison of endorectal US and CT. Radiology 1989;170:319–22.
73. Goldenberg DM, DeLand E, Kim E. Use of radiolabeled antibodies to carcinoembryonic antigen in the detection and localization of diverse cancers by external photoscanning. N Engl J Med 1978;298:1384–88.
74. Holting T, Schlag P, Steinbacher M, Kretzschmar U. The value of immunoscintigraphy for the operative retreatment of colorectal cancer. Cancer 1989;64:830–3.
75. Goldenberg DM, Larson SM. Radioimmunodetection in cancer identification. J Nucl Med 1992;33:803–14.
76. Abdel-Nabi H, Doerr RJ. Clinical applications of indium-111-labeled monoclonal antibody imaging in colorectal cancer patients. Semin Nucl Med 1993;23:99–113.
77. Rutgers EJT. Radioimmunotargeting in colorectal carcinoma. Eur J Cancer 1995;31A:1243–47.
78. Flanagan FL, Dehdashti F, Ogunbigi OA, Kodner IJ, Siegel BA. Utility of FDG-PET for investigating unexplained plasma CEA elevation in patients with colorectal cancer. Ann Surg 1998;227:319–23.
79. Keogan MT, Lowe VJ, Baker ME, McDermott VG, Lyerly HK, Coleman RE. Local recurrence of rectal cancer: evaluation with F-18 fluorodeoxyglucose PET imaging. Abdom Imaging 1997;22:332–37.
80. Schreve RH, Terpstra OT, Ausema L, Lameris JS, Van Seijen AJ, Jeckel J. Detection of liver metastases: a prospective study comparing ultrasonography and computed tomography. Br J Surg 1984;71:947–49.
81. Steele G, Bleday R, Meyer RJ, Linblad A, Petrelli N, Weaver D. A prospective evaluation of hepatic resection for colorectal carcinoma metastases to the liver: Gastrointestinal Tumor Study Group Protocol 6584. J Clin Oncol 1991;9:1105–12.
82. Ward BA, Miller DL, Frank JA. Prospective evaluation of hepatic imaging studies in the detection of colorectal metastases: correlation with surgical findings. Surgery 1989;105:180–87.
83. Bernadino M, Ervin B, Steinberg H. Delayed hepatic CT scanning: increased confidence and improved detection of hepatic metastases. Radiology 1986;159:71–74.
84. Abdel-Nabi HH, Schwartz AN, Goldfogel G. Colorectal tumors: scintigraphy with In-111 anti-CEA monoclonal antibody and correlation with surgical histopathologic and immunohistochemical findings. Radiology 1988;166:744–52.
85. Vitola JV, Delbehe D, Sandler MP, et al. Positron emission tomography to stage suspected metastatic colorectal carcinoma to the liver. Am J Surg 1996;171:21–26.
86. Gupta NC, Bowman BM, Frank AL. PET FDG imaging for follow-up evaluation of treated colorectal cancer [abstract]. Radiology 1991;199:181P.
87. Strauss LG, Clorius JH, Schlag P. Recurrence of colorectal tumors: PET evaluation. Radiology 1989;170:329–32.
88. Howell JD, Wotherspoon H, Leen E, Cooke TC, McArdle CS. Evaluation of a follow-up programme after curative resection for colorectal cancer. Br J Cancer 1999;79:308–10.
89. Okmura S, Kondo H, Tsuboi M, et al. Pulmonary resection for metastatic colorectal cancer: experiences with 159 patients. J Thorac Cardiovasc Surg 1996;112:867–74.
90. Robinson BJ, Rice TW, Strong SW, Rybicki LA, Blackstone EH. Is resection of pulmonary and hepatic metastases

warranted in patients with colorectal cancer? J Thorac
Cardiovasc Surg 1999;117:66–75.

91. Murata S, Moriya Y, Akasu T, Fujita S, Sugihara K. Resection
of both hepatic and pulmonary metastases in patients with
colorectal carcinoma. Cancer 1998;83:1086–93.

92. Kamiyoshihara M, Hirai T, Kawashima O, Morishita Y.
Resection of pulmonary metastases in six patients with
disease free interval greater than 10 years. Ann Thorac Surg
1998;66:231–33.

93. Regnard JF, Gruenwald D, Spaggiari L, et al. Surgical treatment of hepatic and pulmonary metastases from colorectal
cancers. Ann Thorac Surg 1998:66:214–18.

94. Ambiru S, Miyazaki M, Ito H, et al. Resection of hepatic
and pulmonary metastases in patients with colorectal
carcinoma. Cancer 1998;82:274–78.

95. Zanella A, Marchet A, Mainente P, Nitti D, Lise M. Resection
of pulmonary metastases from colorectal carcinoma. Eur J
Surg Oncol 1997;23:424–27.

96. Vigneswaran WT. Management of pulmonary metastases
from colorectal cancer. Semin Surg Oncol 1996;12:264–66.

97. Baron O, Amini M, Deveau D, Despins P, Sagan CA, Michaud
JL. Surgical resection of pulmonary metastases from colorectal carcinoma. Five year survival and main prognostic
factors. Eur J Cardiothorac Surg 1996;10:347–51.

98. Girard P, Ducreux M, Baldeyrou P, et al. Surgery for lung
metastases from colorectal cancer: analysis of prognostic
factors. J Clin Oncol 1996;14:2047–53.

99. Posner JB, Chernik NL. Intracranial metastases from
systemic cancer. Adv Neurol 1978;19:579–92.

100. Alden TD, Gianino JW, Saclarides TJ. Brain metastases from
colorectal cancer. Dis Colon Rectum 1996;39:541–45.

101. Zimm S, Wampler GL, Stablein D, Hazra T, Young HF.
Intracerebral metastases in solid tumor patients: natural
history and results of treatment. Cancer 1981;48:384–94.

102. Sundaresan N, Galicich JH. Surgical treatment of brain
metastases: clinical and computerized tomography
evaluation of the results of treatment. Cancer 1985;55:
1382–88.

103. Cascino TL, Leavengood JM, Kemeny N, Posner JB. Brain
metastases from colon cancer. J Neurooncol 1983;1:203–209.

104. Cairncross JG, Kim JH, Posner JB. Radiation therapy for
brain metastases. Ann Neurol 1980;7:529–41.

105. Smalley SR, Laws ER, O'Fallon JR, Shaw EG, Schray MF.
Resection of solitary brain metastases: role of adjuvant
radiation and prognostic variables in 229 patients. J
Neurosurg 1992;77:531–40.

106. Farnell GF, Buckner JC, Cascino TL, O'Connell MJ,
Schomberg PJ, Suman V. Brain metastases from colorectal
carcinoma. The long term survivors. Cancer 1996;78:711–16.

107. Besbeas S, Stearns MW Jr. Osseous metastases from carcinoma of the colon and rectum. Dis Colon Rectum
1978;21:266–68.

108. Bonnheim DC, Petrelli NJ, Herrera L, Walsh D, Mittleman A.
Osseous metastases from colorectal carcinoma. Am J Surg
1986;151:457–59.

109. Masgagni D, Corbellini L, Urciuoloi P, Di Matteo G. Endoluminal ultrasound for early detection of local recurrence
of rectal cancer. Br J Surg 1989;76:1176–80.

110. Bruinvels DJ, Stiggelbout AM, Kievit J, Van Houwelingen H,
Habbema DF, Van de Velde C. Follow-up of patients
with colorectal cancer: a meta-analysis. Ann Surg 1994;219:
174–82.

111. Kjeldsen B, Kronberg O, Fenger C, Jorgensen O. A prospective randomized study of follow-up after radical surgery for
colorectal cancer. Br J Surg 1997;84:666–69.

112. Makela JT, Laitnen SO, Kairaluoma MI. Five year follow-up
after radical surgery for colorectal cancer: results of a
prospective randomized trial. Arch Surg 1995;130:1062–67.

13. Surgical Approach to Locally Recurrent Disease

C.A. Paterson and H. Nelson

Introduction

Despite advances in both surgical techniques and adjuvant therapies, recurrence after curative resection of rectal cancer remains a significant problem. Recurrences may be localized within the pelvis or may be metastatic to extrapelvic organs such as the liver, lungs or extrapelvic lymph nodes. Local pelvic recurrence after attempted curative resection occurs in up to 50% of patients and, without further therapy, the mean survival is only 7 months [1,2]. The addition of radiation therapy alone only slightly improves this rather dismal outcome, with median survivals reported as 10–17 months [2]. In contrast to single modality approaches, multimodality strategies including surgery have accomplished median survivals of 44.7 months and 5-year survival rates of up to 34% [3]. These results are similar to the benefits of curative surgery for isolated metastases of the liver or lungs, with 5-year survival rates reported between 25% and 47% [4–7]. This chapter describes in detail the multimodality approach to locally recurrent rectal cancer, including clinical manifestations, diagnostic evaluations, operative planning and techniques, adjuvant therapies, and results, as well as future prospects.

Clinical Presentation

The presentation of patients with recurrent rectal cancer is variable and depends on factors such as site of recurrence, type of previous operation, proximity or invasion of vital structures(e.g. nerves or blood vessels), and physical tumor bulk. For example, solitary small metastases to the liver or lungs typically do not produce symptoms, whereas lesions of a similar size occupying the lumen of the rectum or compressing the sciatic nerve may produce marked symptoms, occasionally with physical findings. It is therefore difficult to identify a single symptom or symptom complex as pathognomonic of this condition. Careful attention must be paid to changes that the patient may experience, particularly the development of new pelvic or perineal symptoms.

Reports on the rate of local recurrence of rectal cancer range from as low as 3% to a high of 50% [8–10]. Although some of this variation reflects differences in tumors and surgical techniques, at least part of it reflects the difficulties associated with diagnosing local recurrence. Symptoms, if present, are often vague and non-localizing. In addition, tumor recurrences are typically extraluminal, hampering their access for tissue diagnosis. Even state-of-the-art imaging often cannot differentiate between postoperative radiation fibrosis and pelvic tumor recurrence. Despite these difficulties, a standard evaluation commencing with a history and physical examination is essential.

The presence and types of symptoms may provide clues to the site of recurrence and occasionally point to involvement of other structures. In general, patients presenting with symptoms sooner after initial surgery may have aggressive tumors, or tumor invading or compressing essential structures. Furthermore, those whose presenting symptom is pain have a worse prognosis than those with an asymptomatic recurrence [11]. Based on past experience, several signs and symptoms are considered to be relative contraindications to aggressive re-resection:

Multifocal, extrapelvic disease

Circumferential or extensive pelvic side wall involvement

S1 or S2 involvement (bony or neural)

Poor surgical risk (American Society of Anesthesiology Classification IV-V)

Bilateral ureteral obstruction

Symptoms associated with alterations in bowel habit are dependent, in part, on previous surgical procedures. In patients who have had a sphincter sparing procedure, changes in the caliber or frequency of the stools, or the presence of blood, may imply luminal pathology. It must be kept in mind that the problem may not simply be an anastomotic recurrence but could also represent a missed synchronous or metachronous lesion. Patients with tumor invasion into the urinary bladder may present with symptoms such as difficulty with micturition, hematuria or pneumaturia. Rarely, those who have previously had an abdominoperineal resection may present with draining sinuses or gross tumor in the perineal wound as the first indication of recurrence. Although it is intuitive that close follow-up regimens with or without carcinoembryonic antigen monitoring [12,13] would help to prevent such unfortunate presentations, this is not proven. The merits of such strategies and the role of surveillance regimens are described in Ch. 12.

Diagnostic Evaluation

All patients with recurrent rectal cancer require a complete staging evaluation prior to consideration for reoperation:

Physical examination (abdominal, rectal, vaginal, nodes)

Blood investigations (complete blood count, chemistry)

Endoscopy (check anastomosis and clear proximal colon)

Chest radiograph

Abdominal/pelvic computed tomographic (CT) scan; biopsy for confirmation (histologic confirmation can be accomplished percutaneously under CT guidance or at times using transrectal or transvaginal approaches)

With or without pelvic magnetic resonance imaging (MRI), as indicated

The goal of such an evaluation is to confirm the presence of pelvic disease and the absence of extrapelvic disease. The criteria used to select patients for aggressive reoperation and multimodality therapy are summarized below:

Good surgical risk

Isolated locoregional disease

Resectable for curative indications

Reconstructable

In general, patients in poor health or those who have a high risk of mortality from the procedure are excluded, as are those with lesions beyond the hope of resectability for cure [14,15].

Physical examination is performed in all patients, both as part of a preoperative workup and as a part of routine surveillance. Although the yield from physical examination is generally poor, several important pieces of information can be gained. Inspection of the patient provides some clues about his or her general state of health and nutrition. The sclera and skin surfaces are examined for evidence of jaundice suggesting either biliary obstruction or extensive liver involvement by tumor. Major areas of nodal drainage, especially the groins and supraclavicular areas, are examined to detect possible metastases. The abdomen is carefully palpated to assess for masses, hepatomegaly or wound tumor implants. When the rectum or a rectal stump remains after previous surgery, a rectal examination is performed to assess for the presence of a tumor mass. Digital rectal examination also provides information about the relative fixation of the lesion in the pelvis and its level above the dentate line. If the tumor is within reach of the examining finger then abdominoperineal resection is likely to be necessary. In women, a vaginal examination is also carried out to gain further information about tumor size, location and fixation, and to assess for vaginal involvement.

Colonoscopy or flexible sigmoidoscopy combined with a barium enema should be performed to rule out the possibility of proximal lesions, either missed synchronous or metachronous. Rigid or flexible endoscopy offers advantages over radiographic contrast studies in that it can be used to obtain biopsies of the tumor as well as assess the distance of the lesion from the dentate line. The role of newer modalities such as virtual colonoscopy in postoperative surveillance are as yet unproven.

Chest radiographs are obtained to exclude pulmonary metastases. When confusion exists regarding a suspicious nodule, CT scans may be of benefit and may be used to guide subsequent tissue sampling for confirmation of malignancy. The routine use of chest CT scanning, however, is not advised because this modality is overly sensitive and not specific [16]. The added costs do not seem justified and the confusion generated by "indeterminate" nodules is not easy to manage.

In contrast to pulmonary disease, extrapelvic abdominal disease can be staged by CT scanning with an accuracy of greater than 85% [17]. In a study by Farouk et al. the accuracy of CT scanning was examined by comparing operative findings and resectability to what had been predicted by preoperative imaging [17]. The results indicate that CT was reliable for determining that the disease was confined to one region with an accuracy of 87%. It was also reliable in determining the need for sacrectomy or hysterectomy, but tended to overestimate involvement of the urinary bladder. The results of CT scanning in predicting the unresectability of a fixed lesion after radiation therapy were much less impressive, with an accuracy of only 25%. Certainly, the degree of experience of both the surgeon and the radiologist play a large part in determining the accuracy of CT in this setting.

The role of additional imaging modalities such as MRI, positron emission tomography and monoclonal antibody scans have not yet been established [18]. Specifically, it is not defined when they should be used to complement or supplement the information provided by standard CT scans. There is some suggestion that MRI may be useful for better defining the involvement of bony structures such as the sacrum. This would be most helpful in patients with bony involvement of borderline resectability. A more precise definition of the proximal or lateral extent may predict the inability to obtain tumor-free margins. Its usefulness in differentiating fibrosis from tumor recurrence has been questioned [19].

Radioimmunodetection methods to identify tumor utilize antibodies that react with antigenic markers such as carcinoembryonic antigen, which are produced and expressed by tumor cells. The antibodies are labeled with radioactive tracers, which can then be detected by external scintigraphy. The value of ^{111}In-CYT-103 scanning in resectable, recurrent colorectal cancer has been reviewed in a blinded clinical trial [18]. The aim of this study was to determine whether any improvements in diagnostic accuracy would translate into increased curability or decreased interventional morbidity. The contribution of the scan to the diagnosis and management of the patient was graded by the surgeon from very beneficial to having a very negative influence. The findings were that the scan had a beneficial effect in only 13% of the study patients, a negative effect in 20%, and no effect in 67%. This study represents the opinions of one group of colorectal surgeons as applied to a small group of patients. Perhaps as techniques are refined radioimmunodetection methods will prove to be more useful.

An appropriate and thorough workup is also essential, both for preoperative patient counseling and operative planning. Previous operative notes are a requisite piece of information because they provide details of alterations in blood supply as well as of unusual findings that may have been encountered at initial laparotomy. Operations for recurrent rectal cancer demand a co-ordinated team approach involving many specialists. It is important to ensure that these resources are available. In addition, the patient must be counseled on the extent and complications of proposed surgery as well as the long-term implications and anticipated functional outcomes.

Part of the preoperative planning and counseling also involves the issue of stomas. For those who have had a previous sphincter sparing procedure, the likelihood of a permanent stoma after a second resection is nearly 100%. Ideally, the patient should meet with a stoma therapist to determine the best possible location and discuss both care of the ostomy and lifestyle issues. Patients who are undergoing pelvic exenteration may experience difficulty with the concept of managing two stomas with the creation of an ileal conduit as well as a colostomy. From a technical standpoint, the placement of stomas on the abdominal wall can be difficult. Scars from previous incisions may render the best stoma site unsuitable. This problem is compounded if the patient requires two stomas or if there are multiple scars on the abdominal wall. In planning for stoma location, the possibility of requiring a rectus abdominis flap for placement within the pelvis must also be considered. If such a flap is anticipated the stoma site must be made on the side opposite to the rectus harvest.

Preoperative Therapies

Modalities that lessen the tumor burden or improve resectability are employed preoperatively because the goal at the time of surgery is to achieve a total resection. External beam radiotherapy (EBRT) in combination with radiosensitizing agents such as 5-fluorouracil (5-FU) is used to treat patients with locally recurrent rectal cancer. The dose delivered is dependent upon prior radiation exposure of the field. Patients who received adjuvant radiation after resection of the primary rectal cancer are treated with low-dose radiation (20 Gy) plus 5-FU-based chemotherapy and then proceed promptly to surgery. Those who did not receive radiation to the pelvis as an adjuvant to the original operation receive a full course of external beam radiation, typically 50.4 Gy, with 5-FU-based chemotherapy. After a full course of EBRT, patients are rested for 4 weeks and then restaged just prior to reoperative surgery. In general, surgery is performed as soon as possible after EBRT in order to provide synergy between the EBRT and planned use of intraoperative radiation therapy.

Preoperative Planning

The surgical approach to patients with recurrent rectal cancer is critically dependent on obtaining as much preoperative information as possible. At this point, those who have remaining contraindications to resection are excluded. Considerations at this stage are the presence of metastatic disease, including its location and extent, the timing of resection of isolated metastases if present, fixation of the tumor to other structures, and the need for reconstruction.

Extensive pelvic re-resection is typically reserved for patients with isolated pelvic recurrences rather than those already demonstrating pulmonary or hepatic metastases. However, the presence of metastatic disease does not always preclude resection for an otherwise isolated local recurrence. Isolated liver or lung metastases may be identified preoperatively. CT scans with or without ultrasound are employed to identify the presence, location and number of metastatic deposits. It is essential to determine both their number and location preoperatively in order to determine resectability and to decide if further surgical intervention is warranted in the presence of extrapelvic disease. It may be reasonable to perform one or two wedge-type resections at the time of reoperation for the rectal lesion without significantly increasing the operative risk. Surgically resectable pulmonary metastases are generally treated at a second operation.

Intraoperative ultrasound has proved invaluable in the further assessment of hepatic involvement. It is not uncommon to identify other small metastatic deposits that were not revealed during preoperative imaging studies. This additional information may alter the operative strategy from one of curative intent to palliation. There is also no substitute for palpation of the liver surface early in the assessment of operability, when small superficial lesions that have escaped detection by other methods, including intraoperative ultrasound, may be identified. If lesions detected by palpation are solid then biopsies should be carried out to confirm them as malignant and consistent with colorectal origin. This information is used to determine the nature of the subsequent surgery.

Operative Strategy

The same initial operative steps apply to all patients, regardless of the extent of the tumor and the presence of fixation:

Evaluate for metastatic disease
Determine extent of local disease
    Local adherence
    Need for en bloc resection
        Urologic structures
        Gynecologic structures
        Sacrum
    Need for reconstruction
Determine extent of previous treatments
    If no previous pelvic radiation therapy:
        EBRT 50.4 Gy
        5-FU protracted venous infusion
        Preoperative rest period of 4–6 weeks
    If previous pelvic radiation therapy:
        EBRT (up to 20 Gy)
        5-FU protracted venous infusion
        No preoperative rest period

Attention to detail in the early stages can prevent complications and expedite the procedure. All patients are placed in the supine position with their legs up in stirrups. Bony prominences and superficial nerves such as the ulnar nerve at the elbow and the common peroneal nerve at the knee are carefully padded. Long operation times contribute to potential nerve injuries typically caused by pressure or traction. In the upper extremities the more common potential injuries are to the brachial plexus or ulnar nerve, while in the lower extremities, injury of the common peroneal nerve may lead to foot drop postoperatively. In addition, prolonged pressure on the calves from stirrups may lead to the development of a compartment syndrome.

At this point, the inked stoma markings are confirmed and are scratched so that they can be identified after the abdomen has been prepared. Ureteric stents and a Foley catheter are placed prior to laparotomy when repeat pelvic dissection is planned. The patient is prepared in a synchronous position from the level of the nipples to the thighs. The perineum is also prepared after the rectum is irrigated with dilute iodine solution.

The abdomen is entered through a midline incision extending initially from the pubis to the level of the umbilicus. This incision is extended cephalad as required. Once the peritoneal cavity is entered a careful inspection is made of peritoneal surfaces for metastatic deposits and the small bowel is inspected over its entire length. Lymph nodes in the retroperitoneum, particularly along the iliac vessels and aorta, are palpated. Suspicious nodules are biopsied and histologic diagnosis made by frozen section. The liver is palpated for deep or superficial nodules as already mentioned.

Attention is then turned to the pelvis after packing away the small bowel. Not infrequently, loops of small bowel that are adherent in the pelvis must be mobilized to gain access. Any areas of adherent small bowel that are suspicious for tumor involvement are not mobilized but instead are transected with proximal and distal linear staplers and then later removed en bloc with the specimen, with instatement of an enteroenterostomy for the two free ends. Once the pelvis is exposed, the dissection is commenced at the level of the pelvic brim. The ureters are identified with the help of the stents at or above the level of the pelvic brim and visualized to the level of insertion into the bladder. The ureters often have to be moved out of the working field to avoid injury or have to be partially removed if involved by tumor. Next, the aorta, vena cava and common iliac vessels are exposed. These vessels are traced down beyond the internal–external bifurcation to gain proximal vascular control to identify areas of tumor invasion or encasement and to ensure that they will not be inadvertently damaged during tumor resection.

From this point, the rest of the direction of the operation is dictated by the location of pelvic fixation. The possibilities include the absence of fixation to other structures or fixation that can be considered either resectable or unresectable. Resectable fixed lesions are further characterized as being fixed anteriorly, posteriorly or laterally within the pelvis, as described by Nyam and Nelson [10] (Fig. 13.1). In the presence of extensive pelvic disease when a curative resection is not possible, patients may benefit from a palliative resection or debulking, particularly when compressive symptoms are present. Alternatively, if a palliative resection is not possible, diversion of the fecal and/or urinary streams may be carried out to provide symptomatic relief.

If fixation is not identified on preoperative imaging then the dissection essentially converts a low anterior resection to an abdominoperineal resection. The difficulty in this lies with identifying the tissue planes that have been obliterated by previous surgery and radiation therapy. Not uncommonly, loose areolar tissue has been replaced by dense scar tissue. The suspicion of infiltration of scar tissue by tumor should be confirmed by frozen section evaluation. The difficulty of dissecting the neorectum or colon from the surrounding fibrosis is compounded by the fact that the bowel is often very thin and easily perforated. In men, the dissection of the rectum from the prostate anteriorly can be difficult and care is needed to avoid excessive bleeding or urethral damage. After completing the proctectomy, consideration should be given to pelvic reconstruction by using a flap, particularly if the pelvic defect is wide and if high doses of radiation are to be delivered intraoperatively.

Anterior fixation generally implies involvement of the bladder and/or ureter. In men, anterior fixation may also involve the prostate, while, in women, the uterus, if present, and the vagina provide a mechanical barrier to the bladder. When anterior fixation is detected at the time of laparotomy the mobilization is carried out posteriorly and laterally before attempting the anterior procedure. Once this has been completed the degree of anterior fixation can better be assessed. If the fixation is to a small portion of the bladder that can be removed without compromising outflow then it is removed en bloc and a primary repair carried out. Fixation near the trigone or prostate necessitates the removal of the entire bladder and prostate with the creation of an ileal conduit. Invasion into the posterior vaginal wall in women can be treated by hysterectomy and partial vaginectomy. If the subsequent vaginal defect is small, it can be primarily repaired. Larger defects typically require flap reconstruction.

The management of posterior fixation depends on the level at which the tumor is adherent to the pelvis. Tumors at or above S2 require removal of the anterior table of the sacrum with careful nerve root dissection. Significant blood loss can be encountered and appropriate preparation should be made (discussed below). Tumor fixation below the S2–S3 junction may be removed en bloc with distal sacral resection. If this procedure is anticipated, then appropriate plans are made because this involves repositioning on the operating table to facilitate both the anterior and posterior approaches. Distal sacrectomy is often associated with significant blood loss [20]. In order to minimize hemorrhage with this procedure the branches of the internal iliac vessels are identified and ligated during the pelvic dissection. The surgical approach for distal sacrectomy has previously been described [20,21].

Lateral pelvic fixation may involve structures such as the ureter, internal iliac vessels, piriformis muscle or sacral nerve roots. This often leads to an inability to achieve complete resection. In situations where an attempt at resection for cure is deemed feasible, the en bloc resection of involved structures along with the specimen is required. Resection of a portion of a single ureter requires a reconstructive procedure to drain the urine if the kidney is still viable. With chronic obstruction the kidney may be nonfunctional as evidenced by preoperative evaluations and may be treated by either ligation of the free end of the ureter or nephrectomy. Occasionally the tumor or surrounding reaction involves the internal iliac vessels, the ligation of distal branches of which is generally well tolerated, allowing for the en bloc removal of the involved segment. Major nerves are preserved when possible for obvious reasons.

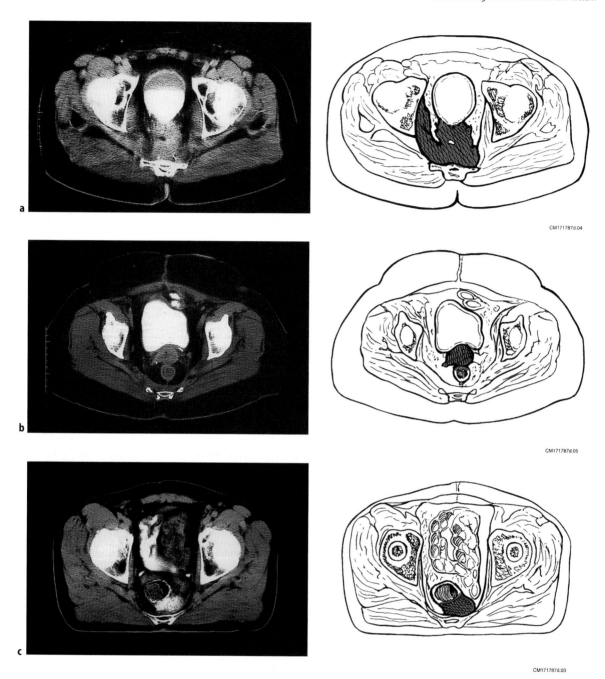

Fig. 13.1. **a** CT scan and representative drawing showing unresectable massive recurrent cancer, which was fixed to vital pelvic organs; **b** CT scan and representative drawing showing anterior recurrent tumor fixed to the base of the bladder; **c** CT scan and representative drawing showing posterior invasion into the sacrum; **d** CT scan and representative drawing showing a resectable lateral recurrence. (Reprinted from reference [10]: Nyam DC, Nelson H. Recurrent colorectal cancer. In: Nichols J, Dozois R, editors. Surgery of the colon and rectum. London: Churchill Livingstone, 1977:511–12, by permission of the publisher, Churchill Livingstone.)

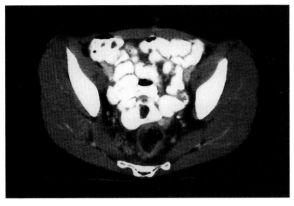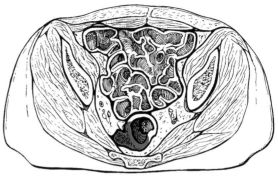

CM171787d.01

d

Fig. 13.1 (*continued*)

Branches directly involved with tumor are isolated from the uninvolved nerves and sacrificed as necessary.

The creation of large perineal wounds, particularly after partial sacrectomy, leads to the potential for serious complications [20,22,23]. Pelvic and perineal tissues have often been irradiated, adding to the potential for the breakdown of surrounding tissues. Myocutaneous flaps have been utilized in an attempt to prevent some of the serious wound complications. In a recent study by Radice et al., myocutaneous flap closure was compared with primary skin and pelvic closure and with primary skin and omental closure [24]. Patients who had primary skin and pelvic floor closure with or without pelvic omental flaps had increased overall morbidity, acute wound complications and delayed wound healing when compared with patients with a myocutaneous flap. A flap closure was not found to add to the length of hospital stay.

Intraoperative Radiation

It is known that surgery alone still leads to a significant rate of local recurrence, particularly when a complete resection has not been achieved. The use of EBRT produces some improvement in the rates of local recurrence, however, doses are kept to less than 60 Gy in order to minimize toxicity to radiosensitive organs such as the large and small bowels. Delivery of radiation therapy to the tumor bed at the time of surgery allows for maximum concentrated doses with less exposure of adjacent structures such as the small bowel because it can be cleared from the field. Two basic approaches can be used; intraoperative electron radiation therapy (IOERT); or intraoperative high-dose brachytherapy (IOHDR).

Intraoperative Electron Radiation Therapy

When using IOERT, a large single dose of radiation delivered intraoperatively produces two to three times the equivalent dose of fractionated EBRT in terms of biologic effectiveness [25]. Intraoperative radiation therapy is typically used as a supplement to EBRT, with or without fluorouracil, but may be used alone for patients with locally recurrent rectal cancer [26,27]. The dose of IOERT is dependent upon the amount of previously received radiation and the amount of residual disease subsequent to surgical resection. According to Martenson and Nelson, a typical dose of 10 Gy is delivered for microscopic residual disease, 15 Gy for gross disease <2 cm in diameter, and 17.5–20 Gy for gross disease ≥2 cm in diameter [28].

The complications of IOERT have been described [29–31]. Factors influencing the type and frequency of complications include the anatomic structures that are present in the field and the dose and energy of radiation delivered [29–31]. Structures such as the ureters, bladder, small bowel and nerves are quite radiosensitive and are subject to damage. Whenever possible these structures are mobilized out of the intended field of radiation to minimize complications.

The dose-limiting factor for IOERT is nerve, which is the most radiosensitive structure, followed by the ureter, which may be narrowed to the point of obstruction [31]. The ureter is not usually dose limiting because it can frequently be mobilized out of the field or at least stented to prevent obstruction. Criteria have been developed by the National Cancer Institute IOERT Contract Group to grade the complications seen after this type of therapy [32]. In a report by Gunderson et al. [30] the complications after treatment with IOERT were reported. Grade 1 toxicity (mild or intermittent paresthesia and/or pain; narcotics not required) was seen in 56% of the patients. The incidence of grade 2 or 3 toxicity was found to have a direct relationship with the IOERT dose, with an incidence of 3% for doses ≤2.5 Gy and 23% for doses >15 Gy. Four patients in their series developed grade 4 toxicities (one gastrointestinal obstruction, one soft tissue abscess, two wound complications) requiring emergency surgery.

Intraoperative High-Dose Brachytherapy

In contrast to the intraoperative delivery of an electron beam that requires a linear accelerator, brachytherapy can be performed using a mobile afterloading machine. Both IOERT and IOHDR require a high degree of technical support and their equipment costs are substantial, and both can be used to optimize tumor to normal tissue exposure ratios. However, there are key differences between IOERT and IOHDR that deserve mention. First of all, the electron beam is typically delivered from the linear accelerator to the tumor resection site by using a Lucite cylinder fixed to the operating table and docked to the accelerator. Approximately 20–45 minutes are required for the process in a radiation-equipped operating room. The ability to focus the beam on the field at risk may be limited by the anatomic location, especially anteriorly. Brachytherapy is performed by placment of a flexible afterloading apparatus. This facilitates direct apposition of radiation from a multichannel high-dose afterloading machine with an iridium-192 [33] or iodine-125 source [34]. Whereas it typically takes longer to perform IOHDR (30–120 minutes), it can in some patients offer better exposure.

Key therapeutic differences between IOERT and IOHDR concern the depth of penetration. IOHDR provides high surface doses (<1 cm tumor thickness) but inadequate penetration beyond 1 cm. IOERT delivers 90% of the maximum dose at the surface (<1 cm tumor thickness) and greater than 90% of the maximum dose beyond 1 cm. Although it would be ideal for institutions to be equipped with both modalities, most prefer, and/or are familiar with, either IOERT or IOHDR. Results with IOHDR are not so established or extensive as with IOERT, although preliminary analyses parallel those reported for IOERT and, overall, show promise.

Results

Without surgical intervention the survival rate of patients with a local recurrence of rectal cancer is less than 4% at 5 years [2]. EBRT with or without chemotherapy provides palliation of pelvic pain in up to 95% of symptomatic patients; however, the duration of this relief is usually only a few months [35–38]. These data clearly indicate that neither surgery nor radiation alone provides either long-term survival or effective palliation. Multimodality therapies combining surgery and radiation with radiosensitizers have shown more promise in an otherwise bleak scenario. The results of a multimodality approach including IOERT applied to 224 patients treated at the Mayo Clinic have been published [39,40]. Patients who underwent curative resections had 5-year survival rates of 34%, whereas those with residual disease after resection still had some improvement with a 5-year survival of 12%. The extent of residual disease influenced the 5-year survival rates, with those having only microscopic disease achieving 33% and those with gross disease achieving 9%. Improved 5-year survivals with multimodality therapy including both external beam radiotherapy and IOERT have also been demonstrated in other major centers using these techniques [29,41]. Although there are no controlled trials demonstrating the benefits of IOERT, retrospective analysis has demonstrated a clear improvement in local control rates when compared with EBRT [26].

Brachytherapy is currently performed in at least four locations, including Munich [42], New York [43], Los Angeles [34] and Rome [44]. Experience ranges from 30 to 56 patients treated [34,42]. Goes and colleagues describe long-term follow-up for 28 of 30 patients treated with IOHDR. They conclude that surgical morbidity and mortality are acceptable and that IOHDR provides good local control (64%) [34].

Extended Resection

The role of sacropelvic resection in the management of recurrent rectal cancer merits discussion. Although 4-year cure rates of up to 33% have been achieved [21], this operation represents the most aggressive local surgical therapy for recurrent disease. The morbidity rates of the procedure range from 25% to 60% and most complications involve the posterior sacral wounds [20]. Accordingly, sacropelvic resection is not recommended for palliation. However it does provide an effective alternative to uncontrolled pelvic tumor growth and the associated problems of pain, urinary tract dysfunction and recurrent sepsis. In a small series of 16 patients most (eight out of nine) of the patients alive at the time of follow-up reported an improved quality of life after sacropelvic resection and two-thirds of these patients were able to return to work. Overall, the potential of complications from uncontrolled pelvic tumor growth must be weighed against the morbidity of the procedure. Newer techniques of perineal wound closure such as myocutaneous flaps show promise in reducing postoperative morbidity, making sacropelvic resection a more attractive alternative [24].

Future Directions

Despite advances in both surgical and adjuvant therapies for the treatment of recurrent rectal cancer, there is still room for improvement. While better local control has been achieved through aggressive multimodality therapy, the majority of failures are still systemic, suggesting the need for more efficacious chemotherapeutic agents. Alternatively, newer agents such as immune modulators or tumor antibodies may provide more effective control both locally and systemically [45].

Novel Therapeutics

Although the conventional approach has been to combine EBRT with chemotherapy and IOERT to increase systemic effects and sensitize and enhance the local effects of radiation, more novel approaches include the use of hyperthermia and neutron therapies. Hyperthermia has been tested as a method of modifying the effects of radiation therapy, based on the fact that it increases cytotoxicity and interferes with DNA repair. Clinically, the application of radiochemotherapy and hyperthermia has been evaluated in a Phase I/II study [46] and in prospective comparisons with conventional EBRT alone [47]. In the Phase I/II study of 24 patients with primary advanced (T3/T4) and six patients with locally recurrent rectal cancer, treatment was with regional hyperthermia weekly prior to radiotherapy. At surgery, 70% were down-staged and, at 30 months' follow-up, actuarial survival was reported as 85% for primary and 60% for recurrent rectal cancer [46]. In a prospective study, 75 patients

were randomized to receive microwave-induced hyperthermia plus radiation therapy or radiation therapy alone. When they were compared, there was no significant difference with respect to survival or extent and duration of local control. Further studies should elucidate the role, if any, that hyperthermia plays in the management of rectal cancer.

Neutron therapy offers the potential advantage of highly ionizing radiation, possessing a high linear energy transfer. A recent review details results from worldwide studies of neutron irradiation over the last 20 years [48]. Data on approximately 350 patients are available. Randomized trials show an advantage for neutrons over photons for local control but not for survival. Side effects and complications are significant, which is discouraging. Perhaps modifications in dose, delivery or technique will improve results with neutron therapy; until that time, it remains experimental.

References

1. Sagar PM, Pemberton JH. Surgical management of locally recurrent rectal cancer. Br J Surg 1996;83:293–304.
2. Gunderson LL, Sosin H. Areas of failure found at reoperation (second or symptomatic look) following "curative surgery" for adenocarcinoma of the rectum. Clinicopathologic correlation and implications for adjuvant therapy. Cancer 1974;34:1278–92.
3. Suzuki K, Dozois RR, Devine RM, et al. Curative reoperations for locally recurrent rectal cancer. Dis Colon Rectum 1996;39:730–36.
4. Nordlinger B, Jaeck D, Guiget M, et al. Multicentric retrospective study by the French Surgical Association. In: Nordlinger B, Jaeck D, editors. Treatment of hepatic metastases of colorectal cancer. Paris: Springer-Verlag, 1992:129–46.
5. Rosen CB, Nagorney DM, Taswell HF, et al. Perioperative blood transfusion and determinants of survival after liver resection for metastatic colorectal carcinoma. Ann Surg 1992;216:493–505.
6. Sauter ER, Bolton JS, Willis GQ, et al. Improved survival after pulmonary resection of metastatic colorectal carcinoma. J Surg Oncol 1990;23:135–38.
7. Goya T, Miyazawa N, Kondo H, et al. Surgical resection of pulmonary metastases from colorectal cancer: 10-year follow-up. Cancer 1989;64:1418–21.
8. Karanjia ND, Schache DJ, North WR, et al. "Close shave" in anterior resection. Br J Surg 1990;77:510–12.
9. Stipa S, Nicolanti V, Botti C, et al. Local recurrence after curative resection for colorectal cancer: frequency, risk factors and treatment. J Surg Oncol 1991;(Suppl 2):155–60.
10. Nyam DC, Nelson H. Recurrent colorectal cancer. In: Nichols J, Dozois R, editors. Surgery of the colon and rectum. London: Churchill Livingstone, 1977:505–23.
11. Suzuki K, Dozois RR, Devine RM, et al. Curative reoperations for locally recurrent rectal cancer. Dis Colon Rectum 1996;39:730–36.
12. Martin EW Jr, Minton JP, Carey LP. CEA-directed second-look surgery in the asymptomatic patient after primary resection of colorectal carcinoma. Ann Surg 1985;202: 310–17.

13. Moertel CG, Flemming TR, Macdonald JS, et al. An evaluation of the carcinoembryonic antigen (CEA) test for monitoring patients with resected colon cancer. JAMA 1993;270:943–47.

14. Beecher HK, Todd DP. A study of the deaths associated with anesthesia and surgery. Ann Surg 1954;140:2–34.

15. Dripps RD, Lamont A, Eckenhoff JE. The role of anesthesia in surgical mortality. JAMA 1961;178:261–66.

16. Povoski SP, Fong Y, Sgouros SC, et al. Role of chest CT in patients with negative chest X-rays referred for hepatic colorectal metastases. Ann Surg Oncol 1998;5:9–15.

17. Farouk R, Nelson H, Radice E, et al. Accuracy of computed tomography in determining resectability for locally advanced primary or recurrent colorectal cancers. Am J Surg 1998;175:283–87.

18. Dominguez JM, Wolff BG, Nelson H, et al. 111In-CYT-103 scanning in recurrent colorectal cancer: does it affect standard management? Dis Colon Rectum 1996;39:514–19.

19. Ebner F, Kressel HY, Mintz ME, et al. Tumor recurrence versus fibrosis in the female pelvis: differentiation with MR imaging at 1.5T. Radiology 1988;166:333–40.

20. Magrini S, Nelson H, Gunderson LL, Sim FH. Sacropelvic resection and intraoperative electron irradiation in the management of recurrent anorectal cancer. Dis Colon Rectum 1996;39:1–9.

21. Wanebo HJ, Koness RJ, Vezeridis MP, et al. Pelvic resection of recurrent rectal cancer. Ann Surg 1994;220:586–97.

22. Touran T, Frost DB, O'Connell TX. Sacral resection: operative technique and outcome. Arch Surg 1990;125:911–13.

23. Wanebo HJ, Gaker DL, Whitehill R, et al. Pelvic recurrence of rectal cancer: options for curative resection. Ann Surg 1987;205:482–95.

24. Radice E, Nelson H, Mercill S, Farouk R, Petty P, Gunderson L. Primary myocutaneous flap closure following resection of locally advanced pelvic malignancies. Br J Surg 1999;86:349–54.

25. Gunderson LL, Martin JK, Beart RW, et al. Intraoperative and external beam irradiation for locally advanced colorectal cancer. Ann Surg 1988;207:52–60.

26. Farouk R, Nelson H, Gunderson LL. Aggressive multimodality treatment for locally advanced irresectable rectal cancer. Br J Surg 1997;84:741–49.

27. Gunderson LL, Nelson H, Martenson JA, et al. Intraoperative electron and external beam irradiation with or without 5-fluorouracil and maximum surgical resection for previously unirradiated, locally recurrent colorectal cancer. Dis Colon Rectum 1996;39:1379–95.

28. Martenson JA Jr, Nelson H. Radiation therapy for locally recurrent rectal cancer. In: Cohen AM, Winawer SJ, Friedman MA, Gunderson LL, editors. Cancer of the colon, rectum and anus. New York: McGraw Hill, 1994: 873–79.

29. Willett CG, Shellito PC, Tepper JE, et al. Intraoperative electron beam radiation therapy for recurrent locally advanced rectal or rectosigmoid carcinoma. Cancer 1991;67:1504–508.

30. Gunderson LL, Nelson H, Martenson JA, et al. Locally advanced primary colorectal cancer: intraoperative electron and external beam irradiation ± 5-FU. Int J Radiat Oncol Biol Phys 1997;37:601–14.

31. Shaw EG, Gunderson LL, Martin JK, et al. Peripheral nerve and ureteral tolerance to intraoperative radiation therapy: clinical and dose-response analysis. Radiother Oncol 1990;18:247–55.

32. Tepper JE, Gunderson LL, Orlow E, et al. Complications of intraoperative radiation therapy. Int J Radiat Oncol Biol Phys 1984;10:1831–39.

33. Stepan R, Zimmerman FB, Huber FT, et al. Clinical and experimental evaluation of the HDR-after-loading-IORT-FLAB-method. Proceedings of the Fifth International Congress in Radio-Oncology ICRO/OGRO. 1995;5:613–17.

34. Goes RN, Beart RW Jr, Simons AJ, et al. Use of brachytherapy in management of locally recurrent rectal cancer. Dis Colon Rectum 1997;40:1177–79.

35. Arnott SJ. The value of combined 5-fluorouracil and X-ray therapy in the palliation of locally recurrent and inoperable rectal carcinoma. Clin Radiol 1975;26:177–82.

36. Allum WH, Mack P, Priestman TJ, et al. Radiotherapy for pain relief in locally recurrent colorectal cancer. Ann R Coll Surg Engl 1987;69:220–21.

37. O'Connell MJ, Childs DS, Moertel CG, et al. A prospective controlled evaluation of combined pelvic radiotherapy and methanol extraction residue of BCG (MER) for locally unresectable or recurrent rectal carcinoma. Int J Radiat Oncol Biol Phys 1982;8:1115–19.

38. Danjoux CE, Gelber RD, Catton GE, et al. Combination chemo-radiotherapy for residual, recurrent, or inoperable carcinoma of the rectum: ECOG study (EST 3276). Int J Radiat Oncol Biol Phys 1985;11:765–7.

39. Suzuki K, Gunderson LL, Devine RM, et al. Intraoperative irradiation after palliative surgery for locally recurrent rectal cancer. Cancer 1995;75:939–52.

40. Gunderson LL. Rationale for and results of intraoperative radiation therapy. Cancer 1994;74:537–41.

41. Kramer T, Share R, Kiel K, et al. Intraoperative radiation therapy of colorectal cancer. In: Abe M, Takahashi M, editors. Intraoperative radiation therapy. New York: Pergamon, 1991:308–10.

42. Huber FT, Stepan R, Zimmerman F, et al. Locally advanced rectal cancer: resection and intraoperative radiotherapy using the FLAB method combined with preoperative or postoperative radiochemotherapy. Dis Colon Rectum 1996;39:774–79.

43. Harrison LB, Enker WE, Anderson LL. High-dose-rate intraoperative radiation therapy for colorectal cancer. Oncology 1995;9:737–41.

44. Sofo L, Ratto C, Valentini V, et al. Intraoperative radiation therapy in treatment of rectal cancers: results of Phase II study [abstract]. Dis Colon Rectum 1996;39:A7.

45. Riethmuller G, Holz E, Schlimok G, et al. Monoclonal antibody therapy for resected Dukes' C colorectal cancer: seven year outcome of a multicenter randomized trial. J Clin Oncol 1998;16:1788–94.

46. Wust P, Rau B, Gellerman J, et al. Radiochemotherapy and hyperthermia in the treatment of rectal cancer. Recent Results Cancer Res 1998;146:175–91.

47. Trotter JM, Edis AJ, Blackwell JB, et al. Adjuvant VHF therapy in locally recurrent and primary unresectable rectal cancer. Australas Radiol 1996;40:298–305.

48. Engenhart-Cabillic R, Debus J, Prott FJ, et al. Use of neutron therapy in the management of locally advanced non-resectable primary or recurrent rectal cancer. Recent Results Cancer Res 1998;150:113–24.

14. Metastatic Rectal Cancer

K. Sumpter and D. Cunningham

Introduction

Carcinomas of the rectum are defined anatomically as tumours arising in the distal 15 cm of the large bowel. The rectum lies below the peritoneal reflection, hence, unlike colonic carcinomas, the growth of rectal tumours is not limited by the serosa. At presentation, 50% of patients with rectal carcinoma are considered to be operable; of these, 50% will have a curative resection. The likelihood of developing local recurrence or metastatic disease after curative surgery increases with Dukes' stage from A to C and with the extent of tumour penetration of the bowel, Gunderson and Sosin Stage 1–3. The 5-year survival rates for patients with rectal carcinoma according to Dukes' stage are as follows: Dukes' A 80%, Dukes' B 55% and Dukes' C 32%. The management of locally recurrent rectal cancer depends upon its extent and whether it is amenable to curative treatment. Ultimately, 25% of patients with B2 disease and 50% of patients with C disease develop local recurrence. In this instance patients should be assessed to establish whether surgical excision is feasible because this offers a chance of cure. Radiotherapy should also be considered, either in an attempt to downstage local recurrence or as a palliative treatment for inoperable disease.

The commonest sites for metastatic disease in rectal cancer are the liver, lungs and peritoneum. A proportion of patients who present with metastatic disease will be potentially curable by surgery and they should be evaluated with this in mind. The main treatment option for the majority of patients with metastatic and inoperable locally advanced rectal cancer is chemotherapy. Owing to the anatomical differences previously stated, primary and locally recurrent rectal tumours should be considered as a disease entity separate from colonic cancer. However, in the metastatic disease setting, rectal and colonic cancer can be considered together and the vast majority of chemotherapeutic trials recruit patients with both diseases. 5-Fluorouracil (5-FU) has been and still remains the main cytotoxic agent used for colorectal cancer but, recently, newer drugs have been developed with encouraging results. This increases the scope for the treatment of this disease in the future. This chapter will review the chemotherapeutic agents used in metastatic rectal cancer and will discuss future directions for the management of the disease. The surgical aspects of metastatic disease will also be briefly discussed.

Surgery for Metastatic Rectal Cancer

In all patients with metastatic disease the possibility of surgical resection should be considered, since this offers the only potential chance of cure. In reality, the number of patients for whom surgery is feasible is small, because selection criteria are strict. Liver and lung metastases are the sites that are most commonly amenable to resection; however, solitary brain metastases can also be considered for surgery. The adrenal gland is an uncommon site of disease in colorectal cancer and there are few data on the role of surgery for adrenal metastases; however, solitary lesions in the absence of other sites of disease can be considered for resection.

Surgical Resection of Liver Metastases

The surgical resection of liver metastases should be performed only with curative intent. A number of recent studies have reported the results of hepatic resections for metastatic colorectal cancer [1–6]. Operative mortality is generally less than 5%, with postoperative morbidity of the order of 20%. The most common postoperative complications are transient liver failure, haemorrhage, subphrenic abscess or biliary fistula. Five-year survival rates vary from 24% to 38%. A number of factors are associated with a poor prognosis, the most important being an involved resection margin and the presence of extrahepatic disease. Other factors include a raised serum carcinoembryonic antigen (CEA) level and a short disease-free interval from primary surgery.

Taylor et al. showed that 5-year survival was also dependent on the number of lesions resected [3]. In a series of 123 patients, overall 5-year survival was 34%. This could be broken down into a 47% 5-year survival in patients with only one lesion, 16% in those with one lesion and satellite nodules, and 17% in the presence of multiple lesions.

Re-resection of hepatic metastases is also of value in selected patients in whom there is no evidence of extrahepatic disease [7–10]. Mortality and morbidity figures are similar to those for the first resection, as are 5-year survival data.

To summarise, liver resection should be considered when macroscopically clear resection margins can be obtained and there is no evidence of extrahepatic disease. After resection, careful follow-up should be performed, as there is a role for re-resection.

Surgical Resection of Lung Metastases

The lungs are another common site of metastatic disease in colorectal cancer as a whole; this is particularly the case for rectal tumours. As with liver metastases, consideration should be given to the possibility of lung resection in patients who have no other sites of metastatic disease and when complete resection of the metastases can be performed. In this situation, the long-term survival rates vary between 20% and 60%, depending on the series reported [11–14].

There are limited data on the resection of both lung and liver lesions when they occur either synchronously or metachronously. Such reports are retrospective and involve small patient numbers [15,16]. The Memorial Sloan-Kettering Cancer Center published a retrospective review of ten patients who had undergone resection of both hepatic and pulmonary metastases from colorectal cancer. The median survivals were 34 months after hepatic resection and 18 months after pulmonary resection. The actuarial 5-year survival was 52%. There does therefore appear to be a role for the resection of both hepatic and pulmonary lesions in selected patients.

Surgical Resection of Brain Metastases

The brain is an uncommon site of metastatic disease in colorectal cancer. The presence of brain metastases in this situation is usually in the context of widespread dissemination of the tumour. The management of brain metastases varies from steroid treatment only, to radiotherapy or surgery, depending on the clinical situation. Alden et al. retrospectively reviewed the case histories of 19 patients with brain metastases from colorectal cancer. The median survival of these patients was 2.8 months, with none surviving >1 year. Survival varied, depending on the treatment but it was still uniformly poor: median survival after craniotomy 4.2 months and after radiotherapy 2.8 months [17]. Patchell et al. reported a randomised trial of patients with solitary brain metastases who were treated with either surgery and postoperative radiotherapy or radiotherapy alone. The surgery arm had significantly longer survival than the radiotherapy arm [18]. For the majority of patients with brain metastasis palliative measures with steroids and/or radiotherapy provide the mainstay of treatment; however, in a small group of patients with solitary lesions and without extracranial disease, surgery remains an option.

Chemotherapy Versus Best Supportive Care for Patients with Advanced Colorectal Cancer

The role of chemotherapy in the management of patients with advanced or metastatic colorectal cancer has been well established by trials comparing chemotherapy with best supportive care. These trials are summarised in Table 14.1. A Nordic study randomised patients with asymptomatic advanced colorectal cancer to receive either chemotherapy (methotrexate (MTX) 250 mg/m^2, 5-FU 500 mg/m^2, leucovorin (LV) 15 mg 2-weekly for eight courses, 3-weekly for two courses, and 4-weekly for two courses) or primary expectancy [19]. Five months after randomisation, 57% of the patients in the primary expectancy arm had developed symptoms and crossed over to receive chemotherapy. The median overall survival (OS) and progression-free survival (PFS) were significantly better for the patients treated initially with chemotherapy (OS: 14 months and 9 months respectively, $p < 0.02$; PFS: 8 months and 3 months respectively, $p < 0.001$). Scheithaeur et al. randomised 40 patients with metastatic colorectal cancer, in a 2:1 fashion, to

Table 14.1. Summary of the critical trials of chemotherapy versus best supportive care in patients with metastatic colorectal cancer

Trial	Reference	Randomisation	No. patients	Median survival	
Nordic	19	Primary expectancy *versus* MTX 250 mg/m^2, 5-FU 500 mg/m^2 (3 + 23 hours), LV 15 mg p.o. × 3 days	183	9 months *versus* 14 months	($p \leq 0.02$)
Scheithaeur et al.	20	Best supportive care *versus* 5-FU 550 mg/m^2 per day, LV 200 mg/m^2 per day + cisplatin 20 mg/m^2 per day days 1–4, 4 weekly	40	5 months *versus* 11 months	($p = 0.006$)
Allen-Mersh et al.	22	Best supportive care *versus* Hepatic artery infusional uoxuridine 0.2 mg/kg per day, heparin 5000 iu/day for 14 days, 4-weekly	100	226 days *versus* 405 days	($p = 0.03$)

MTX, methotrexate; 5-FU, 5-fluoxuracil; LV, leucovorin.

receive either chemotherapy (LV 200 mg/m^2, 5-FU 550 mg/m^2, cisplatin 20 mg/m^2 days 1–4, 4-weekly) or best supportive care [20]. The median time to disease progression and the median survival were again both improved in the patients treated with chemotherapy (median time to disease progression 6 months and 2.3 months respectively, $p = 0.0008$; median survival 11 months and 5 months respectively, $p = 0.006$). There was no difference in quality of life (QOL) between the two groups despite the side effects associated with chemotherapy. Indeed, in patients whose pretreatment QOL scores were abnormal the score was improved after chemotherapy.

A further study of 235 patients looked at the role of 5-FU and LV in advanced gastrointestinal malignancies (3/4 of whom had colorectal cancer). The patients were stratified according to age, and 157 patients aged over 70 years were randomised to receive 5-FU/folinic acid (5-FU 600 mg/m^2 and folinic acid 300 mg/m^2 weekly) or best supportive care [21]. The overall survival was significantly longer in the chemotherapy-treated patients ($p < 0.002$) and chemotherapy-associated side effects were mild. Criticisms of this study would include the fact that no subgroup analysis was performed and that the study has been published only in abstract form.

The role of hepatic artery infusion of floxuridine was established in 100 patients with unresectable liver metastases secondary to colorectal cancer [22]. These patients were randomised to hepatic artery infusion of chemotherapy (0.2 mg/kg per day for 14 days with heparin 5000 iu/day, repeated every 4 weeks) or best supportive care. The median survival of the patients receiving chemotherapy was significantly longer than the best supportive care patients (405 days and 226 days, $p = 0.03$).

These trials clearly demonstrate a survival advantage from the use of palliative chemotherapy in patients with advanced colorectal cancer in all age groups, including those who are elderly. In addition, the Nordic study confirms a benefit from the early use of chemotherapy for metastatic disease, rather than delaying treatment until the onset of symptoms.

5-Fluorouracil

Mechanism of Action

5-FU was first synthesised in 1957 and it has been the major cytotoxic agent used in the management of colorectal cancer since then. It is itself inactive and requires intracellular conversion to form active metabolites. Its three major active metabolites are:

1. 5-fluorodeoxyuridylate (5-FdUMP), which inhibits thymidylate synthase (TS), the rate-limiting step in DNA synthesis
2. 5-fluorouridine triphosphate (5-FUTP), which incorporates into RNA and causes alterations in its processing
3. 5-flourodeoxyuridine triphosphate (5-FdUTP), which incorporates into DNA instead of deoxythymidine triphosphate (dTTP), the usual substrate for DNA polymerase

5-FU degradation is rate limited by the enzyme dihydropyrimidine dehydrogenase (DPD) and, within 24 hours of a bolus injection, 80% of the drug is broken down via this enzyme. The plasma half-life of 5-FU is only 10–12 minutes, but the binding of FdUMP to TS can be for up to 6 hours at physiological doses of reduced folate [23]. It is known that the mechanism by which 5-FU exerts its cytotoxic effect varies depending on the administration scheduling of the drug, with bolus injections acting via the RNA effect and infusional regimens acting predominantly via TS inhibition.

As a single agent, response rates of the order of 10% are seen with bolus 5-FU, with median survival rates of no more than 1 year [24]. In an attempt to improve on these response rates and survival figures, administration schedules have been modified, biochemical modulators have been utilised and other drugs have been used in combination.

Modulation of 5-Fluorouracil with Leucovorin

LV is the most frequently used biochemical modulator of 5-FU. Its mechanism of action is via increasing the intracellular levels of reduced folate. This enhances the formation and retention of the 5-FdUMP/TS complex, thus increasing the inhibition of DNA synthesis. Phase I and II studies have suggested that the addition of LV to 5-FU might enhance its activity [25,26]. Subsequently, a number of randomised trials were set up to test this hypothesis. The Advanced Colorectal Cancer Meta-Analysis Project performed a meta-analysis of nine trials, including data on more than 1500 patients [24]. There was heterogeneity amongst the treatment schedules, so they broadly categorised them into 3 groups:

1. The addition of LV to a weekly 5-FU regimen (average dose of 5-FU 2400 mg/m^2 per month + 200 or 500 mg/m^2 LV weekly)
2. 5-FU given for 5 consecutive days every 28 days (5-FU dose intensity 1850–2000 mg/m^2 per month and LV 20 mg/m^2 per day given)
3. Higher doses of 5-FU used in the control group (2400–2500 mg/m^2 per month compared with 2000 mg/m^2 per month used in the LV arm)

The results of the meta-analysis showed a significant increase in response rates in the 5-FU/LV group compared with 5-FU alone (23% versus 11%, odds ratio 0.45, $p < 10^{-7}$). The median survival times were not significantly different at 11.5 months and 11 months respectively. The meta-analysis, however, did not include data from the North Central Cancer Treatment Group (NCCTG) study, which randomised patients to six arms of treatment to look at the role of MTX, high- or low-dose LV and cisplatin in combination with 5-FU [27]. The results

Table 14.2. Trials comparing high- with low-dose LV

Trial	Reference	No. patients	Treatment schedule	Response rate (%)	Median survival
GITSG (Patreki et al.)	31	318	5-FU (500 mg/m^2 days 1–5, 4-weekly)	12.1	46 weeks
			5-FU (600 mg/m^2 + 500 mg LV/week)	30.3	55 weeks
			5-FU (600 mg/m^2 + 25 mg LV/week)	18.8	45 weeks
PALL1 (Joager et al.)	30	325	5-FU (500 mg/m^2 + 500 mg/m^2 LV/week)	21.6	55.1 weeks
			5-FU (500 mg/m^2 + 20 mg/m^2 LV/week)	17.5	54.1 weeks
NCCTG (Poon et al.)	27	208	5-FU (375–400 mg/m^2 days 1–5, 4-weekly)	10	34 weeks
			5-FU (375–400 mg/m^2 + 200 mg/m^2 LV days 1–5, 4-weekly)	26	52 weeks
			5-FU (375–400 mg/m^2 + 20 mg/m^2 LV days 1–5, 4-weekly)	43	53 weeks
Buroker et al.	29	372	5-FU (375–400 mg/m^2 + 20 mg/m^2 LV days 1–5, 4-weekly)	35	9.3 months
			5-FU (375–400 mg/m^2 + 200 mg/m^2 LV days 1–5, 4-weekly)	31	10.7 months
GISCAD (Valsecchi et al.)	28	422	5-FU 370 mg/m^2 + 6S-FA 100 mg/m^2 days 1–5, 4-weekly	9.3	11 months
			5-FU 370 mg/m^2 + 6S-FA 10 mg/m^2 days 1–5, 4-weekly	10.7	11 months
de Gramont et al.	32	437	5-FU 370 mg/m^2 + 20 mg/m^2 LV days 1–5, 4-weekly LV 200 mg/m^2 1-hour infusion + 5-FU 400 mg/m^2 bolus + 600 mg/m^2 22-hour infusion days 1–2, 2-weekly		
SWOG (Leichmann et al.)	33	178	5 FU 425 mg/m^2 + LV 20 mg/m^2 days 1–5, 4-weekly	27	14 months
			LV 500 mg/m^2 + 5-FU 600 mg/m^2 weekly for 6 out of every 8 weeks	21	13 months

GITSC, Gastrointestinal Tumor Study Group; PALL1, Palliative Treatment of Metastatic Colorectal Cancer Study Protocol 1; NCCTG, North Central Cancer Treatment Group; GISCAD, Italian Group for the Study of Digestive Tract Cancer; SWOG, South West Oncology Group; 5-FU, 5-fluorouracil; LV, leucovorin; 6S-FA, Stereoisomer of folinic acid.

showed that, with either high- (200 mg/m^2) or low- (20 mg/m^2) dose LV, the response rates and survival were significantly improved over the 5-FU alone group. There was no statistically significant difference in the survival rates between high- or low-dose LV, although the low dose did show a higher response rate (43% versus 26%). None of the other treatment arms differed statistically from that of 5-FU alone. After these studies, 5-FU and LV became regarded as the standard treatments for advanced colorectal cancer.

A number of studies have attempted to address the issue of whether high-dose LV is superior to low-dose LV. Table 14.2 summarises these trials, their treatment regimens and results. Three of these trials compared low- or high-dose LV with 5-FU according to the NCCTG protocol (5-FU 375–400 mg/m^2 days 1–5 every 4 weeks) [27–29]. The results of these trials show clearly that no benefit is derived from high-dose over low-dose LV. In the two studies that compared high- with low-dose LV when 5-FU is administered weekly (5-FU 500–600 mg/m^2 per week), the Palliative Treatment of Metastatic Colorectal Cancer Study Protocol 1 (PALL1) study showed no improvement in response rates or survival in the high-dose arm and the Gastrointestinal Tumor Study Group (GITSG) study showed an improvement in response rates with high-dose LV without a survival advantage [30,31]. The de Gramont study compared monthly bolus 5-FU and low-dose LV (NCCTG regimen) with a 48-hour bimonthly schedule of bolus and infusional 5-FU and high-dose LV (de Gramont regimen) in patients with advanced colorectal cancer. The results showed significantly higher response rates with the de Gramont regimen ($p = 0.004$) and a longer PFS ($p = 0.0012$), without a significant improvement in median survival time (monthly regimen 56.8 weeks; bimonthly regimen 62 weeks; $p = 0.067$) [32]. The Southwest Oncology Group Study (SWOG) study is a large randomised Phase II study with seven treatment arms. Two of these schedules compared bolus 5-FU with either low- or high-dose LV. The response rates and survival for both of these groups were comparable [33]. From these studies it can be concluded that low-dose LV is not only as effective as high-dose LV, but it is associated with less toxicity and is more cost-effective. It is therefore recommended that low-dose LV is used to modulate 5-FU.

Modulation of 5-Fluorouracil with Methotrexate

MTX inhibits dihydrofolate reductase, resulting in an increase in the level of cellular phosphate donor phosphoribosyl pyrophosphate (PRPP). PRPP accumulation results in the formation of FUTP, which in turn incorporates into RNA, thus inhibiting its func-

tion. One of the mechanisms of action of 5-FU is via incorporation into RNA. 5-FU is broken down to 5-fluoro-2′-deoxyuridylate (5-FUMP) in the presence of PRPP. 5-FUMP is then incorporated into RNA, altering its maturation and inducing cytotoxicity.

MTX given prior to 5-FU has been shown in experimental models to enhance the effect of 5-FU [34]. Phase II trials were commenced to investigate the combination of 5-FU and MTX. Herrmann et al. treated 56 patients who had previously untreated metastatic colorectal cancer with 5-FU and MTX (MTX 150 mg/m^2 intravenous bolus followed by 150 mg/m^2 intravenous infusion over 4 hours + 5-FU 900 mg/m^2 intravenously 7 hours after commencing MTX + LV 22.5 mg orally q.d.s. for 2 days beginning 24 hours after MTX; 2-weekly for three cycles and then 3-weekly) [35]. The overall median survival was 12.5 months and the overall response rate was 38%. Kemeny et al. reported a trial in which 45 patients were treated with MTX and 5-FU (MTX 40 mg/m^2 days 1 and 8 plus 5-FU 600 mg/m^2 days 2 and 9: 4-weekly) and the overall response rate was 32% [36].

Nine randomised trials have been performed comparing 5-FU alone with 5-FU and MTX. The tumour response rates in most of these trials were better for 5-FU/MTX, but in only one was there a survival advantage [37]. The Advanced Colorectal Cancer Meta-Analysis Project published the results of a meta-analysis using data from eight of these trials [38]. A total of 1178 patients were included in the analysis. The dose of MTX used was generally between 200 and 250 mg/m^2; however, the European Organization for Research on Treatment of Cancer (EORTC) study used 40 mg/m^2 [39]. A highly significant superiority of MTX/5-FU was found for overall response rates (odds ratio 0.51, $p < 0.0001$). The median overall survival in the 5-FU alone arm was 9.1 months and in the 5-FU/MTX arm 10.7 months. This survival advantage for 5-FU/MTX was statistically significant ($p = 0.024$).

On comparing the results of the meta-analyses of 5-FU/LV and 5-FU/MTX, the two appear similar in terms of response rates. In experimental models the addition of LV to 5-FU/MTX has not yielded results superior to either of the two separate combinations [40].

Protracted Venous Infusional 5-Fluorouracil

There are a number of factors that favour the administration of 5-FU as a continuous infusion:

1. It is a cell-cycle-specific agent whose major effects occur during the S phase. However,

it is known that at any one time only 3% of colorectal cancer cells are in S phase.

2. 5-FU has a short plasma half-life of 10–12 minutes and TS inhibition after a bolus dose is short, with a dissociation half-life of 6 hours.

3. An increased duration of exposure to 5-FU has been observed to result in significantly increased cellular toxicity.

For these reasons the infusional delivery of 5-FU has been developed, with the aim of increasing the binding to TS.

In 1981, Lokich et al. reported a Phase I study of continuous 5-FU [41]. The maximum tolerated dose in this study was 300 mg/m^2 per day. The main toxicities observed were stomatitis and palmar plantar erythema. This is in contrast to myelosuppression, which is seen commonly with bolus 5-FU schedules. These findings suggested a different mechanism of action for the drug when administered infusionally. After this, a number of Phase II studies were conducted, which reported response rates in the order of 31–53%.

In 1989 a randomised study comparing bolus 5-FU (500 mg/m^2 days 1–5, 5-weekly) with protracted venous infusional (PVI) 5-FU (300 mg/m^2 per day) was published [42]. A total of 174 patients were evaluable. In the bolus 5-FU group 7% responded compared with 30% in the PVI 5-FU group ($p < 0.001$). The toxicity profiles in the two groups were also significantly different, in that a greater number of patients in the bolus group developed neutropenia ($p < 0.001$), with four patients dying of neutropenic sepsis. In contrast, a significantly greater number of patients in the PVI group developed palmar plantar erythema ($p < 0.001$). The median survival times were similar: 11 months with bolus 5-FU and 10 months with PVI 5-FU. However, 32% of the patients treated with bolus 5-FU crossed over to receive PVI 5-FU when they progressed. The survival time was much better than that typically observed for the bolus group and this may mask a potential survival advantage for the PVI 5-FU group.

There have been further trials comparing bolus with infusional 5-FU. The Eastern Cooperative Oncology Group (ECOG) reported response rates of 28% for patients treated with PVI 5-FU (300 mg/m^2 per day) and 18% for patients who received bolus 5-FU (500 mg/m^2 days 1–5 followed after 2 weeks by weekly bolus 5-FU at 600 mg/m^2) [43]. This improved response rate in the PVI group was statistically significant ($p = 0.045$). When survival was compared in the 312 patients treated with PVI 5-FU (with or without cisplatin) with the 153 patients treated with bolus 5-FU (with or without cisplatin), there was a significant improvement in PFS

($p = 0.003$). The National Cancer Institute of Canada randomised 184 patients to receive either bolus or infusional 5-FU with resulting response rates of 6% and 12% respectively, which were not statistically different [44]. Rougier et al. reported a response rate of 8% for bolus 5-FU-treated patients and 19% for PVI 5-FU ($p = 0.02$) [45]. Again there was no overall survival difference.

There have been no randomised Phase III trials comparing PVI 5-FU with bolus 5-FU modulated by LV. In a randomised Phase II study performed by the SWOG, two of the seven arms involved continuous infusional 5-FU [33]. One of these consisted of continuous infusional 5-FU (300 mg/m^2, days 1–28 of a 5-weekly cycle). The other arm comprised continuous infusional 5-FU (200 mg/m^2, days 1–28 of a 5-weekly cycle) with LV 20 mg/m^2 weekly. The objective response rates were 29% and 27% respectively. This was not significantly different from either the bolus 5-FU arm with high-dose LV or the bolus 5-FU arm with low-dose LV (21% and 27% respectively). There was no survival advantage associated with any of the treatments.

Most of these randomised studies confirm an increase in tumour response with continuous infusional 5-FU. However, the magnitude of this is not clear, nor is its impact on survival. A meta-analysis has recently been published using data from six of the seven published randomised trials comparing continuous infusional 5-FU with bolus 5-FU (in one of the trials, comprising 70 patients, data could not be retrieved) [46]. The analysis included data on 1219 patients. Details of the trials and the chemotherapy regimens are shown in Table 14.3. The ECOG trial was a three-armed study and the continuous infusional 5-FU and cisplatin arm was excluded from the analysis [43]. The SWOG study, as previously stated, consisted of two arms in which continuous infusional 5-FU was administered; these have been compared separately with bolus 5-FU. In two cohorts of patients, the 5-FU in both treatment arms was administered with LV [33,47]. The results of this meta-analysis showed an improved overall response rate with continuous infusion 5-FU (22% continuous infusion versus 14% bolus, $p = 0.0002$), which translated into a survival advantage (median survival time continuous infusion 12.1 months versus 11.3 months bolus, $p = 0.04$). The incidence of grade 3 or 4 toxicity was highly significantly reduced in the continuous infusion-treated patients (4% continuous infusion versus 31% bolus, $p = <10^{-7}$). There were 145 assessable patients in the two trials that used LV as a biochemical modulator. When only these trials are used to compare continuous infusional with bolus 5-FU, the overall response is improved in the continuous infusional patients but

Table 14.3. Summary of trials comparing continuous infusional with bolus 5-FU

Trial	No. patients	Reference	Chemotherapy schedules	
			Continuous infusion	Bolus
ECOG (Hauran et al.)	324	43	5-FU 300 mg/m^2 per day	5-FU 500 mg/m^2 days 1–5 then 600 mg/m^2 weekly
NCIC (Weinerman et al.)	184	44	5-FU 350 mg/m^2 days 1–15 every 4 weeks	5-FU 400–450 mg/m^2 days 1–5 every 4 weeks
MAOP (Lokich et al.)	174	42	5-FU 300 mg/m^2 per day	5-FU 500 mg/m^2 days 1–5 every 5 weeks
Rougier et al.	155	45	5-FU 750 mg/m^2 days 1–7 every 3 weeks	5-FU 500 mg/m^2 days 1–5 every 4 weeks
Isacson et al.	26	47	5-FU 600 mg/m^2 + FA 15 mg q.d.s. p.o. days 1–5 every 3 weeks	5-FU 600 mg/m^2 + folinic acid 15 mg q.d.s. p.o. days 1–5 every 3 weeks
SWOG (Leichmann et al.)	181	33	5-FU 300 mg/m^2 days 1–28 every 5 weeks	5-FU 500 mg/m^2 days 1–5 every 5 weeks
SWOG (Leichmann et al.)	175	33	5-FU 200 mg/m^2 days 1–28 every 5 weeks and FA 20 mg/m^2 intravenously weekly	5-FU 425 mg/m^2 + FA 20 mg/m^2 intravenously days 1–5 every 4 weeks for two courses and then every 5 weeks

ECOG, Eastern Cooperative Oncology Group; NCIC, National Cancer Institute of Canada; MAOP, Mid-Atlantic Oncology Program Study; SWOG; South West Oncology Group; 5-FU, 5-fluorouracil; FA, Folinic acid.

it does not reach statistical significance, probably due to the fact that the number of patients is too small.

A randomised study is ongoing at the Royal Marsden Hospital, comparing 6 months' bolus 5-FU/LV (NCCTG regimen) with 12 weeks' PVI 5-FU 300 mg/m^2 as adjuvant chemotherapy for patients with Dukes' C or high-risk Dukes B' colorectal cancer.

Few studies have assessed the role of LV modulation with continuous infusional 5-FU. In a Phase II trial, 41 patients received PVI 5-FU (200 mg/m^2 per day) for 4 weeks, with a 2-week rest period, and then monthly cycles of 3 weeks PVI 5-FU with 1 week's rest, and LV (20 mg/m^2) by intravenous bolus every week of treatment [48]. Forty-six per cent of the patients responded to this regimen and the median survival time was 16 months. In the previously mentioned SWOG trial, two of the arms comprised PVI 5-FU (300 mg/m^2 per day) and PVI 5-FU (200 mg/m^2 per day) with bolus LV (20 mg/m^2) weekly [33]. The response rates and survival times were similar (response rates: 29% and 26% respectively). On the basis of these studies there is no evidence that benefit is derived from the biochemical modulation of PVI 5-FU with LV.

Other Continuous Infusional 5-Fluorouracil Schedules

In an attempt to improve response rates, various other regimens have been developed involving continuous infusional 5-FU. They have largely centred on varying the duration of the infusion. In a Phase I–II study, the maximum tolerated dose of continuous infusional 5-FU was found to be 3.5 g/m^2, given over 48 hours every week [49]. The dose-limiting toxicities observed were diarrhoea and mucositis, and the response rate in previously untreated patients was 43%. These results were confirmed in a further Phase II study performed by the Spanish Cooperative Group for Gastrointestinal Tumour Therapy, when response rates of 38.5% were reported [50]. The same group then reported a trial concerning continuous infusional 5-FU with LV modulation [51]. The original dose of 5-FU used (3 g/m^2 continuous infusion over 48 hours) was associated with high levels of toxicity and the dose was therefore modified to 2 g/m^2 over 48 hours weekly, with 60 mg/m^2 LV 6-hourly for the duration of the infusion. A total of 110 patients were treated in this regimen and the median dose intensity of 5-FU was 1.6 g/m^2 per week. The overall response rate was 37.5%, with a median survival time of 14.5 months. The incidences of grade 3 diarrhoea and vomiting were 24.5% and 12.6% respectively. This is higher than that seen with protracted infusional 5-FU regimens.

The "de Gramont" regimen is commonly used in France and the United Kingdom. This combines the bolus and infusional administration of 5-FU with LV (LV 200 mg/m^2 per day as a 2-hour infusion, 5-FU 400 mg/m^2 per day intravenous bolus, and a 22-hour infusion of 600 mg/m^2 per day for 2 consecutive days every 2 weeks). This regimen was compared in a randomised study to the Mayo NCCTG regimen

(LV 20 mg/m^2 and 5-FU 425 mg/m^2 days 1–5, repeated every 4 weeks) [32]. A total of 448 patients were randomised. The overall response rate for the monthly treatment was 14.5% and for the bimonthly treatment 32.6% (p = 0.0004). PFS was also significantly longer in the bimonthly group (27.6 weeks versus 22 weeks, p = 0.001). Median survival was longer with the bimonthly regimen, although this did not reach statistical significance (62 weeks versus 56.8 weeks, p = 0.067).

Chronomodulated Chemotherapy

The suprachiasmatic nucleus maintains biological functions on a 24-hour time frame. The main circadian rhythm is the rest–activity cycle, but cellular mechanisms also display circadian changes. For example, there is a wide variation in the activity of several enzymes, such as DPD. It was discovered that the toxicity of 5-FU in mice varied 2–3-fold according to the dosing time; this is as a result of circadian rhythms [52]. In addition to this, the dosing time producing least toxicity was found in the main to be associated with a high antitumour effect in transplanted tumours. The least toxic circadian time for 5-FU is early in the rest span (i.e. 00:00–04:00 hours). The proliferative activity of human bone marrow, oral and intestinal mucosa, and skin differ by 50% according to a circadian rhythm, with a trough early in the rest span and a peak from 12:00 to 20:00 [53]. The circadian modulation of drugs therefore offers the possibility of decreased toxicity and increased dose intensity.

Phase I studies on the circadian delivery of 5-FU, oxaliplatin and floxuridine have confirmed this potential. Levi et al. treated 35 patients with metastatic colorectal cancer with continuous infusional 5-FU for 5 days, with delivery rates varying sinusoidally (highest at 04:00 and null from 18:00 to 22:00) [53]. Intrapatient dose escalation was performed (1 g/m^2 per course to 5–9 g/m^2 per course) and treatment cycles were 3-weekly. The maximum tolerated dose was 7.5 g/m^2 per course. The dose-limiting toxicities were predictably mucositis, diarrhoea and palmar plantar erythema.

Phase II trials assessing the chronomodulation of 5-FU alone or with LV have shown encouraging antitumour activity. A multicentre Phase II trial was used to treat 36 patients with metastatic colorectal cancer (17 of whom had been pretreated) with chronomodulated 5-FU and LV (5-FU 600–800 mg/m^2 per day; LV 300 mg/m^2 per day: peaks at 04:00 × 5 days 3-weekly). No grade 3/4 toxicity was observed. The objective response rate was 35% in chemonaive patients and 5% in pretreated patients [54].

The chronomodulated combination of oxaliplatin, 5-FU and LV was initially studied by Levi et al. They treated 93 patients (half of whom had received previous chemotherapy) with a 5-day infusion of the three drugs (oxaliplatin 25–30 mg/m^2 per day infused for 12 hours from 10:15 to 21:45 hours, with a sinusoidally varying delivery rate and peak delivery at 16:00; and 5-FU 700–800 mg/m^2 per day + LV 300 mg/m^2 per day from 22:15 to 09:45 hours, with peak delivery at 04:00). The objective response rate was 58% (6.4% complete responses) and 33% of patients achieved stabilisation of their disease. An objective response of 58% was seen in the 19 patients who had progressed while on 5-FU-based chemotherapy. The main toxicities associated with the treatment were nausea and vomiting, diarrhoea and peripheral sensitive neuropathy (grade 3/4 in 8%, 5% and 11% of treatment cycles respectively) [55].

Two randomised trials have been published to date, comparing constant-rate infusional oxaliplatin, 5-FU and LV, utilising a chronotherapy regimen. The first randomised 92 patients with previously untreated metastatic colorectal cancer to receive either a constant rate infusion of the three drugs (oxaliplatin 20–25 mg/m^2 per day, 5-FU 600–700 mg/m^2 per day, and LV 300 mg/m^2 per day for 5 days every 3 weeks) or a chronomodulated regimen (details as for the previously mentioned Phase II study) [56]. The median dose of oxaliplatin administered was similar in both treatment arms but, with chronomodulation, the median dose of 5-FU was 700 mg/m^2 per day compared with 500 mg/m^2 per day when the drug was delivered as a constant rate infusion (p < 0.0001). The objective response rates were 53% for chronotherapy and 32% for the constant rate infusion (p = 0.038). This translated into a prolonged median survival favouring chronotherapy (19 months versus 14.9 months, p = 0.03). The main toxicity reported was stomatitis; and grade 3/4 stomatitis was 8.7 time more likely to occur with the constant rate treatment (p < 0.0001). Peripheral sensory neuropathy was the main side effect with chronotherapy and grade 2 toxicity was four times more likely in these patients. The trial was terminated early owing to a risk of partial chemical inactivation of oxaliplatin with the basic pH of 5-FU in the constant rate arm [57].

A second multicentre randomised trial was then commenced, in which the risk of chemical drug interaction was avoided. The results of this were published in 1997 [58]. One hundred and eighty-six patients with previously untreated metastatic colorectal cancer were randomised to receive constant rate or chronomodulated oxaliplatin, 5-FU and LV (details of doses and delivery as for previous study [57]). The study was interrupted early owing to the results. Objective responses were seen in 51% of patients treated with chronotherapy and in 29% of those treated with constant rate treatment. Complete responses were seen in 22% and 14% of the patients respectively. The improved response rate seen with chronotherapy did not convey an improvement in progression-free or median survival (median survival 16.9 months for chronotherapy and 15.9 months for constant rate infusion). This may be attributable in part to the fact that 24% of patients in the constant rate infusion arm were subsequently treated with chronotherapy on progression of their disease. The incidences of all toxicities were either similar or significantly reduced in the chronotherapy group (peripheral sensory neuropathy and mucositis were significantly reduced; $p = 0.01$ and $p = 0.0001$).

Chronomodulation therefore offers an exciting new development in the treatment of metastatic colorectal cancer; the combination of 5-FU, LV and oxaliplatin appears to be particularly effective.

5-Fluorouracil and Mitomycin C

Mitomycin C (MMC) has been used for over 30 years as a single agent in the management of metastatic colorectal cancer. Response rates have varied from 0% to 33% [59,60]. In human colon carcinoma cell lines MMC has been shown to enhance the effect of a 5-day infusion of 5-FU and this was seen maximally when the MMC was administered prior to the 5-FU [61]. Early Phase II studies on the combination of 5-FU and MMC demonstrated response rates of between 33% and 39%, which suggested a synergistic effect [62,63]. Two randomised trials that investigated the potential benefits of a 5-FU/MMC combination over 5-FU treatment alone failed to show any improvement in response or survival [64,65]. In the first study, 274 patients were randomised to a 4-day infusion of 5-FU (1000 mg/m^2 per day) with either MMC (15–20 mg/m^2) or methyl CCNU (N-(2-chloroethyl)-N′-cyclohexyl-N-nitrosourea, 150–175 mg/m^2 p.o.). The second randomised 140 patients to weekly bolus 5-FU alone or bolus 5-FU, MMC and methyl CCNU (5-FU 400 mg/m^2 intravenously weekly, methyl CCNU 70 mg/m^2 p.o. 6-weekly and MMC 10 mg/m^2 intravenously 6-weekly). More recently, the results of a randomised trial have been published in which 200 patients were randomised to receive either PVI 5-FU alone (300 mg/m^2 per day for 24 weeks) or PVI 5-FU +

MMC (10 mg/m^2 6-weekly × 4) [66]. The MMC dose was reduced to 7 mg/m^2 every 6 weeks because of the development of haemolytic uraemic syndrome in two patients. At a cumulative maximum dose of 56 mg, no patients developed the haemolytic uraemic syndrome. The response rates for the combination of 5-FU and MMC were significantly better (54% 5-FU/MMC, 38% 5-FU alone; $p = 0.024$) and this translated into an improved DFS (7.9 months versus 5.4 months respectively, $p = 0.033$). A recently updated analysis has demonstrated a survival benefit associated with the 5FU/MMC arm (unpublished data). The same group then performed a further phase III study comparing the previously described PVI 5FU/MMC regimen with chronomodulated 5FU (600–450 mg/m^2 infused at a flat rate between 10.15 pm and 9.45 am) and MMC 7 mg/m^2 6 weekly. Three hundred and twenty patients were included in this study and response rates were 40% and 29% respectively, with similar overall survivals (17.6 months versus 16 months respectively)[67]. This confirms the efficacy of PVI 5FU/MMC which remains a good reference treatment in colorectal cancer.

Oral Fluoropyrimidines

Oral fluoropyrimidines offer several potential advantages over 5-FU. They provide prolonged 5-FU exposure at lower peak concentrations than those seen with bolus intravenous 5-FU and the incidence of toxic effects can be reduced. They also have the advantage of having a more convenient administration route. Four main oral fluoropyrimidines will be discussed here: uracil-tegafur (UFT) and oral LV; capecitabine; S-1; and eniluracil plus oral 5-FU.

Uracil-Tegafur and Oral Leucovorin

Tegafur (1-(2-tetrahydrofuranyl)-5-fluorouracil) is an oral 5-FU prodrug. It is hydroxylated and converted to 5-FU in the liver by microsomal p450. Uracil is a biochemical modulator of 5-FU. Its mechanism of action is via inhibition of DPD, thus reducing the degradation of 5-FU. Uracil and tegafur have been combined in a 4:1 molar ratio to produce the drug UFT.

Phase I studies using UFT as a single agent, administered in three divided daily doses, have established the dose-limiting toxicities to be neutropenia when a 5-day schedule is employed and diarrhoea when a 28-day schedule is used [68]. Further Phase I studies have concerned the combination of UFT with the biochemical modulator LV.

Studies have been performed using high- and low-dose oral LV modulation. A dose of UFT 300–350 mg/m^2 per day with LV 150 mg/day in three divided doses for 28 days, with 1 week rest, was the recommended dose for the high-dose LV regimen; UFT 350 mg/m^2 plus LV 15 mg/day using the same schedule was recommended for low-dose LV combinations. The dose-limiting toxicity in both cases was diarrhoea [69].

Twenty-one patients with previously untreated metastatic colorectal cancer were treated in a Phase II study with UFT and LV (UFT 350 mg/m^2 per day in three divided doses, with LV 5 mg t.d.s. for 28 days every 5 weeks) [70]. Twenty-five per cent of evaluable patients achieved an objective response and the median survival had not been reached at the time of reporting, but it was longer than 12 months. The main toxicity encountered was diarrhoea, with 20% of patients experiencing grade 3/4 toxicity. Forty-five patients were treated in a Phase II study combining UFT (350 mg/m^2 per day, reduced to 300 mg/m^2 per day after 5/7 patients developed prolonged diarrhoea) and LV (150 mg/day) in three divided doses for 28 days every 5 weeks. The overall response rate was 42.2% [71].

Two phase III trials have compared UFT and oral LV with bolus intravenous 5FU/LV regimens. In the first, 380 patients were randomised to receive either oral UFT (300 mg/m^2/day) and oral LV (90 mg/day for 28 days every 35 days or intravenous 5FU (425 mg/m^2/day) and LV (20 mg/m^2/day) for 5 days every 35 days. The median survival times were comparable, 12.2 and 11.9 months respectively. The incidence of stomatitis and haematological toxicity were significantly lower in the oral UFT/LV group [72]. The second study enrolled 816 patients who were randomised to receive either oral UFT (300 mg/m^2/day) and LV (75–90 mg/day) for 28 days every 35 days or either intravenous 5FU (425 mg/m^2) and LV (20 mg/m^2) for 5 days every 28 days. Early results suggest no difference in survival but again there were significantly lower incidences of neutropenia and mucositis in the oral group [73].

Capecitabine

Doxifluridine (5'-deoxy-5-fluorouridine, dFUR) is a synthetic fluoropyrimidine that was designed as an oral 5-FU prodrug. The conversion of doxfluoridine to 5-FU is catalysed by thymidine phosphorylase. This enzyme is found in greater amounts in tumours than in normal tissues; hence doxifluoridine was felt to have the potential for being tumour specific. Unfortunately, in clinical trials, this selectivity of action has not been shown to lead to a reduction in side effects. The major dose-limiting side

effect of dFUR is diarrhoea and this is attributable to the fact that the small intestine has high levels of thymidine phosphorylase. Therefore, the oral administration of dFUR results in the production of 5-FU within the intestinal tract.

A dose of 1000–1400 mg/m^2 of dFUR was established in early studies to exhibit antitumour activity with acceptable side effects [74]. Bajetta et al. treated 108 patients with metastatic colorectal cancer with oral dFUR 1200 mg/m^2 preceded by LV 25 mg on days 1–5 every 10 days [75]. Fifty-seven per cent of the patients entered in the study had received no previous chemotherapy; the remainder had received 5-FU with or without LV as adjuvant (17%) or first line metastatic treatment (26%). A median number of 15 cycles of treatment were administered per patient. The response rate in previously untreated patients was 32% compared with 13% in those who had received previous treatment. The median survival in the two groups was 14 and 12 months respectively. The main documented side effect was diarrhoea; 29% of patients experienced grade 3/4 toxicity. These results were encouraging and the fact that 13% of the patients who had been previously treated with 5-FU responded indicates the possibility of non-cross-resistance. The role of dFUR in patients with 5-FU resistant metastatic colorectal cancer was investigated in a subsequent trial (progressive disease (PD) on or within 8 weeks of 5-FU treatment) [76]. Response rates of 16% were observed, with a median duration of response of 6 months. Although doxifluridine has shown promising activity in metastatic colorectal cancer, the incidence of diarrhoea associated with its use remains a problem.

Capecitabine was developed as an oral tumour-selective fluoropyrimidine. It passes through the intestinal mucosa as an intact molecule and the incidence of diarrhoea should therefore be reduced. It is primarily metabolised in the liver and then further metabolised at the tumour site to 5-FU by thymidine phosphorylase. Preclinical studies have demonstrated that it is cytotoxic only on its conversion to 5-FU. It has also been shown to be more active than 5-FU and to have some activity in 5-FU-resistant cell lines. Phase I studies have established doses for the administration of capecitabine in a continuous schedule (maximum tolerated dose (MTD) 1657 mg/m^2 per day in two divided doses) and an intermittent schedule (MTD 3000 mg/m^2 per day for 2 weeks with 1 week rest) [77,78]. The dose-limiting toxicities were diarrhoea and vomiting in both of these studies. The combination of capecitabine and oral LV (60 mg/day) has also been investigated in Phase I studies. The MTD for the continuous schedule with LV 60 mg/day was capecitabine 1004 mg/m^2 per day and for the intermittent schedule 2000 mg/m^2 per day.

A randomised open-label Phase II trial has been carried out to evaluate three schedules of capecitabine as first line treatment in 109 patients with metastatic colorectal cancer: capecitabine administered twice daily continuously, intermittently or intermittently with oral LV. Response rates were comparable in all arms at between 21% and 24%. The PFSs were 17 weeks in the continuous arm, 30 weeks in the intermittent arm and 24 weeks in the intermittent arm with LV [79]. Two randomised phase III trials have been performed comparing Capecitabine with intravenous 5FU/LV, Mayo regimen. In one, 602 patients with previously untreated colorectal cancer were randomised to receive either Capecitabine 2500 mg/m^2/day × 14 days every 3 weeks or 5FU/LV intravenously (5FU 450 mg/m^2 and LV 20 mg/m^2 D1-5 every 4 weeks) [80]. The response rate in the Capecitabine arm was significantly higher (26% versus 17.9%, p = 0.013) but PFS was similar in both treatment arms (5.3 versus 4.8 months). In the second study 605 patients were randomised to the same two treatment arms [81]. Response rates in the Capecitabine arm was again increased significantly (23% versus 15.5%, p = 0.02) but no PFS advantage was seen. The most common toxicities seen with Capecitabine in these studies were hand-foot syndrome and diarrhoea. Oral Capecitabine is now being evaluated in a phase III study as adjuvant treatment for patients with Dukes C colon cancers.

Eniluracil

Eniluracil is a potent inhibitor of DPD. In animal models it has been shown to increase the therapeutic index of 5-FU by up to sixfold. A Phase I trial using a twice-daily regimen of oral 5-FU and eniluracil confirmed that this combination can produce plasma concentrations of 5-FU comparable with PVI 5-FU [82]. The dose recommended for Phase II studies was 5-FU 1 mg/m^2 and eniluracil 10 mg/m^2 orally twice daily for 28 days with 1 week rest. A multicentre phase II study has been published which evaluated a 28 day regimen of oral 5FU and Eniluracil in patients with previously untreated metastatic colorectal cancer [83]. Patients received either 1.00 mg/m^2 or 1.15 mg/m^2 oral 5FU and Eniluracil at a 1:10 ratio twice daily for 28 days every 5 weeks. A total of 55 patients were included and there was a 25% response rate with a further 36% having disease stabilisation. Phase III studies have been undertaken in metastatic colorectal cancer comparing an oral eniluracil and 5FU regimen with the conventional Mayo regimen. Results are as yet unpublished.

S-1

S-1 is a new oral fluoropyrimidine combining tegafur with two modulators of 5-FU: chloro-2,4-dihydroxypyridine (CDHP) and potassium oxonate, in a molar ratio of 0:0.4:1. CDHP is a DPD inhibitor that is 200 times more potent than uracil; potassium oxonate blocks 5-FU phosphorylation. 5-FU phosphorylation is responsible for both the antitumour activity of 5-FU and its gastrointestinal toxicity. Potassium oxonate selectively inhibits 5-FU phosphorylation in the gastrointestinal tissue while minimising its inhibition in tumour tissue. In an EORTC Phase I study, S-1 was administered twice daily for 4 weeks with 1 week rest. The MTD was 45 mg/m^2 twice daily and the dose-limiting toxicity was diarrhoea [84]. A phase II study has evaluated S1 at a standard dose of 8.0 mg/m^2/day in 63 patients with metastatic colorectal cancer [85]. All patients were previously untreated for metastatic disease. 35% had a partial response and median survival was 12 months, suggesting equivalence with an infusional 5FU regimen.

Irinotecan

Irinotecan (CPT11) is a semisynthetic water-soluble camptothecan. Its mechanism of action is via inhibition of the nuclear enzyme DNA topoisomerase I, which allows the relaxation of supercoiled DNA to occur so that replication and transcription can proceed. Inhibition of this enzyme results in an accumulation of single-strand DNA breaks in the cell, with resultant cell death. In vivo irinotecan is esterified in the liver into 7-ethyl-10-hydroxy-camptothecan (SN-38), which is 1000 times more potent in its action as a topoisomerase inhibitor. Colorectal cancer cells have levels of topoisomerase 14–16 times higher than those of normal tissues [86]. In preclinical studies, irinotecan has demonstrated activity against a broad range of tumours including colorectal cancer, mesothelioma and ovarian cancer. It has also been shown to have activity in cell lines expressing the multidrug resistance phenotype, often found in colorectal cancer [87].

Phase I clinical trials have been performed in the USA, Japan and Europe [88]. These have established the major dose-limiting toxicities of irinotecan to be diarrhoea and myelosuppression. The diarrhoea encountered can be divided into two distinct types, early and delayed onset. Early onset diarrhoea occurs within the first 24 hours after the administration of irinotecan. It is associated with an acute cholinergic-like syndrome and the symptoms

Table 14.4. Summary of Phase II trials of irinotecan (CPT 11)

Trial	Reference	CPT11 regimen	No. patients: evaluable	Prior treatment	% Response rates (evaluable patients)
Rothenburg et al.	84	125–150 mg/m^2 per week × 4 every 6 weeks	48:43	All patients PD on or within 6 months of 5 FU	23
Shimada et al.	82	100 mg/m^2 per week or 150 mg/m^2 per 2 weeks	67:63	52 prior chemo/radiotherapy 11 chemonaïve	25 36
Rougier et al.	83	350 mg/m^2 3-weekly	213:178	165 prior chemo 48 chemonaïve	17.7 18.8
NCCTG (Pitot et al.)	88	125 mg/m^2 per week × 4 every 6 weeks	66:33	41 prior chemo 25 chemonaïve	24 15
van Cutsem et al.	85	350 mg/m^2 3-weekly	107:95	All prior chemo	13.7
Conti et al.	87	125 mg/m^2 per week × 4 every 6 weeks	41:41	All no prior chemo	32
Ychou et al.	86	350 mg/m^2 3-weekly	136:99	All 5 FU-resistant disease	12.1

NCCTG, North Central Cancer Treatment Group; CPT11, irinotecan; PD, progressive disease; 5-FU, 5-fluorouracil.

resolve after the administration of atropine sulphate. The delayed diarrhoea is more severe and it typically occurs between 4 and 8 days after irinotecan. It can, however, be controlled by using intensive loperamide regimens. The results of Phase I trials are unified in establishing diarrhoea and myelosuppression to be the dose-limiting toxicities; however, the MTD and the scheduling of the drug varied between the continents involved in the trials. In the European studies the greatest dose intensity was achieved with irinotecan administered 3-weekly and doses of 350 mg/m^2 could be tolerated. In contrast, in Japan and the USA, the MTD for 3-weekly administered irinotecan was 240–250 mg/m^2. The reason for these differences could be due to the fact that the definition of MTD varied. In the European trials it was defined as the dose level at which more than 50% of patients developed grade 3/4 toxicity during the first cycle. In the USA and Japan it was defined as the dose at which no more than one in six patients developed grade 3/4 toxicity and the dose level above which severe or life-threatening toxicities were observed respectively. European groups have therefore tended to use a 3-weekly regimen of irinotecan (350 mg/m^2) for subsequent studies, and in American and Japanese studies weekly regimens were used (150 mg/m^2 per week × 4 with a 2-week rest, or 100 mg/m^2 per week).

Seven Phase II studies have been published evaluating the role of irinotecan in patients with metastatic colorectal cancer. A summary of these trials is shown in Table 14.4. The first trial reported was from Japan [89], where patients were treated with either weekly or 2-weekly irinotecan (100 mg/m^2 per week or 150 mg/m^2 per 2 weeks). Of the 67 patients included in the study, 63 were evaluable for response and 81% had received previous chemotherapy. An overall response rate of 27% was observed (17/63 patients partial response) and this could be broken down into a response rate of 25% in patients who had received previous chemotherapy and 36% in chemonaive patients. In the largest published trial to date, 213 patients received irinotecan 350 mg/m^2 every 3 weeks [90]. The overall response rate was 18%; there was no difference in the response rates between patients who had or had not received previous chemotherapy. Indeed, when looking at the subset of patients who had undergone previous treatment with 5-FU, those who had progressed while receiving 5-FU were as likely to respond as those who had progressed after the 5-FU (response rates 16.1% and 19.1% respectively). Administering irinotecan at a dose of 150 mg/m^2 per week × 4 every 6 weeks, Rothenburg et al. reported 23% response rates in the 43 evaluable patients who had progressed on or within 6 months of stopping 5-FU [91]. A study using a similar regimen in which all patients had 5-FU-resistant disease reported similar results [92]. A further European study, using the same dose regimen of irinotecan (350 mg/m^2 3-weekly), was performed to assess both the efficacy of the drug and to assess the role of Tiorfan (an antisecretory enkephalinase inhibitor) [93]. Patients were randomly assigned to receive Tiorfan or not, to assess its role in the prevention of irinotecan-associated delayed diarrhoea. One hundred and thirty-six patients with 5-FU-resistant disease were enrolled, of whom 99 were evaluable for response. A 12.1% response rate was obtained. Tiorfan was found not to have an effect on CPT11-associated delayed diarrhoea. Conti et al. reported data on 41 patients with metastatic colorectal cancer who received irinotecan 125 mg/m^2 per week × 4 every 6 weeks [94]. None of these patients had received any previous chemotherapy. An overall response rate of 32% was seen. This is consistent with the response rates of 15–36% reported in other trials for subgroups of patients who had not received previous cytotoxic therapy.

These Phase II studies confirm that irinotecan is an active agent in metastatic colorectal cancer, in patients who are either chemonaive or pretreated [95]. The lack of cross-resistance with 5-FU is also highlighted in the encouraging response rates observed in patients with genuine 5-FU-resistant disease. These results have led to the development of combination regimens of irinotecan with either 5-FU, Tomudex or oxaliplatin to ascertain if first line treatment regimens can be optimised.

Two randomised trials have recently been reported that support the role of irinotecan as a second line agent for metastatic colorectal cancer. In the first, 279 patients with progressive metastatic colorectal cancer, who had received previous 5-FU-based chemotherapy, were randomised to receive either supportive care and irinotecan (350 mg/m^2 over 90 minutes 3-weekly) or supportive care alone [96]. The median survival times were 9.2 months and 6.5 months respectively ($p = 0.0001$); 1-year survival was 2.6 times greater in the irinotecan treated patients. This survival benefit was associated with an improvement in quality of life scores in the irinotecan group (survival without performance status deterioration $p = 0.0001$; without weight loss >5% $p = 0.018$; and PFS $p = 0.003$). This study clearly establishes the role of irinotecan as a second line agent in metastatic colorectal cancer. The second was a Phase III study in which 267 patients with progressive metastatic colorectal cancer who had failed to respond to, or progressed on, 5-FU were randomised to receive either irinotecan (350 mg/m^2 over 90 minutes every 3 weeks) or infusional 5-FU [97]. Any one of three infusional regimens could be used:

1. LV 200 mg/m^2 + 5-FU 400 mg/m^2 bolus with 600 mg/m^2 continuous infusion over 22 hours on days 1 and 2 every 2 weeks
2. PVI 5-FU 250–300 mg/m^2 per day
3. 5-FU 2.6–3.0 g/m^2 per day over 24 hours ± 20–500 mg/m^2 LV every week for 4 weeks with 2 weeks rest

The 1-year survival rates were 45% in the irinotecan-treated patients and 32% in the 5-FU-treated patients. The overall survival for the irinotecan group was significantly better ($p = 0.035$). There was no difference in the quality of life scores in the two groups. In the light of these studies, the use of irinotecan as a second line agent in patients with metastatic colorectal cancer should be considered standard practise.

A number of trials assessing the combination of irinotecan and 5-FU are either under way or have been completed. Two Japanese studies have looked at this combination. In the first, irinotecan (50–250 mg/m^2 dose escalation, as a 90-minute infusion day 1) and 5-FU (400 mg/m^2 per day continuous infusion for 7 days, repeated every 3–4 weeks) was administered to 36 patients [98]. The maximum tolerated dose of irinotecan was 250 mg/m^2. The second study evaluated the sequential administration of irinotecan and 5-FU (CPT11 100–175 mg/m^2 days 1 and 15 + 5-FU 600 mg/m^2 per day continuous infusion days 3–7 every 4–5 weeks) [99]. At a dose of 150 mg/m^2 the maximum tolerated dose of irinotecan has not yet been reached in this study.

Saltz et al. also confirmed the feasibility of the combination of irinotecan and 5-FU in patients with advanced solid tumours, 90% of whom had colorectal cancer [100]. They reported on 42 patients treated with 5-FU with dose escalation and irinotecan, also with dose escalation once the maximum dose of 5-FU had been achieved safely (5-FU 210–500 mg/m^2 and LV 20 mg/m^2 weekly for 4 weeks every 6 weeks + irinotecan 100–150 mg/m^2 weekly for 4 weeks, with dose escalated only when the dose of 5-FU had safely reached 500 mg/m^2). These authors found the maximum tolerated dose of irinotecan to be125 mg/m^2 when 5-FU was administered at a dosage of 500 mg/m^2. The design of the study also enabled pharmacokinetic data to be obtained on irinotecan alone and on irinotecan followed or preceded by 5-FU/LV. Small reductions in the SN-38 peak plasma concentration (13.7%) and the area under the curve 0–24 (8.2%) were observed when irinotecan was followed by 5-FU/LV, but not vice versa. This is not considered to be of clinical importance and it supports the evidence that 5-FU does not exert a substantial effect on the conversion of irinotecan to its active metabolite. A French study is ongoing, in which the combination of irinotecan and 5-FU are given 4-weekly (CPT11 200–350 mg/m^2 and 5-FU 375 mg/m^2 – previously 500 mg/m^2 days 1–5 4-weekly) [101].

Two randomised studies have now been reported, one European and one North American in which the combination of 5FU and Irinotecan has been compared to 5FU alone as first line treatment for metastatic colorectal cancer. In the European study 387 patients with previously untreated advanced colorectal cancer were randomised to receive either a combination of Irinotecan, 5FU and LV or the same 5FU/LV schedule (Group A: Irinotecan 180 mg/m^2 D1 + 5FU 400 mg/m^2 iv bolus + 600 mg/m^2/day as a

22 hour infusion + LV D1 + 2 2 weekly or Irinotecan 80 mg/m^2 + 5FU 2.3 g/m^2 as a 24 hour infusion + LV weekly × 6 every 7 weeks versus Group B: the same regimen of 5FU/LV alone) [102]. Results show a progression free survival of 35.1 weeks in the Irinotecan/5FU/LV treated group versus 18.6 weeks in the 5FU/FA group. Response rates were 39% and 22% respectively. Grade 3/4 toxicities were neutropenia 40% versus 13% and diarrhoea 20% versus 10%.

The North American Study used a 3 way randomisation: Irinotecan 125 mg/m^2 + LV 20 mg/m^2 bolus weekly × 4 q 6 weekly versus LV 20 mg/m^2 + 5FU 425 mg/m^2 D1-5 q 4 weekly versus Irinotecan 125 mg/m^2 weekly × 4 q 6 weekly. Six hundred and eighty three patients, who had not received previous chemotherapy for advanced disease, were included in the study [103]. Response rates were higher in the Irinotecan/5FU/LV treated group compared to the 5FU/LV treated group (39% versus 21%, p <0.001). This translated into an overall survival advantage (14.8 months versus 12.6 months, p = 0.04). These trials both confirm the benefit of an Irinotecan/5FU/LV combination over 5FU/LV alone as first line treatment in advanced colorectal cancer. This combination is currently being evaluated in the adjuvant setting.

Raltitrexed

Raltitrexed (Tomudex) is a direct and specific TS inhibitor. It is incorporated into the cell via the reduced folate membrane carrier system. Once raltitrexed is intracellular, it is polyglutamated. This has two benefits: first, it extends the intracellular retention of the drug and secondly it prolongs TS inhibition. Consequently, it can be administered as a single dose 3-weekly. In-vitro studies have shown raltitrexed to be a potent inhibitor of human cancer cells in culture, with a potency 94-fold greater than 5-FU alone and 56-fold greater than 5-FU modulated with LV [104].

As a result of these encouraging preclinical findings, Phase I studies were performed in both Europe and the USA. In the American study, 50 patients with progressive solid tumours who had received previous 5-FU therapy were recruited [105]. The dose range of raltitrexed was 0.6–4.5 mg/m^2, administered as a 15-minute infusion every 3 weeks. Seventy-six per cent of the patients included had colorectal cancer. The maximum tolerated dose was 4.5 mg/m^2. The dose-limiting toxicities were asthenia and neutropenia in 56% of the patients at 4.5 mg/m^2 and in 27% at 4 mg/m^2. The European study recruited 61 patients from two centres [106]. These patients also had refractory solid tumours, with the

largest group (26%) having colorectal cancer. The dose escalation range was 0.1–3.5 mg/m^2 as a 15-minute infusion every 3 weeks. At least three patients were treated at each dose level and dose escalations for individual patients were not allowed. No significant toxicity was seen at doses below 1.6 mg/m^2. The maximum tolerated dose was 3.5 mg/m^2 but, of the six patients treated at this dose level, four developed malaise, asthenia, anorexia and nausea, and two developed grade 3/4 neutropenia. At a dose of 3 mg/m^2 no patients experienced severe malaise, but grade 3/4 neutropenia and thrombocytopenia were seen in 22% and 9% of patients respectively. At this dosage, 26% of the patients had grade 3/4 hepatic dysfunction but this did not result in any treatment delay; liver function tests normalised on cessation of therapy. No drug-related nephrotoxicity was observed.

Based on these findings, the dosage of raltitrexed in European Phase II studies was 3 mg/m^2 every 3 weeks. The North American group developed a Phase II programme in which 3 mg/m^2 and 4 mg/m^2 arms are being compared to evaluate further the optimum dosage.

The pivotal raltitrexed Phase II study on colorectal cancer involved 15 centres in Europe, Australia and South Africa [107]. A total of 176 patients with advanced/metastatic colorectal cancer who had not previously received chemotherapy, other than in the adjuvant setting, were recruited. Raltitrexed was administered at a dose of 3 mg/m^2 every 3 weeks to a total of 848 courses. Overall response rates were 26%, with an additional 49% achieving disease stabilisation. The median time to progression was 4.2 months and the median survival time 11.2 months. In the main, the drug was well tolerated.

The results of this study led to the setting up of two large randomised international trials, which compared raltitrexed with 5-FU. In one trial, also conducted in Europe, South Africa and Australia, 439 patients were randomised to either raltitrexed (3 mg/m^2 every 3 weeks) or 5-FU/LV (NCCTG regimen) [108]. Overall response rates were similar for both groups (raltitrexed 19.3%, 5-FU 16.7%, p = 0.48), as was the proportion of patients whose disease stabilised (raltitrexed 35%, 5-FU 32.4%). It is not surprising that the median survival time was also the same for both raltitrexed- and 5-FU-treated patients (10.1 and 10.2 months respectively, p = 0.42). In the other, a European-based study, the same dose schedule of raltitrexed was compared with 5-FU and high-dose LV (5-FU 400 mg/m^2 + LV 200 mg/m^2 days 1–5 every 4 weeks). Four hundred and ninety-five patients were entered into this trial. Again, both overall response rates and the percentage of patients with disease stabilisation were similar in the raltitrexed and 5-FU arms (overall response rate 18.6% and 18.1% respectively, $p = 0.896$; stable disease 51.4% and 52.4% respectively). There was no difference in the median survival times (raltitrexed 10.7 months and 5-FU/LV 11.8 months, $p = 0.36$).

In North America, a Phase III trial followed on from the Phase I studies. Four hundred and twenty-seven patients were randomised in a three-arm design to receive raltitrexed 3 or 4 mg/m^2 every 3 weeks or 5-FU/LV (NCCTG regimen). Owing to unacceptable toxicity, the raltitrexed 4 mg/m^2 dose arm was discontinued and the study proceeded as a two-arm trial. The response rates and disease stabilisation rates were similar for both treatment arms and comparable with the European studies (overall response rate: 5-FU 15.2%, raltitrexed 14.3%; stable disease: 5-FU 40%, raltitrexed 33.2%). The median survival time, however, was significantly longer in the 5-FU/LV-treated group (12.7 versus 9.7 months, $p = 0.01$). This discrepancy compared with the European trials may be explained by the heightened awareness of the investigators for discontinuing treatment in the raltitrexed group because of the toxicity seen at the dose of 4 mg/m^2 [109].

The studies carried out to date show that raltitrexed had response rates comparable with a 5-FU/LV combination and, in two out of three Phase III trials, a similar survival time. This, combined with the fact that raltitrexed has a simple dose schedule, represents an advance in the management of colorectal cancer. Phase II trials are underway looking at the combination of Raltitrexed with 5FU, Oxaliplatin and Irinotecan.

Oxaliplatin

Oxaliplatin is a third generation platinum compound whose major toxicities are peripheral sensory neuropathy and nausea. As a single agent, response rates in patients with 5-FU-resistant disease are 10% [110,111] and 25% for those receiving first line treatment [112]. Synergy between oxaliplatin and 5-FU has been demonstrated both preclinically and clinically. Garufi et al. and de Gramont et al. demonstrated this phenomenon by proceeding with the same schedule of 5-FU/LV on progression of disease, but with the addition of oxaliplatin [113,114]. Rather than the expected response rate of 10%, the observed response rates in these trials were 27% and 46% respectively. The regimen used in the de Gramont study was FOLFOX 2 (oxaliplatin 100 mg/m^2 as a 2-hour infusion day 1; LV 500 mg/m^2 as a 2-hour infusion followed by 5-FU 1.5–2 g/m^2 over 24 hours for 2 days every 2 weeks).

In this study 46 patients were treated, all of whom had progressed on 5-FU/LV administered for metastatic disease or had relapsed within 6 months of adjuvant treatment. The response rate was 46% and the PFS 7 months. Overall, the incidence of grade 3/4 toxicity was 46%, with 9% peripheral neuropathy. Forty-four patients have been evaluated in a Phase II study using a similar schedule of oxaliplatin/5-FU/LV (FOLFOX 6) as second or third line treatment for metastatic colorectal cancer. Twenty-three per cent of these patients responded and a further 48% had disease stabilisation. The incidence of grade 3 peripheral neuropathy was 13% [115].

Two large Phase III trials have assessed the role of oxaliplatin in addition to 5-FU and LV as first line treatment for advanced colorectal cancer. Four hundred and twenty patients were randomised to receive a regimen of LV and 5-FU bolus plus a 24-hour infusion on 2 consecutive days every 2 weeks with or without oxaliplatin 85 mg/m^2 on day 1 every 2 weeks. The median PFS was superior in the oxaliplatin arm (9.0 versus 6.2 months, p = 0.0003). The improvement in overall survival did not however reach significance (median survival 16.2 versus 14.7 months, p = 0.12) [116]. The second study assessed the role of oxaliplatin in addition to chronomodulated 5-FU/LV. Two hundred patients were randomised to receive chronomodulated 5-FU (700 mg/m^2 per day × 5) and LV (300 mg/m^2 per day × 5) with peaks at 04:00 hours, with or without oxaliplatin (125 mg/m^2 day 1). The median PFS was 7.9 months in the oxaliplatin arm and 4.3 months in the control arm ($p = 0.05$). There was no significant difference in the median overall survival between the two arms (17.6 months oxaliplatin; 19.4 months control; p = 0.82) [117]. An analysis of the use of second line chemotherapy and surgery for metastasis in the two arms showed that the incidence of both of these modalities was more frequently employed in the control group. This may account for the lack of a significant survival benefit in the oxaliplatin arm [118].

As previously mentioned, oxaliplatin can be administered in a chronomodulated fashion. The least toxic circadian time for its delivery is in the second half of the activity span (i.e. 16:00–22:00 hours). In a randomised Phase I study, 25 patients (none with colorectal cancer) received either oxaliplatin administered as a 5-day continuous or chronomodulated infusion [119]. Doses were escalated by 25 mg/m^2 per course. Patients treated with the chronomodulated regimen had a 15% greater maximum tolerated dose than those who received continuous infusional treatment (175 mg/m^2 versus 150 mg/m^2 per course). Furthermore, toxicities were significantly reduced in the patients treated with chronotherapy. Chronomodulated oxaliplatin had response rates of 10% in a Phase II study of 29 patients, the majority of whom had received previous treatment [120]. Randomised trials comparing chronomodulated with continuous infusional chemotherapy combinations of 5-FU, oxaliplatin and LV have been mentioned earlier in this chapter.

Intra-Arterial Hepatic Chemotherapy for Isolated Liver Metastases

The liver is the commonest site of metastatic disease in colorectal cancer. As previously discussed, surgical excision should be considered in all patients with metastatic disease isolated to the liver. However, approximately 70% have disease that is inoperable. Another approach to the management of these patients, rather than by systemic chemotherapy, is the delivery of chemotherapy via the hepatic artery. In the early development of metastatic disease in the liver, the blood supply of micrometastases is via the portal vein. Once lesions become approximately 1 mm in size the main blood supply switches to the hepatic artery. For this reason, and also because of the fact that the liver has the capability of eliminating in the order of 80% of the infused drug, with a resultant reduction in systemic concentration and thus toxicity, the concept of intra-arterial hepatic chemotherapy was developed. When 5-FU is administered via the hepatic artery, the concentration of the drug in the liver is higher than that achieved when it is administered systemically. Floxuridine (5-fluoro-2′deoxyuridine; FUDR) achieves a higher concentration than 5-FU when given via the hepatic artery [121].

Phase II trials of intra-arterial hepatic chemotherapy using 5-FU and external pumps gave encouraging results, with response rates between 30% and 80%. With the development of implantable pumps and the use of FUDR, response rates of the order of 30–60% have been reported. Five randomised trials have been published comparing hepatic arterial infusion of chemotherapy with intravenous chemotherapy (FUDR 0.2–0.3 mg/kg per day for 14 days every 4 weeks via the hepatic artery; FUDR 0.075–0.125 mg/kg per day for 14 days every 4 weeks intravenously, or 5-FU bolus regimens intravenously). Two further trials compared hepatic arterial chemotherapy with no treatment. The majority of these trials confirmed improved response rates with chemotherapy administered via the hepatic artery; however, the impact on survival was not consistently established in the individual trials. A meta-analysis

was therefore carried out using data from the 654 patients included in these seven trials [122]. For the five trials (391 patients) comparing intra-arterial hepatic with intravenous chemotherapy, response rates of 41% versus 14% were reported; this improvement, in favour of hepatic artery chemotherapy, was highly statistically significant ($p < 10^{ms10}$). This translated into a median survival of 16 months versus 12.2 months in the two groups respectively, which was not statistically significant ($p = 0.14$). A survival benefit for hepatic arterial chemotherapy was clearly demonstrated in the two trials in which the control arm was best supportive care. There are, however, problems in interpreting these results, namely because the systemic treatment arm involves fluoropyrimidine treatment alone without biochemical modulation, which is not the standard systemic treatment for metastatic colorectal cancer. Another potential factor influencing the results is that in some of the trials there was a crossover from intravenous to intrahepatic arterial chemotherapy and this may have had some bearing on the lack of survival benefit, despite improved response rates.

Obviously, one of the major concerns associated with hepatic artery infusional chemotherapy is its potential toxicity. Although this route of administration reduces the systemic toxicity associated with fluoropyrimidines, it is associated with an increased risk of chemical hepatitis and sclerosing cholangitis [123]. In an attempt to overcome these problems, short infusions of 5-FU have been used with some success. Another adverse effect is that of catheter thrombosis, the incidence of which seems to be operator dependent, with a reduction in its occurrence in the hands of an experienced surgeon.

These results clearly demonstrate a role for intra-arterial hepatic chemotherapy in patients with inoperable isolated liver metastases. Future developments are being focused on the combined modality of intra-arterial hepatic and systemic chemotherapy, but the results of randomised trials are awaited to establish if this approach is superior to either treatment alone.

Biological Therapy

Immunotherapy

A number of tumour-associated antigens have been identified on colorectal cancer cells: CEA, cathepsin B, 17-1, CA19-9 and TAG-72. Monoclonal antibodies (mAb) targeting these antigens result in antibody-dependent cell-mediated cytotoxicity. MAb 17-1A is a murine IgG class 2A immunoglobulin that detects tumour-associated antigen CO17-1A. Trials have been performed using mAb 17-1A in patients with advanced colorectal cancer. They have reported response rates of the order of 5% but this has not been statistically significant [124,125]. Reithmuller et al., however, have shown a 30% reduction in mortality with mAb being used in the adjuvant setting for patients with Dukes' C colorectal cancer [126]. Other mAb are currently being investigated in advanced and adjuvant trials.

The major problem with the use of murine mAb is the development of a human antimurine response. This limits the therapeutic effect and shortens the antibody half-life. Chimeric antibodies have been developed in an attempt to overcome these problems. They have the variable antigen binding region of a mouse mAb but with the human constant region. This combination provides specificity with reduced immunogenicity and hence a longer half-life. Trials have not been reported comparing murine with chimeric mAb. Anti-idiotypic antibodies mimic the structure of tumour antigen. They may continue to act as a stimulus for the immune response after the mAb has been cleared and thus provide long-term immunity. Foon et al. reported on 23 patients with advanced colorectal cancer who were treated with a murine anti-idiotype antibody against a mAb specific for CEA epitope. Seventeen of 23 patients had an anti-anti-idiotypic response and 11 resulted in antibody-dependent cell-mediated cytotoxicity. Thirteen patients had true anti-CEA responses. Although there were no objective clinical responses, the overall survival time was 11.3 months [127].

Cytokines

Cytokines with potential antitumour activity include interleukin 2, interferon alpha, interferon beta, and tumour necrosis factor alpha. Cytokines are produced by lymphocytes in response to antigenic recognition by T cells. They induce an immune reaction, which can lead to the rejection of cancer cells. The use of interleukin 2 and interferon alpha, beta or gamma alone or in combination has not been shown to be effective in the management of advanced disease and in addition to this they are associated with significant toxicity.

There are convincing in-vitro data suggesting the biomodulation of 5-FU by interferon [128,129]. In addition, in vitro the modulation of 5-FU by LV plus interferon has been shown to be synergistic [130]. Randomised trials have been performed to assess the role of interferon as a lone modulator of 5 FU [131,132] or in addition to LV [133,134]. None of these trials has demonstrated any benefits from the clinical use of interferon in this situation.

Gene Therapy

Gene therapy involves the insertion of genes into cells with the intent of correcting an inborn genetic error or creating a new cellular function. The molecular basis of colorectal cancer is being intensively researched and much is known about the numerous genes involved in the carcinogenesis of this disease. Gene therapy does not necessarily constitute the replacement of a mutated gene; there are a number of different approaches:

1. Enzyme or prodrug systems (gene directed enzyme prodrug therapy). In this situation the transferred gene converts a non-toxic prodrug to an active cytotoxic agent. This can be a tumour-specific action if the gene or prodrug is targeted at the tumour cells.
2. Tumour suppressor gene replacement with wild-type p53.
3. Immune gene therapy (e.g. a polynucleotide tumour vaccine of CEA complementary DNA).

A number of clinical trials are currently under way to evaluate these methods.

Conclusion

Significant advances have been made in the management of metastatic colorectal cancer since the early 1990s. Patients who present with or develop metastatic disease should always be evaluated to establish whether they have potentially operable disease, either before or after chemotherapy. With the development of improving imaging techniques (magnetic resonance imaging and positron emission tomography scanning) patient selection for the surgical management of metastatic disease is improving. For the majority of patients whose disease is inoperable, chemotherapy is the main treatment modality. 5-FU continues to be the major cytotoxic agent used and, although bolus regimens such as the NCCTG schedule, which include LV as a biochemical modulator, have been clearly shown to improve survival and quality of life, infusional 5-FU is increasingly becoming the preferred delivery route. This is based on the higher response rates and reduced toxicity observed with infusional delivery. Chrono-modulation of infusional regimens has shown impressive results but further trials are required to evaluate such schedules.

Oral 5-FU analogues and specific TS inhibitors, such as raltitrexed, are unlikely to improve on efficacy when compared with intravenous 5-FU, but they offer a more convenient route of administration. This is of particular importance in rectal cancer, which is predominantly a disease of elderly people.

Irinotecan has now been clearly shown to prolong survival and quality of life in patients with metastatic disease who have failed on 5-FU. This now provides a second line agent of proven benefit and its use should be adopted as standard practice in patients who maintain a good performance status.

Both irinotecan and oxaliplatin in combination with 5FU have shown higher response rates than single agent 5FU in patients with previously untreated colorectal cancer, with irinotecan conveying a survival advantage. The question, which has not yet been answered, is which combination of treatment is the best first line treatment and what the subsequent lines of therapy should be.

The scope of treatment for metastatic rectal cancer has broadened significantly since the early 1990s, with current regimens offering improved survival and quality of life for these patients. A number of genetic alterations are know to play a role in the development of colorectal cancer such as *ras* mutations, loss of p53 expression and loss of deleted in colon cancer gene (a tumour suppressor gene). Increased understanding of the molecular biology of colorectal cancer has implications for screening in the disease and the future development of targeted therapies.

References

1. Bakalakos EA, Kim JA, Young DC, et al. Determinants of survival following hepatic resection for metastatic colorectal cancer. World J Surg 1998;22:299–304.
2. Ohlsson B, Stenram U, Tranberg KG. Resection of colorectal liver metastases: 25 year experience. World J Surg 1998;22:268–76.
3. Taylor M, Forster J, Langer B, et al. A study of prognostic factors for hepatic resection for colorectal metastases. Am J Surg 1997;173:467–71.
4. Fong Y, Cohen AM, Fortner JG, et al. Liver resection for colorectal metastases. J Clin Oncol 1997;15:938–46.
5. Waneble HJ, Chu QD, Veqeridis MP, et al. Patient selection for hepatic resection of colorectal metastases. Arch Surg 1996;131:322–29.
6. Pedersen IK, Burchart F, Roikjaer O, et al. Resection of liver metastases from colorectal cancer. Indications and results. Dis Colon Rectum 1994;37:1078–82.
7. Tuttle TM, Curley SA, Roh MS. Repeat hepatic resection as effective treatment of colorectal liver metastases. Ann Surg Oncol 1997;4:125–30.
8. Adam R, Bismuth H, Castaing D, et al. Repeat hepatectomy for colorectal liver metastases. Ann Surg 1997;225:51–60.
9. Bismuth H, Adam R, Navarro F, et al. Re-resection for colorectal liver metastasis. Surg Oncol Clin North Am 1996;5:353–64.
10. Vaillant JC, Balladur P, Nordlinger B, et al. Repeat liver resection for recurrent colorectal metastases. Br J Surg 1993;80:340–44.
11. Zanella A, Marchet A, Mainente P, et al. Resection of pulmonary metastases from colorectal carcinoma. Eur J Surg Oncol 1997;23:424–27.
12. Girard P, Ducreux M, Baldeyrou P, et al. Surgery for lung metastases from colorectal cancer: analysis of prognostic factors. J Clin Oncol 1996;14:2047–53.
13. Shirouzu K, Isomoto H, Hayashi A, et al. Surgical treatment for patients with pulmonary metastases after resection of primary colorectal carcinoma. Cancer 1995;76: 393–98.
14. Van Halteren HK, Van Geel AN, Hart AA, et al. Pulmonary resection for metastases of colorectal origin. Chest 1995;107:1526–31.
15. Robinson BJ, Rice TW, Strong SA, et al. Is resection of pulmonary and hepatic metastases warranted in patients with colorectal cancer? J Thorac Cardiovasc Surg 1999;117:66–75.
16. Smith JW, Fortner JG, Burt M. Resection of hepatic and pulmonary metastases from colorectal cancer. Surg Oncol 1992;1:399–404.
17. Alden TD, Gianino JW, Saclarides TJ. Brain metastases from colorectal cancer. Dis Colon Rectum 1996;39:541–45.
18. Patchell RA, Tibbs PA, Walsh JW, et al. A randomised trial of surgery in the treatment of single metastases to the brain. N Engl J Med 1990;322:494–500.
19. Nordic Gastrointestinal Tumour Adjuvant Therapy Group. Expectancy or primary chemotherapy in patients with advanced asymptomatic colorectal cancer: a randomised trial. J Clin Oncol 1992;10:904–11.
20. Scheithauer W, Rosen R, Kornek G, et al. Randomised comparison of combination chemotherapy plus best supportive care with supportive care alone in patients with metastatic colorectal cancer. BMJ 1993;306:752–55.
21. Beretta G, Bollina R, Martignoni G, et al. Fluorouracil and folates (FUFO) as standard treatment for advanced/metastatic gastrointestinal carcinomas (AGC) [abstract]. Ann Oncol 1994;5 Suppl 8:239.
22. Allen-Mersh G, Earlam S, Fordy C, et al. Quality of life and survival with continuous hepatic artery floxuridine infusion for colorectal liver metastases. Lancet 1994;344:1255–59.
23. Macmillan WE, Wolberg WH, Welling PG, et al. Pharmacokinetics of 5 fluorouracil in humans. Cancer Res 1978;38: 3479–82.
24. Advanced Colorectal Cancer Meta-analysis Project. Modulation of 5 fluorouracil by leucovorin in patients with advanced colorectal cancer: evidence in terms of response. J Clin Oncol 1992;10:896–903.
25. Madajewicz S, Petrelli N, Rustmum YM, et al. Phase I–II trial of high dose calcium leucovorin and 5 fluorouracil in advanced colorectal cancer. Cancer Res 1984;44:4667–69.
26. Luporini G, Labianca R, Pancera G, et al. Treatment of metastatic colorectal cancer: improvement of 5 fluorouracil activity with modulating agents. Forum 1991;1:246–56.
27. Poon M, O'Connell M, Moertel C, et al. Biochemical modulation of fluorouracil: evidence of significant improvement of survival and quality of life in patients with advanced colorectal carcinoma. J Clin Oncol 1989;7:1407–18.
28. Valsecchi R, Labianca R, Cascinu S, et al. High-dose versus low-dose l-leucovorin as a modulator of 5 days 5 fluorouracil in advanced colorectal cancer: a GISCAD Phase III study [abstract]. Proc ASCO 1995;14:457.
29. Buroker TR, O'Connell MJ, Wieand HS, et al. Randomised comparison of two schedules of fluorouracil and leucovorin in the treatment of advanced colorectal cancer. J Clin Oncol 1994;12:14–20.
30. Jaeger E, Heike M, Bernhard H, et al. Weekly high-dose leucovorin versus low-dose leucovorin combined with fluorouracil in advanced colorectal cancer. J Clin Oncol 1996;14:2274–79.

31. Petrelli N, Douglas HD, Herrera L, et al. The modulation of fluorouracil with leucovorin in metastatic colorectal carcinoma. A prospective randomised Phase III trial. J Clin Oncol 1989;7:1419–26.

32. De Gramont A, Bosset JF, Milan C, et al. A prospective randomised trial comparing 5 fluorouracil bolus with low-dose folinic acid (FUFOLld) and 5 fluorouracil bolus plus continuous infusion with high-dose folinic acid (LV5FU2) for advanced colorectal cancer [abstract]. Proc ASCO 1995;14:455.

33. Leichmann C, Fleming T, Muggia F, et al. Phase II study of fluorouracil and its modulation in advanced colorectal cancer: a Southwest Oncology Group Study. J Clin Oncol 1995;13:1303–11.

34. Cadman E, Hemier R, Davis L. Enhanced 5 fluorouracil nucleotide formation after methotrexate administration: explanation for drug synergism. Science 1979;205:1135–37.

35. Herrmann R, Spehn J, Beyer J, et al. Sequential methotrexate and 5 fluorouracil: improved response rates in metastatic colorectal cancer. J Clin Oncol 1984;2:591–94.

36. Kemeny N, Ahmed T, Michaelson R, et al. Activity of sequential low-dose methotrexate and fluorouracil in advanced colorectal carcinoma: attempt at correlation with tissue and blood levels of phosphoribosylpyrophosphate. J Clin Oncol 1984;2:311–15.

37. Nordic Gastrointestinal Tumour Adjuvant Therapy Group. Superiority of sequential methotrexate, fluorouracil and leucovorin to fluorouracil alone in advanced symptomatic colorectal carcinoma: a randomised trial. J Clin Oncol 1989;7:1437–46.

38. The Advanced Colorectal Cancer Meta-analysis Project. Meta-analysis of randomised trials testing the biochemical modulation of fluorouracil by methotrexate in metastatic colorectal cancer. J Clin Oncol 1994;12:960–69.

39. Blijham GH, Stellestags J, Sahmound T, et al. The modulation of high-dose 5 fluorouracil with low-dose methotrexate in metastatic colorectal cancer: a Phase III study of the EORTCGI Cancer Cooperative Group [abstract]. Proc ASCO 1993;12:586.

40. Van Der Wilt C, Braeklinis B, Pinedo H, et al. Addition of leucovorin in modulation of 5 fluorouracil with methotrexate: potentiating or reversing effect? Int J Cancer 1995;61:672–78.

41. Lokich J, Bothe A, Fine N, et al. Phase I study of protracted venous infusion 5 fluorouracil. Cancer 1981;48:2565–68.

42. Lokich J, Ahlgren J, Gullo J, et al. A prospective randomised comparison of continuous infusion fluorouracil with a conventional bolus schedule in metastatic colorectal carcinoma: a Mid-Atlantic Oncology Program Study. J Clin Oncol 1989;7:425–32.

43. Hansen R, Ryan L, Anderson T, et al. Phase III study of bolus versus infusional fluorouracil with or without cisplatin in advanced colorectal cancer. J Natl Cancer Inst 1996;88:668–74.

44. Weinerman B, Shah A, Fields A, et al. Systemic infusion versus bolus chemotherapy in measurable colorectal cancer. Am J Clin Oncol 1992;15:518–23.

45. Rougier P, Paillot B, Laplanche A, et al. End results of a multicenter randomised trial comparing 5FU in continuous systemic infusion to bolus administration in measurable metastatic colorectal cancer [abstract]. Proc ASCO 1992;11:465.

46. The Meta-analysis Group in Cancer. Efficacy of intravenous continuous infusion of fluorouracil compared with bolus administration in advanced colorectal cancer. J Clin Oncol 1998;16:301–308.

47. Isacson S. 5-Fluorouracil and folinic acid in the treatment of colorectal carcinoma: a randomised trial of two differ- ent schedules of administration. Second International Conference on Gastro-intestinal Cancer, Jerusalem, Israel 1989.

48. Leichman C, Leichman L, Spears P, et al. Prolonged continuous infusion of fluorouracil with weekly bolus leucovorin: a Phase II study in patients with disseminated colorectal cancer. J Natl Cancer Inst 1993;85:41–44.

49. Diaz-Rubio E, Aranda E, Martin M, et al. Weekly high-dose infusion of 5-fluorouracil in advanced colorectal cancer. Eur J Cancer 1990;26:727–29.

50. Diaz-Rubio E, Aranda E, Camps C, et al. A Phase II study of weekly 48-hour infusion with high-dose fluorouracil in advanced colorectal cancer: an alternative to biochemical modulation. J Infus Chemother 1994;4:58–61.

51. Aranda E, Cervantes A, Carrato A, et al. Outpatient weekly high-dose continuous infusion 5 fluorouracil plus oral leucovorin in advanced colorectal cancer. A Phase II trial. Ann Oncol 1996;7:581–85.

52. Levi F. Chronopharmacology of anticancer agents. In: Redfern PH, Lemmer B, editors. Handbook of experimental pharmacology: physiology and pharmacology of biological rhythms. Cancer chemotherapy. Berlin: Springer-Verlag, 1997:299–331.

53. Levi F. Chronotherapy for gastrointestinal cancers. Curr Opin Oncol 1996;8:334–41.

54. Chollet PH, Cure H, Garufi C, et al. Phase II trial with chronomodulated 5-fluorouracil (5-FU) and folinic acid (FA) in metastatic colorectal [abstract]. Proceedings of the 6th International Conference on Chronopharmacology and Chronotherapy; 1994 Jul 5–9; Amelia Island, FL: VIIIb-4

55. Levi F, Perpoint B, Garufi C, et al. Oxaliplatin activity against metastatic colorectal cancer. A Phase II study of 5-day continuous venous infusion at circadian rhythm modulated rate. Eur J Cancer 1993;29A:1280–84.

56. Levi F, Misset J, Brienza S, et al. A chronopharmacologic Phase II clinical trial with 5 fluorouracil, folinic acid and oxaliplatin using an ambulatory multichannel programmable pump. Cancer 1992;69:893–900.

57. Levi F, Zidani R, Vannetzel J, et al. Chronomodulated versus fixed-infusion rate delivery of ambulatory chemotherapy with oxaliplatin, fluorouracil and folinic acid (leucovorin) in patients with colorectal cancer metastases: a randomised multi-institutional trial. J Natl Cancer Inst 1994;86:1608–17.

58. Levi F, Zidani R, Misset J. Randomised multicenter trial of chronotherapy with oxaliplatin, fluorouracil and folinic acid in metastatic colorectal cancer. Lancet 1997;350:681–86.

59. Petrelli N, Mittelman A. An analysis of chemotherapy for colorectal carcinoma. J Surg Oncol 1984;25:201–206

60. Poplin E, Lorusso P, Lokich J, et al. Randomised clinical trial of mitomycin C with or without pre-treatment with WR-2721 in patients with advanced colorectal cancer. Cancer Chemother Pharmacol 1994;33:415–19.

61. Russell O, Romanini A, Civalleri D, et al. Time dependent interactions between 5 fluorouracil and mitomycin C on human colon carcinoma cell line, HCT-8, in vitro. Eur J Cancer Clin Oncol 1989;25:571–72.

62. Buroker T, Kim P, Baker L, et al. Mitomycin C alone and in combination with infused 5 fluorouracil in the treatment of disseminated gastrointestinal carcinomas. Med Pediatr Oncol 1978;4:35–42.

63. Krauss S, Sonoda T, Solomon A. Treatment of advanced gastrointestinal cancer with 5 fluorouracil and mitomycin C. Cancer 1979;43:1598–603.

64. Buroker T, Kim P, Groppe C, et al. 5 Fluorouracil infusion with mitomycin C versus 5 fluorouracil infusion with methyl CCNU in the treatment of advanced colon cancer. A Southwest Oncology Group Study. Cancer 1978;42:1228–33.

65. Richards F, Case L, White D, et al. Combination chemotherapy (5 fluorouracil, methyl CCNU, mitomycin C) versus 5 fluorouracil alone for previously untreated colorectal carcinoma. A Phase III study of the Piedmont Oncology Association. J Clin Oncol 1986;4:565–70.

66. Ross P, Norman A, Cunningham D, et al. A prospective randomised trial of protracted venous infusion 5 fluorouracil with or without mitomycin C in advanced colorectal cancer. Ann Oncol 1997;8:995–1001.

67. Price T, Cunningham D, Hickish T, et al. Phase III study of chronomodulated versus protracted venous infusional 5-fluorouracil both combined with mitocycin in first line therapy for advanced colorectal carcinoma. Proc Am Soc Clin Oncol 1999;18:233a.

68. Padzur R, Lassere Y, Diaz-Canton E, et al. Phase I trials of uracil tegafur (UFT) using 5 and 28 day administration schedules: demonstration of schedule dependent toxicities. AntiCancer Drugs 1996;7:728–33.

69. Padzur R, Lassere Y, Diaz-Canton E, et al. Phase I trial of uracil-tegafur (UFT) plus oral leucovorin: 28-day schedule. Cancer Invest 1998;16:145–51.

70. Saltz L, Leichmann C, Young C, et al. A fixed-ratio combination of uracil and ftorafur (UFT) with low dose leucovorin: an active oral regimen for advanced colorectal cancer. Cancer 1995;75:782–85.

71. Padzur R, Lassere Y, Rhodes V, et al. Phase II trial of uracil and tegafur plus oral leucovorin: an effective oral regime in the treatment of metastatic colorectal cancer. J Clin Oncol 1994;12:2296–300.

72 Carmichael J, Popiela T, Radstone D, et al. Randomised Comparative study of ORZEL (Oral Uracil/Tegafur (UFT)) Plus Leucovorin (LV) versus Parentral 5Fluorouracil (5FU) Plus LV in patients with Metastatic Colorectal cancer [abstract]. Proc ASCO 1999;18:264a.

73 Pazdur R, Doulliard J-Y, Skillings JR, et al. Multicenter Phase III Study of 5-fluorouracil (5FU) or UFT in combination with Leucovorin (LV) in patients with Metastatic Colorectal Cancer. Proc ASCO 1999;18:263a.

74. Alberto P, Winkelmann J, Paschono N, et al. Phase I study of oral doxifluridine using two schedules. Eur J Cancer Clin Oncol 1989;25:905–908.

75. Bajetta E, Colleoni M, Di Bartolomeo M, et al. Doxifluridine and leucovorin: an oral treatment combination in advanced colorectal cancer. J Clin Oncol 1995;13:2613–19.

76. Bajetta E, Di Bartolomeo M, Somma L, et al. Doxifluridine in colorectal cancer patients resistant to 5 fluorouracil (5FU) containing regimens. Eur J Cancer 1997;33:687–90.

77. Merepol NG, Budman DR, Creaven PJ, et al. A Phase I study of continuous twice daily treatment with capecitabine in patients with advanced and or metastatic solid tumours [abstract]. Ann Oncol 1996;7 Suppl 1:87.

78. Hughes M, Planting A, Twelves C, et al. A Phase I study of intermittent twice daily oral therapy with capecitabine in patients with advanced and or metastatic solid cancers [abstract]. Ann Oncol 1996;7 Suppl 1:87.

79. Findlay M, van Cutsem E, Kocha W, et al. A randomised Phase II study of Xeloda (capecitabine) in patients with advanced colorectal cancer [abstract]. Proc ASCO 1997;16:227a.

80 Twelves C, Harper P, Van Cutsem E, et al. A phase III Trial (S014796) of Xeloda (Capecitabine) in previously Untreated advanced/Metastatic Colorectal Cancer. Proc ASCO 1999;18:263a.

81 Cox J, Pazdur R, Thibault A, et al. A phase III Trial of Xeloda (Capecitabine) in previously Untreated advanced/Metastatic Colorectal Cancer. Proc ASCO 1999;18:265a.

82. Baker SD, Khor SP, Adjei AA, et al. Pharmacokinetic oral bioavailability and safety study of fluorouracil in patients treated with 776C85 an inactivator of DPD. J Clin Oncol 1996;14:3085–96.

83 Mani S, Hochster H, Beck T, et al. Multicenter phase II study to evaluate a 28-day regimen of oral fluorouracil plus eniluracil in the treatment of patients with previously untreated metastic colorecal cancer. J Clin Oncol 2000;18:2894–2901.

84. Peters GJ, Van Groeningen CJ, Schomage JH, et al. Phase I clinical and pharmacokinetic study of S-1, an oral 5-fluorouracil (5FU)-based antineoplastic agent [abstract]. Proc ASCO 1997;16:227a.

85 Ohtsu A, Baba H et al. Phase II study of S-1, a novel oral fluoropyrimidine derivative, in patients with metastatic colorectal carcinoma. British J Cancer 2000;83:141–145.

86. Giovanella B, Stehlin J, Wall M, et al. DNA topoisomerase 1 targeted chemotherapy of human colon cancer in xenografts. Science 1989;246:1046–48.

87. Tsuro T, Matsuzaki T, Matsushita M, et al. Antitumor effect of CPT11, a new derivative of camptothecin, against pleiotrophic drug resistant tumours in vitro and vivo. Cancer Chemother Pharmacol 1988;21:71–74.

88. Armand J. CPT11: clinical experience in Phase I studies. Semin Oncol 1996;23:27–33.

89. Shimada Y, Yoshino M, Wakin A, et al. Phase II study of CPT11, a new camptothecin derivative in metastatic colorectal cancer. J Clin Oncol 1993;11:909–13.

90. Rougier P, Bugat R, Douillard J, et al. Phase II study of irinotecan in the treatment of advanced colorectal cancer in chemotherapy naive patients and patients pretreated with fluorouracil-based chemotherapy. J Clin Oncol 1997;15:251–60.

91. Rothenberg M, Eckardt J, Kuhn J, et al. Phase II trial of irinotecan in patients with progressive or rapidly recurrent colorectal cancer. J Clin Oncol 1996;14:1128–35.

92. Van Cutsem E, Cunningham D, Ten-Bokkel Huiniuk W, et al. Irinotecan (CPT11) multicenter Phase II study in colorectal cancer patients with documented progressive disease on prior 5FU: preliminary results [abstract]. Proc ASCO 1996;15:A562.

93. Ychou M, Douillard J, Rougier P, et al. Randomised comparison of prophylactic antidiarrheal treatment versus no prophylactic antidiarrheal treatment in patients receiving CPT-11 (irinotecan) for advanced 5FU resistant colorectal cancer: an open-label multicenter Phase II study. Am J Clin Oncol 2000;23:143–48.

94. Conti J, Kemeny N, Saltz L, et al. Irinotecan is an active agent in untreated patients with metastatic colorectal cancer. J Clin Oncol 1996;14:709–15.

95. Pitot H, Wender D, O'Connell M, et al. A Phase II trial of CPT-11 (irinotecan) in patients with metastatic colorectal carcinoma: a North Central Cancer Treatment Group (NCCTG) study [abstract]. Proc ASCO 1994;13:573.

96. Cunningham D, Pyrhonen S, James R, et al. Randomised trial of irinotecan plus supportive care versus supportive care alone after fluorouracil failure for patients with metastatic colorectal cancer. Lancet 1998;352:1413–18.

97. Rougier P, van Cutsem E, Baguette E, et al. Randomised trial of irinotecan versus fluorouracil by continuous infusion after fluorouracil failure in patients with metastatic colorectal cancer. Lancet 1998;352:1407–12.

98. Shimada Y, Sasaki Y, Sugano K, et al. Combination Phase I study of CPT11 (irinotecan) with continuous infusion 5-FU in metastatic colorectal cancer [abstract]. Proc ASCO 1993;12:575.

99. Yamao T, Shimada Y, Shirao K, et al. Phase I study of CPT11 combined with sequential 5FU in metastatic colorectal cancer [abstract]. Proc ASCO 1996;15:A1527.

100. Saltz L, Kanowitz J, Kemeny N, et al. Phase I clinical and pharmacokinetic study of irinotecan, fluorouracil and leucovorin in patients with advanced solid tumors. J Clin Oncol 1996;14:2959–67.

101. Grossin F, Barbault H, Benhammouda A, et al. A Phase I pharmacokinetic study of concomitant CPT11 (C) and 5FU (F) combination. Proceedings of the Annual Meeting of the AACR; 1996 Apr 23; Washington, DC.

102. Douillard JY, Cunningham D, Roth AD, et al. Irinotecan combined with fluorouracil alone as first line treatment for metastic colorectal cancer: a multicenter randomised trial. Lancet 2000;355:1041–1047.

103. Saltz LB, Cox JV, Blanke C, et al. Irinotecan fluorouracil and leucovorin for metastatic colorectal cancer. Irinotecan Study Group. N Engl J Med 2000;343:905–914.

104. Jackmann A, Farrugia D, Gibson W, et al. ZD1694 (Tomudex): a new thymidylate synthase inhibitor with activity in colorectal cancer. Eur J Cancer 1995;31A:1277–85.

105. Sorenson J, Jordan E, Crem J, et al. Phase I trial of ZD1694 (Tomudex) a direct inhibitor of thymidylate synthase [abstract]. Ann Oncol 1994;5 Suppl 5:132.

106. Clarke S, Hanwell J, de Boer M, et al. Phase I trial of ZD 1694, a new folate-based thymidylate synthase inhibitor, in patients with solid tumours. J Clin Oncol 1996;14:716–21.

107. Zalcberg J, Cunningham D, van Cutsem E, et al. ZD 1694: a novel thymidylate synthase inhibitor with substantial activity in the treatment of patients with advanced colorectal cancer. J Clin Oncol 1996;14:716–21.

108. Cunningham D, Zalcberg J, Rath U, et al. Final results of a randomised trial comparing Tomudex (raltitrexed) with 5 fluorouracil plus leucovorin in advanced colorectal cancer. "Tomudex" Colorectal Cancer Study Group. Ann Oncol 1996;7:961–65.

109. Kerr D. Clinical efficacy of "Tomudex" (raltitrexed) in advanced colorectal cancer. Anticancer Drugs 1997;8 Suppl 2:S11–15.

110. Levi F, Perpoint B, Garufi B, et al. Oxaliplatin activity against metastatic colorectal cancer. A Phase II study of 5 day continuous venous infusion at circadian rhythm modulated rate. Eur J Cancer 1993;29A:1280–84.

111. Machover D, Diaz-Rubio E, de Gramont A, et al. Two consecutive Phase II studies of oxaliplatin (L-OHP) for treatment of patients with advanced colorectal cancer who were resistant to previous treatment with fluoropyrimidines. Ann Oncol 1996;7:95–98.

112. Diaz-Rubio E, Zaniboni A, Gastiabuni J, et al. Phase II multicentric trial of oxaliplatin (L-OHP) as first line chemotherapy in metastatic colorectal cancer [abstract]. Proc ASCO 1996;15:207.

113. Garufi B, Brienza S, Bensmain MA, et al. Addition of oxaliplatin to chronomodulated 5 fluorouracil and folinic acid for reversal of acquired chemoresistance in patients with advanced colorectal cancer [abstract]. Proc ASCO 1995;14:446.

114. De Gramont A, Vignoud J, Tournigand C, et al. Oxaliplatin with high-dose leucovorin and 5-fluorouracil 48-hour continuous infusion in pre-treated metastatic colorectal cancer. Eur J Cancer 1997;33:214–19.

115. Maindrault-Goebel F, De Gramont A, Louvet C, et al. Bimonthly oxaliplatin with leucovorin and 5-fluorouracil in pre-treated metastatic colorectal cancer (FOLFOX 6) [abstract]. Proc ASCO 1998;17:273a.

116. de Gramont A, Figer A, Seymour M, et al. Leucovorin and Fluorouracil with or without Oxaliplatin as first line treatment in advanced Colorectal Cancer. J Clin Oncol 2000;18:2938–2947.

117. Giachetti S, Zidani R, Perpoint B, et al. Phase III trial of 5-fluorouracil, folinic acid, with or without oxaliplatin in previously untreated patients with metastatic colorectal cancer [abstract]. Proc ASCO 1997;16:229a.

118. Giachetti S, Brienza S, Focan C, et al. Contribution of second line oxaliplatin-chronomodulated 5 fluorouracil–folinic acid and surgery to survival in metastatic colorectal cancer patients [abstract]. Proc ASCO 1998;17:273a.

119. Caussanel J, Levi F, Brienza S, et al. Phase I trial of 5-day continuous venous infusion of oxaliplatin at circadian rhythm-modulated rate compared with constant rate. J Natl Cancer Inst 1990;82:1046–50.

120. Levi F, Soussan A, Adams R, et al. A Phase I-II trial of 5 day continuous intravenous infusion of fluorouracil delivered at circadian rhythm modulated rate in patients with metastatic colorectal cancer. J Infus Chemother 1995;5:153–58.

121. Ensminger W, Gyves J. Regional chemotherapy of neoplastic diseases. Pharmacol Ther 1983;21:277–93.

122. Meta-Analysis Group in Cancer. Reappraisal of hepatic arterial infusion in the treatment of nonresectable liver metastases from colorectal cancer. J Natl Cancer Inst 1996;88:252–58.

123. Rougier P, Laplanche A, Hughier M, et al. Hepatic arterial infusion of floxuridine in patients with liver metastases from colorectal carcinoma: long-term results of a prospective randomised trial. J Clin Oncol 1992;10: 1112–18.

124. Wadler S. The role of immunotherapy in colorectal cancer. Semin Oncol 1991;18:27–38.

125. Mellstedt H, Frodin JE, Masucci G, et al. The therapeutic use of monoclonal antibodies in colorectal carcinoma. Semin Oncol 1991;18:462–77.

126. Reithmuller G, Holz E, Schilmok G, et al. Monoclonal antibody therapy for resected Dukes' C colorectal cancer: seven-year outcome of a multicentre randomised trial. J Clin Oncol 1998;16:1788–94.

127. Foon KA, John WJ, Chakraborty M, et al. Clinical and immune responses in advanced colorectal cancer patients treated with anti-idiotype monoclonal antibody vaccine that mimics carcinoembryonic antigen. Clin Cancer Res 1997;3:1267–76.

128. Chu E, Zinn S, Boarman D, et al. Interaction of gamma interferon and 5-fluorouracil in the H630 human colon carcinoma cell line. Cancer Res 1990;50:5834–40.

129. Wadler S, Schwartz EL. Antineoplastic activity of the combination of interferon and cytotoxic agents against experimental and human malignancies: a review. Cancer Res 1990;50:3473–86.

130. Houghton JA, Adkins DA, Rahman A, et al. Interactions between 5-fluorouracil, [6RS] leucovorin and recombinant human interferon α-2a in cultured colon adenocarcinoma cells. Cancer Commun 1991;3:220–24.

131. Corfu-A Study Group. Phase III randomised study of two fluorouracil combinations with either interferon alpha-2a or leucovorin for advanced colorectal cancer. J Clin Oncol 1995;13:921–28.

132. York M, Greco FA, Figlin RA, et al. A randomised Phase III trial comparing 5-FU with or without interferon alfa-2a for advanced colorectal cancer [abstract]. Proc ASCO 1993;12:200.

133. Kohne CH, Schoffski P, Wilke H, et al. Effective biomodulation by leucovorin of high-dose infusion fluorouracil given as weekly 24-hour infusion: results of a randomised trial in patients with advanced colorectal cancer. J Clin Oncol 1998;16:418–26.

134. Seymour MT, Slevin ML, Kerr DJ, et al. Randomised trial assessing the addition of interferon α-2a to fluorouracil and leucovorin in advanced colorectal cancer. Colorectal Cancer Working Party of the United Kingdom Medical Research Council. J Clin Oncol 1996;14:2280–88.

15. Rare Histiotypes

E.M. Grossmann, R.A. Audisio, J.G. Geraghty and W.E. Longo

Introduction

Although the overwhelming majority of malignancies of the rectum are adenocarcinomas, a number of rare histiotypes will undoubtedly be encountered in clinical practice. Owing to their infrequent occurrence, one must be familiar with the tumor biology, natural history and treatment options for such lesions. These disease entities often present difficulties with diagnosis, staging, management, pathology and follow-up. In this chapter we will discuss the rare histiotypes most commonly encountered, including carcinoid tumors, rectal lymphoma, anorectal melanoma, neuroendocrine (NE) carcinoma of the rectum, vascular lesions, squamous cell carcinoma of the rectum and its variants, and, finally, rectal sarcoma. Although the ultimate management of such lesions may still be controversial in different physician's eyes, often due to lack of experience with these tumors, we hope to provide an evidence-based approach to support decisions regarding appropriate therapy.

Carcinoid Tumors of the Rectum

The term "Karzinoide" was originally used to describe small "cancer-like" neoplasms thought to have minimal malignant potential [1]. Current use of the term carcinoid refers to a group of neoplasms with NE differentiation capable of synthesizing and secreting a variety of biogenic amines and peptide hormones. Many of these products are putative neurotransmitters; hence the term "neuro" endocrine. The gastrointestinal (GI) tract is the site of 90% of carcinoids, and the rectum accounts for 16–55% of GI carcinoids [2–5]. Carcinoid tumors are thought to arise from the enterochromaffin cells in the crypts of Lieberkuhn. These enterochromaffin cells (named for their resemblance to the chromaffin cells of the adrenal medulla) are part of the intrinsic endocrine system of the GI tract. These cells have been classified with similar cells from other sites (e.g. thyroid, adrenal medulla, pancreas) as part of the amine precursor uptake and decarboxylation (APUD) system.

Traditional teaching has been that the appendix represents the most common site of carcinoid tumors. Some have suggested, however, that, with the increasing use of proctosigmoidoscopy as a screening tool, the rectum is rapidly becoming the most commonly identified site of this disease [5]. Carcinoid histiotypes represent 0.1–1% of all rectal cancers [4,6–8]. The majority of tumors referred to as carcinoid are slow growing and have minimal potential for metastasis. Considerable debate, however, exists regarding the use of the term carcinoid. Some 10–20% of rectal lesions traditionally labeled carcinoid will demonstrate the ability to metastasize and are associated with a very grave prognosis [2,3,5,6,8–11]. Some have suggested that the term should be reserved for the subset of NE tumors that are small, well-differentiated and have minimal invasive potential [12]. It has also been suggested that large carcinoids, invasive carcinoids and carcinoids with atypical features should be grouped with other tumors that display NE features (e.g. small cell, anaplastic) into a broader category simply termed NE intestinal tumors (see later in this chapter: "Neuroendocrine carcinoma of the rectum"). Although this change in categorization may be useful for discussion purposes, in clinical practice there remains no reliable method for differentiating carcinoid tumors that will follow a benign course from those that will behave in a malignant manner. All carcinoids, therefore, must be considered to have some metastatic potential.

Clinical Presentation and Diagnosis

Although patients in virtually every age range have been described with this condition, the majority are in their fifth or sixth decade of life [2–11]. Meta-analysis has suggested that there may be a slight male preponderance [10]. The majority of rectal carcinoids are asymptomatic, and are discovered during screening examinations or are discovered incidentally at the time of evaluation of other anorectal conditions. (e.g. hemorrhoids, fissures) [3,5,6,8,13,14]. Carcinoid tumors of the rectum are discovered in 0.04–0.06% of patients undergoing screening proctoscopic evaluation [6,15]. Although symptoms related to other concomitant conditions (e.g. fissures) are common, symptoms directly referable to the tumor itself are rare and, when present, are associated with advanced disease [2–7,13,14]. Carcinoid lesions typically appear as small, firm, yellow, submucosal nodules, although occasionally they may appear macroscopically as pedunculated, sessile or ulcerated lesions. Metachronous or synchronous carcinomas (often, but not exclusively, found in the GI tract) may be present in up to 30% of patients [2,3,6,10,13,14], mandating a thorough physical examination and evaluation of the entire colon.

A "carcinoid syndrome" (comprising diarrhea, flushing, telangiectasia, dyspnea and right-sided valvular heart disease) has been described in relation to carcinoid tumors. This syndrome is thought to be the result of the systemic release of the NE products of these neoplasms (serotonin has been implicated as the primary mediator). The liver appears to exhibit a first pass effect on these products because carcinoid syndrome is seldom seen until the tumor metastasizes to the liver and thus bypasses the portal system. Elevated urinary levels of 5-hydroxyindole-acetic acid (5-HIAA, a breakdown product of serotonin), in conjunction with classic symptoms, confirm the diagnosis of carcinoid syndrome. Patients with rectal carcinoids (including those with liver metastasis) rarely exhibit elevations of urinary 5-HIAA [11,16] and the carcinoid syndrome itself is encountered in only 0.7% of patients with rectal carcinoids [10]. It remains unclear why rectal carcinoids and their metastases generally seem incapable of producing this syndrome.

Histologically, carcinoids are composed of small uniform cells with few mitotic figures. These cells are arranged in a variety of patterns, variously described as ribbon like, trabecular, rosette, tubular, acinar and nests of cells [17]. None of these patterns clearly correlates with invasive potential. Overall, 80% of intestinal carcinoids demonstrate the ability to take up silver stains (argyrophilic) and many are able to reduce silver stains (argentaffinic) [10]. For this reason, carcinoid lesions have at times been referred to as argentaffinomas. Only 50–60% of rectal carcinoids, however, display argyrophilic reactions, and few are argentaffinic [9,10,15,17–19]. Electron microscopy may demonstrate neurosecretory granules, but this has not found widespread clinical application. Instead, the development of specific antibodies directed at NE markers and products has greatly facilitated the correct identification of carcinoid tumors. Non-specific markers of NE differentiation, such as neuron specific enolase and chromogranin, can be demonstrated by immunohistochemistry in the majority of rectal carcinoids [9,10,15,16]. Immunohistochemistry is also useful to demonstrate the synthesis of specific hormonal products. The most common peptides synthesized by rectal carcinoids are pancreatic polypeptide, carcinoembryonic antigen, and prostate specific antigen [9,10,18]. Also frequently demonstrated are serotonin, glucagon and somatostatin. Single tumors can often synthesize more than one product, and metastases may not synthesize the same product as the primary tumor [9,10,18]. Although identification of these products is helpful in confirming the histologic diagnosis of carcinoid, no correlation between any specific product and tumor behavior has been demostrated. Flow cytometric DNA analysis has not proved to be a useful prognostic indicator [14].

Treatment and Prognosis

The treatment of rectal carcinoids remains controversial and specific guidelines continue to be developed. The size of these lesions has clearly been demonstrated to correlate with their malignant potential (Table 15.1). The majority of lesions found (65–80%) [3,6,8,10,13] will be less than 1 cm in diameter. Metastatic disease associated with lesions of this size occurs in only 3–5% of patients [3,10]. Transanal endoscopic resection has repeatedly been demonstrated to be safe and curative for the vast majority of patients with these small carcinoids [15,20–22]. Appropriate follow-up to detect local

Table 15.1. Metastatic potential of rectal carcinoids

Diameter (cm)	Metastatic potential (%)
<1	3–5
1.0–1.9	10–30
≥2	>75

recurrence or metastatic disease is warranted. Rectal carcinoids ranging from 1 to 1.9 cm in diameter are associated with a 10–30% chance of metastases [3,10,16]. Invasion of the tumor into the muscularis propria appears to be the most significant histologic prognosticator of metastatic potential [3,8,10], prompting most experts to recommend full thickness transanal excision for lesions of this size to allow proper histologic evaluation. Some have suggested that transrectal ultrasound may provide an alternative approach to gauging the depth of invasion [7]. Most authorities recommend that patients with tumors of 1–1.9 cm in size, with invasion of the muscularis propria and no evidence of metastatic disease, should undergo low anterior resection (LAR) or abdominoperineal resection (APR) with curative intent. Other studies have also found correlation of metastatic potential with tumor ulceration, mitotic ratio, vascular and lymphatic invasion, and high nuclear grade [5,9,11,14]. It is unclear whether the former represent independent risk factors or are simply characteristics common to large and invasive carcinoids. For 1–1.9 cm tumors without histologic risk factors, transanal full thickness excision appears to be a reasonable alternative to APR and LAR. Lesions >2 cm have a 75% chance of metastasizing [3,16], a median survival of

7 months [4], and a 10-year mortality of 60% [14]. Most authorities believe that APR or LAR provides good palliation for these large tumors and the best chance for cure. Aggressive surgical intervention, however, has never been demonstrated to improve survival compared with local excision in tumors >2 cm. Some investigators, citing the dismal prognosis regardless of treatment and the existence of long-term survivors after local resection, have suggested that APR and LAR are unwarranted in the majority of patients with large rectal carcinoids [4,11]. This controversy remains unresolved. Adjuvant chemotherapy and radiotherapy has occasionally been used for large carcinoids, without clear evidence of benefit [5]. Our algorithm for the treatment of rectal carcinoids based on size is depicted in Fig. 15.1.

Regional lymph nodes and the liver are the most common sites of metastasis, with less frequent sites including brain, bone, peritoneum and lung [4,7,10]. Various combinations of chemotheraputic agents have been used for metastatic rectal carcinoids, with little evidence of improved survival [3,4]. The carcinoid syndrome is seldom an issue for tumors originating in the rectum, therefore the debulking of liver metastases from a primary rectal carcinoid has not been discussed in the literature.

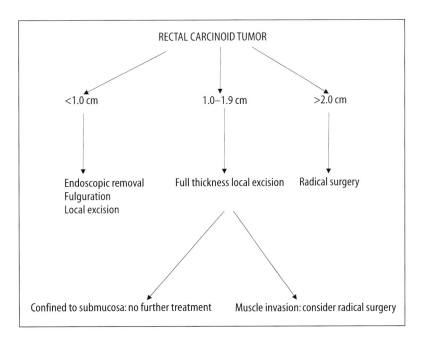

Fig. 15.1. Suggested algorithm for management of rectal carcinoid based on tumor size.

Lymphoma of the Rectum

Primary Lymphoma of the Rectum

Lymphoma involving the rectum may represent a primary rectal malignancy (primary rectal lymphoma) or metastases from a nodal origin (secondary rectal lymphoma). The GI tract is the most common site of origin for primary lymphomas arising in extranodal locations. The large intestine is the site of 8–15% of primary GI lymphomas [23–25] and approximately one-half of these are located in the rectum [24]. This rare form of cancer represents only 0.2% of all primary colorectal malignant neoplasms [26]. Virtually all described primary colorectal lymphomas have been designated as being of the non-Hodgkin's type. Originally, any lymphoma that presented with primarily GI symptoms was considered to be of GI origin. Strict criteria for the diagnosis of primary GI lymphoma were introduced in 1961 by Dawson et al. [27]. They suggested that, in order for a lesion of the GI tract to be considered a primary lymphoma, a number of criteria must be satisfied. These include: no palpable superficial lymphadenopathy, no mediastinal enlargement on chest radiography, normal peripheral blood smear, only mesenteric lymph nodes adjacent to the tumor are involved at laparotomy, and the liver and spleen are free of disease. Most authorities would now add a normal bone marrow biopsy and no involvement of the spleen, liver or mediastinum by computed tomographic (CT) scan to the necessary criteria. The accurate differentiation of primary from secondary intestinal lymphoma is necessary because the prognosis and treatment of these two entities are quite distinct. However, it is apparent that use of this system will misclassify a certain number of patients with a primary GI lymphoma who present with widely metastatic disease. The clinical significance of such misclassifications is uncertain.

Clinical Presentation and Diagnosis

Prototype patients with primary rectal lymphoma are in their 50s or 60s [24,28,29]. Presentation is similar to that of adenocarcinoma of the rectum, with rectal bleeding being the most frequent complaint. Low rectal lesions may be palpable during digital rectal examination. Higher lesions require contrast enema or colonoscopy for identification. There are no characteristic radiologic or colonoscopic features to differentiate this lesion reliably from more common rectal neoplasms. Histologic patterns are variable and correlate poorly with the classification patterns developed for lymphoma of nodal origin. Multiple biopsies and immunohisto-

chemistry are often necessary for definitive diagnosis [24,29–31]. After histologic confirmation of a lymphoma involving the rectum, a thorough physical examination, peripheral smear, chest radiograph, bone marrow biopsy and CT scan of the chest/abdomen/pelvis should be performed to determine if the lesion in fact meets the criteria for a primary colonic lymphoma. Synchronous colonic adenocarcinoma has been described [26], so examination of the entire colon is necessary.

Primary rectal lymphoma has been associated with a number of conditions, including longstanding ulcerative colitis [26,32], pelvic irradiation [33], and solid organ transplantation [34]. Owing to the rare nature of this lesion, it is impossible to demonstrate definitively a relationship between these conditions and the development of the neoplasm. A number of investigators have recently described primary rectal lymphomas arising in homosexual men [35–39]. These authors have proposed possible relationships between the development of rectal lymphoma and ano-receptive intercourse, HIV or the human T-cell lymphotropic virus type III. The prevalence of AIDS continues at epidemic proportions; therefore, if a relationship exists with HIV, it is possible that primary rectal lymphoma will become a more common entity.

Prognosis and Treatment

The treatment for potentially resectable disease remains controversial. It has been clear for some time that resection offers the best chance of cure for the more common primary gastric lymphomas [40]. There is some evidence to indicate that this relationship holds true for primary colonic lymphoma [28]. Primary radiotherapy for unresectable lesions, high-risk surgical candidates, and patients who are unwilling to undergo surgery, has also been described, with some success [41,42]. High rectal lesions have been successfully treated with LAR, while low rectal lesions have been treated both by APR and transanal excision. No formal analysis of APR versus local excision has been performed. Most authors advocate adjuvant radiotherapy or chemoradiotherapy [26,28,29,41,43,44], although this cancer remains too rare to demonstrate clearly the benefit of such intervention. Our algorithm for the management of rectal lymphoma is depicted in Fig. 15.2.

Overall 5-year survival for primary colorectal lymphoma is 30–50% [28,41], with better survival for patients presenting with localized disease (50% 5-year survival) compared with those presenting with regional lymph node metastasis (24% 5-year survival) [41]. The histologic grade of the lesion may also have some impact on prognosis [26].

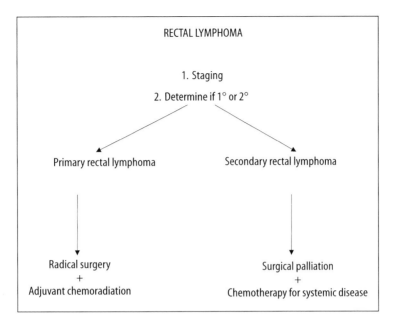

Fig. 15.2. Suggested algorithm for management of rectal lymphoma based on primary or secondary involvement.

Plasmacytoma of the Rectum

Plamacytomas are well-differentiated neoplasms of plasma cells, commonly found in the nasopharynx. Primary rectal plasmacytoma is an exceedingly rare condition, with only a handful of cases being reported in the literature. Although aggressive segmental resection has been used to treat these lesions, they appear to be as radiosensitive as plasmacytomas arising in other locations. Anecdotal experience has demonstrated long-term survival after local excision combined with radiotherapy [45], and after radiotherapy alone [46].

Secondary Lymphoma of the Rectum

Autopsy series have demonstrated that 46% of patients with metastatic lymphoma of nodal origin have some degree of involvement of the GI tract [23]. Rectal involvement of metastatic lymphoma typically presents with hematochezia and weight loss [28]. Secondary lymphoma can imitate inflammatory bowel disease [47]. Primary therapy for metastatic lymphoma remains chemotherapy. Surgical intervention is reserved for the complications of GI involvement such as intussusception, perforation, obstruction or uncontrollable hemorrhage. Overall 5-year survival is only 15% [28] despite such interventions.

Anorectal Melanoma

Although melanocytes do not normally occur in the rectal mucosa, malignant melanoma arising in the rectum well above the dentate line has occasionally been reported in the literature [48–52]. These lesions are sometimes found arising in areas of normal-appearing melanocytes, suggesting that certain individuals may have melanocytes present in the mucosa of the rectum [48,49]. Many malignant melanomas, however, involve the anal canal and/or the anorectal junction. It is often difficult to define exactly where these lesions arise, so most researchers have placed all these tumors under the term "anorectal" for purposes of analysis. Therefore we will also consider this rare rectal cancer under the more general category of anorectal melanoma.

The anorectum is the third most common site for melanoma (after cutaneous and ocular lesions), and represents 0.2–0.7% of all melanomas [52–54]. When considering only the anal canal, melanoma accounts for 4% of malignant lesions [55], but when considering the entire anorectum, however, melanoma represents only 0.2–0.8% of all malignancies in this area [52,54].

Clinical Presentation and Diagnosis

Rectal bleeding has consistently been reported as the most common presenting symptom of anorectal melanoma [51,52,56–58]. The average age of these patients is commonly in the sixth and seventh decades of life [51–53,56,57,59–61]. The mean duration of symptoms before presentation is 5–6 months [57,61]. Although a number of investigators have reported a female preponderance [51,52,57,58,60], recent meta-analysis has disputed this finding [61]. The diagnosis of unsuspected malignant melanoma during histologic examination of hemorrhoidectomy specimens has often been reported [51,56,57,59,61]. Up to 30% of anorectal melanomas will lack visible melanin (i.e. they are amelanotic) [51,56,58,61]. Immunohistochemistry may be useful in identifying lesions with questionable histology because the majority will react with conventional antibodies directed towards markers of malignant melanoma (e.g. vimentin, S-100, HMB-45) [58]. Immunohistochemistry may also be useful in the differentiation of these lesions from other rare tumors with similar morphology such as NE carcinomas. Malignant melanoma has been known to metastasize to the GI tract, so a thorough cutaneous and ocular examination to rule out a primary neoplasm at these locations must be performed. Metastases to regional lymph nodes or distant sites will be present in 20–60% of patients at initial diagnosis [52,53,57,60–62]. Inguinal lymph nodes are frequently involved and pelvic metastases are common even for anal canal lesions. Frequent distant metastases include liver, lung and bone [51,56,57, 60,62], so initial workup should include chest radiography and an abdominal CT scan.

Treatment and Prognosis

The outlook for this rare cancer remains dismal. Although occasional long-term survivors (>10 years) have been reported [52,56,59,63], median survival after diagnosis is 12–16 months [52,60]. Mean survival is better for those with local disease (29 months) compared with those with regional or distant metastasis (6 months) [57]. Overall 5-year survival is 6–20% [53,56,57,59,60,64], and 5-year survival for patients presenting with metastasis may approach 0% [56]. Tumor size, lymph node status and invasive depth of the primary lesion appear to have some prognostic significance [52,59]. For cutaneous melanomas, the thickness of the lesion has clearly been associated with survival. Although this same relationship has been difficult to demonstrate for anorectal melanoma [57], long-term (>5 years) survivors described in the literature (in which the measurement was reported) have had tumors with a depth of invasion of 7 mm or less [56,58,59]. The administration of palliative radiotherapy and chemotherapy (usually dacarbazine) for unresectable and metastatic disease have been reported [51,52,57,59]. Response appears to be poor, although the rare nature of this lesion precludes formal analysis.

The surgical approach for patients with potentially resectable disease remains quite controversial. These lesions almost invariably occur in the distal rectum or the anal canal, and thus the debate has centered on APR (with or without elective inguinal node dissection) and wide local excision. APR offers the theoretical advantage of removing draining pelvic lymph nodes. Lymph node metastases are found in APR specimens from 40–60% of patients [56,60,61]. Long-term survival after APR with removal of metastatic mesenteric disease has been reported [56]. A number of studies have demonstrated lower rates of local recurrence with APR [51,52,56,60,62]. This has led some investigators to conclude that APR (possibly with elective lymphadenectomy of the inguinal region) offers the best chance for cure. However, APR has never been demonstrated to provide a statistically significant difference in overall or disease-free survival [51,52,56–59,61,62] when compared with wide local excision. This lack of demonstrable benefit and the attendant morbidity of a permanent colostomy has led many experts to recommend performing wide local excision when possible, and reserving APR for large lesions.

The search continues for effective adjuvant therapy for anorectal melanoma. Adjuvant radiotherapy, chemotherapy and immunotherapy with Bacillus Calmette Guerin (BCG) have been described [56,60,62,63]. Owing to the rare nature of the lesion, it has been hard to demonstrate clear benefit. Recent advances in the treatment of cutaneous melanoma give some hope for effective adjuvant therapy. Interferon-alpha has been demonstrated to decrease recurrence rates and perhaps improve survival in intermediate depth cutaneous melanomas without nodal metastases [65,66]. The utility of interferon-alpha in the treatment of anorectal melanoma is undetermined at this time. If this adjuvant therapy proves useful in anorectal disease, it will undoubtedly renew the debate concerning the proper primary surgical resection of these lesions.

Neuroendocrine Carcinoma of the Rectum

NE neoplasms have been described in the lungs, genitourinary tract and endocrine organs, as well as the GI system. They share the ability to synthesize and secrete a variety of amines and peptide hormones (hence the designation "endocrine"), many of which are putative neurotransmitters (hence the prefix "neuro"). Historically, for the GI system, this ability was attributed only to carcinoid tumors (see previously in this chapter: "Carcinoid tumors of the rectum"). The development of specific antibodies to markers of NE differentiation and NE products has made immunohistochemistry an important tool in identifying these carcinomas. With the widespread use of these immunohistochemical techniques it has become apparent that a number of rectal neoplasms (including carcinoids, small-cell cancers and some anaplastic tumors) display NE differentiation. Some researchers have suggested that a combination of light microscopy, electron microscopy and immuno histochemistry will reveal NE features in up to 4% of colorectal neoplasms [67]. They have suggested that all of these carcinomas should be grouped under the general title of NE GI tumors, and the term carcinoid reserved for small, minimally invasive, well-differentiated lesions. This classification scheme remains controversial because even well-differentiated carcinoids may occasionally metastasize.

Pathology

Rectal NE tumors are thought to arise within the crypts of Lieberkuhn from enterochromaffin cells. These cells are a part of the intrinsic endocrine system of the GI tract and have been classified with similar cells found in the thyroid, adrenal medulla and pancreas as a part of the APUD system. Originally it was thought that all APUD cell lines originated from ectodermal neural crest. Considerable evidence exists, however, which indicates that intestinal APUD cells are of endodermal origin [68–71]. It has been postulated that multipotential stem cells exist within the colonic epithelium and that malignant transformation of these cells can lead to NE differentiation. An alternative hypothesis is that, during malignant transformation, some adenocarcinomas may develop NE characteristics. DNA analysis has also demonstrated that loss of heterozygosity for the APC (adenomatous polyposis coli), DCC (deleted in colorectal carcinoma), or p53 genes is common for poorly differentiated NE tumors, but is not present in well-differentiated carcinoid lesions [69]. This may indicate that the relatively benign rectal carcinoids do not share a common origin with the highly aggressive NE carcinomas, despite ultrastuctural and immunohistochemical similarities. This controversy remains unresolved.

Clinical Presentation and Diagnosis

On average, these patients are in ther sixth decade of life (range 28–90 years) and presentation is similar to adenocarcinoma of the rectum [67,72,73]. Microscopically, cells are arranged in sheets, trabeculae, rosettes and nests of cells [68,69]. Three cell types have been described: small cell (closely resembling small cell carcinoma of the lung), intermediate cell, and well-differentiated cell (representing carcinoid-like lesions). The resemblance of small cell NE carcinoma of the rectum to small cell carcinoma of the lung mandates that a search for a pulmonary primary neoplasm be performed in any patient with this diagnosis from rectal biopsy. Microscopically, small cell NE rectal carcinoma may also be confused with melanoma, basaloid lesions, lymphoma and various sarcomas. Further studies, such as electron microscopy or immunohistochemistry, are often required for definitive diagnosis. Electron microscopy of rectal NE tumors demonstrates dense-core NE-type granules [68,72,73]. Immunohistochemistry has become the most important tool in the correct identification of these lesions. It has been suggested that as many as 50% of the colorectal cancers identified by microscopic and ultrastructural techniques as poorly differentiated carcinomas would be reclassified as NE by proper immunohistochemistry [67]. Non-specific markers of NE differentiation, such as neuron specific enolase and chromogranin are often present [67,69,72,73]. Other NE markers and products often demonstrated by immunohistochemistry include serotonin, vasoactive intestinal peptide, substance P, somatostatin, cytokeratin and epithelial membrane antigen [67,72,73]. Rectal NE carcinomas, like rectal carcinoids, seem relatively incapable of producing carcinoid syndrome (even with liver metastases).

Treatment and Prognosis

This aggressive cancer is associated with a 58% 6-month survival rate, and a 6% 5-year survival rate [67]. Intermediate-cell and well-differentiated subtypes appear to share the same dismal prognosis as small cell cancer [67,72]. Rectal malignancies with combinations of glandular, squamous and NE differentiation have a prognosis similar to pure NE cancers [67,72,73].

These tumors have a high propensity for nodal and distant metastasis. More than 80% of patients will have nodal or distant metastasis at presentation [67,72]. Metastasis to regional lymph nodes and the liver are most common, although lung, peritoneal and brain metastases have been reported [67–69,72,73–76]. Treatment for the majority of patients reported in the literature has included resection of the tumor through a low anterior approach or an APR. Most authorities suggest that this offers the best palliation and the best chance for cure. Some authors have recommended, owing to the aggressive nature of these lesions, that all patients without evidence of metastatic disease should undergo aggressive resection, systemic chemotherapy and radiotherapy [68]. No formal analysis concerning the survival advantage of this approach has been performed. Palliative radio-chemotherapy has reportedly been used in un-resectable lesions, with some suggestion of efficacy [75]. Various chemotherapeutic agents have been suggested for adjuvant therapy and for treatment of metastatic disease [68,73,75]. Several authors have recommended that the chemotherapeutic agents typically used in oat cell lung carcinoma (such as cyclophosphamide, doxorubicin, vincristine) should be considered in patients with small cell NE carcinoma of the rectum. Although there has been some suggestion of response in isolated cases, the rare nature of this lesion has precluded any formal analysis and no form of treatment has demonstrated any clear survival advantage.

Recent improvements in immunohistochemical techniques will undoubtedly allow us to identify correctly a greater number of rectal NE tumors. Tertiary centers will hopefully obtain sufficient experience with this rare and aggressive neoplasm to define optimal treatment strategies.

Vascular Lesions

Diffuse Cavernous Hemangioma

Diffuse cavernous hemangioma is an unusual entity affecting the rectum, of which only 100 cases have been reported [77]. It is unusual to face such a rare condition in everyday practice, although the colorectal specialist should be aware of this disease in defining the diagnosis of such a rectal lesion in young adults, and occasionally in infants. This entity was first described by Phillips [78] in 1839, and has been associated with the Klippel–Trenaunay–Weber syndrome [79] and the Kasabach–Meritt syndrome [80]. The rectosigmoid is the most common site involved by this disease in the GI tract. The predominant presenting symptom is rectal bleeding, which can be acute recurrent or chronic. Associated hematuria has also been reported [81], while pain is a rare presentation. There is often a substantial delay in diagnosis such that a long history of rectal bleeding is frequently encountered before a correct diagnosis is made [82,83], often 20 years after the onset of symptoms [84,85].

It is interesting that a number of patients have previously undergone hemorrhoidectomy or other surgical treatment for the misdiagnosed condition. The clinical examination often reveals a circumferential, obvious rectal malignant lesion, although a polypoid aspect has also been reported. In a number of instances, an association with angiomas at different sites has been reported [84]. One previously reported patient died of massive intra-cerebral bleeding 10 months after a successful operation on the primary rectal tumor [81].

Imaging plays an important role not only in diagnosis but also in staging and treatment planning. The main features of diffuse cavernous hemangioma have been reported with plain radiography, barium enema, CT, magnetic resonance imaging and endoscopy [84,86]. The presence of extensive phleboliths seen on plain radiographs, a filling defect on barium enema, and a CT scan that reveals a thickened mesentery containing large vacuoles, often suggest the presence of this lesion, but these features are not diagnostic. CT is useful in that it may provide information regarding the diameter of the lesion, its local extent, and involvement of the adjacent structures. Magnetic resonance imaging utilizing endorectal coils reveals specific diagnostic features [84,87,88]. The rectosigmoid thickening can be homogeneous, hypointense on T1-weighted images. The perirectal fat is usually abnormally heterogeneous, with serpiginous hypointense structures in it. Both the rectal wall and the perirectal tissue such as the vulva, clitoris, gluteal and pelvic muscles, urinary bladder, seminal vesicles, and uterus may be synchronously involved. The presence of a rectovaginal or rectovesical fistula has been reported [87]. Tan et al. reported a patient presenting with erosion of the pelvic ureter and iliac vessels [89]. At times the tumor might extend from the sigmoid in continuity with the left colon and, rarely, reach to the transverse colon [77].

Colonoscopy often reveals an irregularly enlarged tortuous submucosal vascular network with a dark and friable overlying mucosal covering [90]. For this reason the lesion has often been described as bluish or plum colored [91]. Although massive bleeding may occur, endoscopic or percutaneous biopsy is often feasible with a moderate attendant risk [92]. When preoperative pathological confirmation cannot be achieved, a conservative approach is recommended. A number of surgical treatments have been proposed and a sphincter saving procedure should be attempted. Most often the patient has undergone some sort of surgical management, such as hemorrhoidectomy/injection of hemorrhoids, laparotomy, bilateral internal iliac artery ligation, cautery of the mucosa, stitching of a rectal prolapse, or local resection at the anal canal [77]. LAR or a coloanal anastomosis is the treatment of choice, often associated with partial cystectomy [81], or any extended procedure aimed at radical removal of the tumor. The final pathologic evaluation may necessitate an APR, which can be performed as a second step.

Although surgical management requires adequate skill, particularly in the presence of multivisceral involvement, the long-term outcome can be favorable, and most patients recover from bleeding. Coloanal sleeve anastomosis was described by Jeffery et al. [93] and a series of 15 patients were treated accordingly at St Mark's Hospital in London [77]. This sphincter saving procedure is based on the division of the rectum just distal to the peritoneal reflection. The mucosa is then infiltrated with normal saline containing adrenaline 1:300 000 using the perianal route. This infiltration lifts the mucosa away from the underlying hemangioma and muscular coats, enabling the mucosa to be stripped from the intact submucosal layers. The mobilized portion of the colon is drawn through the denuded rectum and sutured per anally to the dentate line. The hemangiomatous vessels remaining in the rectal wall are no longer subject to local trauma, which is considered to cause the bleeding; the hemorrhage is thus controlled [77]. Side effects of the surgical management may be further bleeding, incontinence, frequent bowel movements, and sexual dysfunction among those subjects with multiple hemangiomas around the penis, urethra, scrotum or bladder.

Lymphangiomas

Lymphangiomas arise in the lymphatic plexus within the submucosa of the bowel. The widespread use of fibroscopy has increased the detection rate of lymphangiomas affecting the large bowel. Since their initial description in the rectum in 1932 [94], a number of investigators have disputed whether these lesions actually represent vascular malformations. They frequently appear as numerous extramucosal cysts that are often pedunculated; thus, a snare biopsy is often feasible. Endoscopic management of lymphangiomas smaller than 2 mm is recommended [95]. Large (sessile and infiltrative) and symptomatic lesions may require a surgical approach intended to preserve anorectal function, when technically feasible.

Hemangiopericytoma

Hemangiopericytoma is a much more aggressive disease, a very rare capillary tumor that was first described by Stout and Murray in 1942. Abdominal pain, rectal bleeding and intestinal obstruction are common presenting symptoms. Dysuria has been reported as a major complaint, due to retro-

peritoneal invasion and involvement of the ureters. Surgical removal is mandatory, when feasible. Patients may benefit from adjuvant chemotherapy with adriamycin to reduce the local recurrence rate and to prevent distant metastases [96].

Squamous Cell and Adenosquamous Carcinoma of the Rectum

Squamous Cell Carcinoma of the Rectum

Primary squamous cell carcinoma of the colorectum is an extremely rare entity, with less than 100 cases reported in the English language literature [97]. The rectum is the site of almost half of all primary colorectal squamous cell cancers [98]. A population-based study has indicated that as many as 0.4% of rectal cancers are squamous cell [99]; however, this study made no attempt to identify which of these cancers arose in the anal epithelium and simply extended into the rectum. Most authorities estimate that approximately 0.02–0.2% of rectal cancers are primary squamous cell carcinomas [98,100] using the following criteria to identify such lesions correctly: no evidence exists of a squamous cell cancer in another location that could spread (through direct extension or metastasis) to the rectum; the affected bowel does not contain a squamous lined fistula tract (squamous cell cancer arising from these fistulas is well described [101]); and the lesion is not in continuity with the anal epithelium.

Squamous cells do not normally exist within the rectal mucosa. A number of theories have been presented to explain the development of squamous cell cancer in this location:

1. Undifferentiated cells exist within the crypts of the colonic mucosa [102]. It is possible that these represent uncommitted stem cells. Repeated mucosal injury could lead to proliferation and eventual malignant transformation of these multipotential cells into a squamous cell cancer.

2. Squamous metaplasia of the colonic mucosa could occur in response to chronic inflammation, and squamous cell carcinoma could develop in such a setting. Rectal squamous metaplasia has seldom been reported [103], but rectal squamous cancers are likewise rare.

3. Careful examination of colonic adenomatous polyps will reveal some areas of squamous differenti-

ation in 0.4% of specimens [104]. It is possible that squamous cell cancer develops in these adenomatous polyps, and the subsequent development of the tumor obliterates the original adenomatous components.

4. Rectal carcinomas with a combination of adenomatous and squamous cell characteristics have been described [105] (see "Adenosquamous carcinoma of the rectum" later in this chapter). It is possible that during malignant transformation and development some adenocarcinomas may begin to display squamous cell characteristics. If this occurred early enough in tumor development then the squamous histology could come to dominate the lesion.

Clinical Presentation and Diagnosis

On average, these patients are in the fifth decade of life (range 30–90 years) [98,106]. Abdominal pain and hematochezia are the most common presenting symptoms [98,106,107]. The average duration of symptoms before presentation is 6 months [106]. Males and females are affected equally [98,106]. The majority of these lesions are in the lower rectum and more than 80% are detectable by digital rectal examination [98]. Half of these patients will have lymph node metastasis and more than 15% will have distant metastasis at presentation [98]. Reported metastatic sites have included liver, lungs, bone, omentum, peritoneum and adrenals [98,106], prompting some authorities to recommend chest radiography and abdominopelvic CT scanning as part of the initial evaluation.

Squamous cell carcinoma of the colorectum has been reported in the presence of a number of conditions such as colonic duplication, schistosomiasis, ulcerative colitis, amebiasis, ovarian carcinoma and colonic adenocarcinoma [98,100,104,106]. The possible relationship between any of these conditions and the development of rectal squamous cell carcinoma is uncertain. Although human papillomavirus has been implicated in the development of anal squamous cell cancer, there is no current evidence that such a relationship also extends to rectal lesions.

Prognosis and Treatment

Although occasional longterm survivors (>10 years) have been reported, the average survival after diagnosis is approximately 30 months [106]. Overall 5-year survival is 30% [100]. Average survival is somewhat better for patients who present with node-negative disease (39.6 months) compared with those with lymph node metastasis at presentation (29.4 months) [98,108].

Primary chemotherapy has been used to palliate patients with distant metastatic disease; however, no standard treatment regimen has been developed

[107]. Primary chemoradiotherapy for patients who are unwilling or unable to tolerate surgery has also been reported, with some suggestion of a palliative effect [107]. The optimal management of potentially resectable disease remains controversial. Historically, owing to the aggressive nature of this lesion, resection of the involved rectum with the possible addition of adjuvant chemotherapy was often advocated. Nigro and others have demonstrated that chemoradiotherapy combined with local excision is effective treatment for appropriately selected anal squamous cell cancers [109,110]. Several authors have described treating rectal squamous cell cancer with chemoradiation and local excision in a manner similar to anal canal squamous cell cancer, reporting disease-free patients followed up for 6 months [97], 1 year [98] and 2 years [108]. Other authors have described using chemoradiation as an adjuvant to APR for locally invasive rectal squamous cell cancer, reporting a disease-free patient followed up for 13 months [111]. The rare nature of this lesion, however, has precluded formal analysis of the efficacy of chemoradiotherapy and local excision compared with rectal resection.

Adenosquamous Carcinoma of the Rectum

Rarely, malignant tumors with a combination of adenomatous and squamous features will be found in the GI tract. Adenosquamous carcinoma has been estimated to represent 0.06–0.18% of all colorectal malignancies [112–113]. The majority of such lesions occur in the descending colon and rectum. The mean age of these patients is 67 years [112]. An association between this disease and ulcerative colitis has been suggested by several studies [113]. At presentation, disease is localized in 11% of patients and regional in 44%; distant metastases are present in 41% [112]. Common sites of distant metastases include the liver, lungs and peritoneum [113]. Mean survival is 12 months, with 5-year survival estimated to be 30% [112]. Stage for stage survival appears to be generally worse when compared with adenocarcinoma [112]. The primary treatment modality is surgical resection. Adjuvant chemotherapy is commonly used, although its efficacy remains unknown. Commonly used agents include semustine, 5-fluorouracil, carmustine and methotrexate [113]. Postoperative chemoradiotherapy as the Nigro protocol has also been reported [112]. Distant metastases from this disease often appear to contain a greater squamous component than the parent tumor [114], suggesting that it is this portion of the tumor that may account for its more aggressive course.

Sarcomas of the Rectum

Leiomyosarcoma

Although fibrosarcoma, angiosarcoma and other rare stromal malignancies of the colon have been described, leiomyosarcoma comprises 95% of colorectal sarcomas [115]. Leiomyosarcoma of the rectum is rare and accounts for 0.07–0.3% of all rectal malignancies [116,117]. These tumors commonly present in the fifth and sixth decades, and are most commonly found in the lower third of the rectum [117]. They remain difficult to diagnose and are very aggressive. Surgery remains the mainstay of therapy, but controversy exists regarding treatment of these lesions with wide local excision versus radical surgery. In selected patients, conservative surgery (possibly accompanied by adjuvant radiotherapy) may provide a reasonable alternative to radical surgery.

Pathology

Rectal sarcomas arise from smooth muscle cells of the intestinal wall. Grossly, they may remain submucosal, demonstrate superficial ulceration, or extend into the lumen in a polypoid fashion. Occasionally there is a dumb-bell type of extension, with portions of the mass extending into the lumen and other parts encroaching on structures surrounding the rectum. Histologically these tumors are composed of elongated cells that grow in fascicles. Immunohistochemical techniques to examine for the presence of vimentin and desmin may be useful in establishing the diagnosis [118]. Differentiating between benign leiomyomas and leiomyosarcomas based upon histologic criteria can be very challenging to the pathologist. Benign lesions tend to arise in the muscularis mucosa, are often less than 1 cm in diameter, and demonstrate <1 mitosis per 50 high power miscroscopic fields [119,120]. Lesions that follow a malignant course tend to arise in the muscularis propria, have a mean diameter of 4.6 cm, are associated with superficial ulceration, and typically demonstrate 5–58 mitosis per 50 high power microscopic fields [117,119,120]. Malignancy is best determined by an increased mitotic index. Malignant lesions are further categorized as either high or low grade. Even small lesions with benign histologic features have been known to recur, so all patients require vigilant follow-up.

Clinical Presentation and Diagnosis

The most common presenting symptoms of rectal sarcoma are rectal pain, constipation and hematochezia [115,117,119]. Rarely, patients will present with bladder outlet obstruction [119] or a rectal abcess [121,122]. Benign leimyomas may have similar clinical manifestations. Pain is more common in the malignant lesions. Endoscopically these tumors may appear as a submucosal mass, a polypoid lesion or an irregular mucosal pattern. Repeated biopsy may be necessary to obtain a histologic diagnosis.

Treatment and Prognosis

Leiomyosarcoma of the rectum has a high recurrence rate and a less favorable prognosis than adenocarcinoma. Optimal surgical management remains controversial. Wide local excision of these lesions is accompanied by a local recurrence rate as high as 60–67% [117,120]. Radical surgery is associated with only a 20% local recurrence rate [117]. Despite this difference, radical resection has not been demonstrated to provide any survival benefit over wide local excision [117,120,123]. Tumor grade has been shown to co-relate with survival [115,117,120,121], therefore some authors have suggested that small tumors (<2.5 cm) with favorable histology should be treated with wide local excision [123]. Local recurrence has been demonstrated as late as 7 years after wide local excision, so vigilant follow-up is required [119]. Recurrent tumor should be resected whenever possible. The use of adjuvant chemotherapy and radiotherapy for this condition has been described [115]. Although there is some evidence to indicate that adjuvant radiotherapy may decrease local recurrence rates [121], neither adjuvant radiotherapy nor chemotherapy has clearly been demonstrated to affect overall survival. For patients who refuse radical surgery, or those who are unable to tolerate such a procedure, some have suggested various combinations of local excision, brachytherapy and/or external beam radiation [124]. The efficacy of such treatment regimens remains unknown.

The mean survival from diagnosis is 33 months [115], and the overall 5-year survival is 40% [121]. Twenty-four per cent of patients have metastases at presentation [115], the most common sites being the liver and the peritoneum [115]. Lymph node metastases are present in the surgical specimens of radical resections in only 12% of these patients [115]. Liver metastases have been reported as late as 17 years after the initial diagnosis [115].

Kaposi's Sarcoma

The acquired immune deficiency syndrome (AIDS) epidemic has been associated with a number of malignancies, Kaposi's sarcoma being the most common of these. Although this is most often a cutaneous neoplasm, in AIDS patients it has been known to involve the GI tract. Cases of primary

rectal Kaposi's sarcoma, as well as of wide metastatic disease, including the rectum, have been reported
[125–127]. The average age of these patients is
34 years [125]. The most common presenting symptoms are rectal pain, hematochezia and diarrhea.
These tumors are well known to be radiosensitive,
and primary radiotherapy has been the treatment
described for most patients [125–127]. This appears
to offer adequate local control, but subsequent
metastatic disease has been desribed [125], suggesting that this treatment may not provide the optimal
chance for cure. A response to chemotherapy has
also been described [125], although this does not
appear to be as effective as radiotherapy. Because
most of the patients described have suffered from
advanced AIDS, treatment has centered on palliation. As more effective treatments for AIDS are
developed, and thus the life expectancy of the condition lengthens, a re-evaluation of treatment
goals for primary rectal Kaposi's sarcoma may be
required in the future.

References

1. Oberndorfer S. Karzinoide tumoren des dunndarms. Frank-
   furter Z Patol 1907;1:425–32.
2. Aranha GV, Greenlee HB. Surgical management of carcinoid
   tumors of the GI tract. Am Surg 1980;46:429–35.
3. Naunheim KS, Zeitels J, Kaplan EL, et al. Rectal carcinoid tumors – treatment and prognosis. Surgery 1983;94:
   670–76.
4. Sauven P, Ridge JA, Quan SH, Sigurdson ER. Anorectal carcinoid tumors: is aggressive surgery warranted? Ann Surg
   1990;211:67–71.
5. Jetmore AB, Ray JE, Gathright JB, McMullen KM, Hicks TC,
   Timmcke AE. Rectal carcinoids: the most frequent carcinoid
   tumor. Dis Colon Rectum 1992;35:717–25.
6. Quan SH, Bader G, Berg JW. Carcinoid tumors of the
   rectum. Dis Colon Rectum 1964;7:197–206.
7. Teleky B, Herbst F, Langle F, Neuhold N, Niederle B. The
   prognosis of rectal carcinoid tumours. Int J Colorectal Dis
   1992;7:11–14.
8. Burke M, Shepherd N, Mann CV. Carcinoid tumors of the
   rectum and anus. Br J Surg 1987;74:358–61.
9. Federspiel BH, Burke AP, Sobin LH, Shekitka KM. Rectal and
   colonic carcinoids: a clinicopathologic study of 84 cases.
   Cancer 1990;65:135–40.
10. Soga J. Carcinoids of the rectum: an evaluation of 1271
    reported cases. Jpn J Surg 1997;27:112–19.
11. Koura AN, Giacco GG, Curley SA, Skibber JM, Feig BW, Ellis
    LM. Carcinoid tumors of the rectum: effect of size,
    histopathology, and surgical treatment on metastasis free
    survival. Cancer 1997;79:1294–98.
12. Saclarides TJ, Szeluga D, Staren ED. Neuroendocrine cancers
    of the colon and rectum: results of a ten-year experience.
    Dis Colon Rectum 1994;37:635–42.
13. Mani S, Modlin IM, Ballantyne G, Ahlman H, West B.
    Carcinoids of the rectum. J Am Coll Surg 1994;179:231–48.
14. Fitzgerald SD, Meagher AP, Moniz-Pereira P, Farrow GM,
    Witzig TE, Wolff BG. Carcinoid tumor of the rectum: DNA
    ploidy is not a prognostic factor. Dis Colon Rectum
    1996;39:643–48.

15. Matsui K, Iwase T, Kitagawa M. Small, polypoid-appearing
    carcinoid tumors of the rectum: clinicopathologic study of
    16 cases and effectiveness of endoscopic treatment. Am J
    Gastroenterol 1993;88:1949–53.
16. Schindl M, Niederle B, Hafner M, et al. Stage-dependent
    therapy of rectal carcinoid tumors. World J Surg 1998;22:
    628–34.
17. Soga J, Tazawa K. Pathologic analysis of carcinoids: histo-
    logic reevaluation of 62 cases. Cancer 1971;28:990–98.
18. Yang K, Ulich T, Cheng L, Lewin KJ. The neuroendocrine
    products of intestinal carcinoids: an immunoperoxidase
    study of 35 carcinoid tumors stained for serotonin and eight
    polypeptide hormones. Cancer 1983;51:1918–26.
19. Shirouzu K, Isomoto H, Kagegawa T, Morimatsu M. Treat-
    ment of rectal carcinoid tumors. Am J Surg 1990;160:
    262–65.
20. Ishikawa H, Imanishi K, Otani T, Okuda S, Tatsuta M,
    Ishiguro S. Effectiveness of endoscopic treatment of carci-
    noid tumors of the rectum. Endoscopy 1989;21:133–35.
21. Higaki S, Nishiaki M, Mitani N, Yanai H, Tada M, Okita K.
    Effectiveness of local endoscopic resection of rectal carci-
    noid tumors. Endoscopy 1997;29:171–75.
22. Inada-Shirankata Y, Sakai M, Kajiyama T, et al. Endoscopic
    resection of rectal carcinoid tumors using aspiration
    lumpectomy. Endsocopy 1996;28:34–38.
23. Herrmann R, Panahom AM, Barcos MP, Walsh D, Stutzman
    L. Gastrointestinal involvement in non-Hodgkin's lym-
    phoma. Cancer 1980;46:215–22.
24. Heule BV, Taylor CR, Terry R, Lukes RJ. Presentation of
    malignant lymphoma in the rectum. Cancer 1982;49:
    2602–607.
25. Contreary K, Nance FC, Becker WF. Primary lymphoma of
    the gastrointestinal tract. Ann Surg 1980;191:593–98.
26. Shepherd NA, Hall PA, Coates PJ, Levison DA. Primary
    malignant lymphoma of the colon and rectum: a histo-
    pathological and immunohistochemical analysis of 45 cases
    with clinicopathological correlations. Histopathology
    1988;12:235–52.
27. Dawson IMP, Cornes JS, Morson BC. Primary malig-
    nant lymphoid tumours of the intestinal tract. Br J Surg
    1961;49:80–89.
28. Devine RM, Beart RW, Wolff BG. Malignant lymphoma of
    the rectum. Dis Colon Rectum 1986;29:821–24.
29. Aozasa K, Ohsawa M, Soma T, et al. Malignant lymphoma of
    the rectum. Jpn J Clin Oncol 1990;20:380–86.
30. Ohri SK, Keane PF, Sackier JM, Hutton K, Wood CB. Primary
    rectal lymphoma and malignant lymphomatous polyposis.
    Dis Colon Rectum 1989;32:1071–74.
31. Keane PF, Scott R, Wood CB, Stewart I. Primary rectal
    lymphoma. Br J Clin Pract 1990;44:511–12.
32. Teare JP, Greenfield SM, Slater S. Rectal lymphoma after
    colectomy for ulcerative colitis. Gut 1992;33:138–39.
33. Sibly TF, Keane RM, Lever JV, Southwood WFW. Rectal lym-
    phoma in radiation injured bowel. Br J Surg 1985;72:879–80.
34. Fan CW, Chen JS, Wang JY, Fan HA. Perforated rectal lym-
    phoma in a renal transplant recipient: report of a case. Dis
    Colon Rectum 1997;40:1258–60.
35. Gottlieb CA, Meiri E, Maeda KM. Rectal non-Hodgkin's lym-
    phoma: a clinicopathologic study and review. Henry Ford
    Hosp Med J 1990;38:255–58.
36. Burkes RL, Meyer PR, Gill PS, Parker JW, Rasheed S, Levine
    AM. Rectal lymphoma in homosexual men. Arch Intern
    Med 1986;146:913–15.
37. Lee MH, Waxman M, Gillooley JF. Primary malignant lym-
    phoma of the anorectum in homosexual men. Dis Colon
    Rectum 1986;29:413–16.
38. Levine AM, Gill PS, Meyer PR, et al. Retrovirus and ma-
    lignant lymphoma in homosexual men. JAMA 1985;254:
    1921–25.

39. Ziegler JL, Beckstead JA, Volberding PA, et al. Non-Hodgkin's lymphoma in 90 homosexual men. N Engl J Med 1984;311:565–70.

40. Fleming ID, Mitchell S, Dilawari RA. The role of surgery in the management of gastric lymphoma. Cancer 1982;49:1135–41.

41. Freeman C, Berg JW, Cutler SJ. Occurrence and prognosis of extranodal lymphomas. Cancer 1972;29:252–60.

42. Loehr WJ, Mujahed Z, Zahn D, Gray GF, Thorbjarnarson B. Primary lymphoma of the gastrointestinal tract: a review of 100 cases. Ann Surg 1969;170:232–38.

43. Shimono R, Mori M, Kido A, Adachi Y, Sugimachi K. Malignant lymphoma of the rectum treated preoperatively with hyperthermia and radiation. Eur J Surg Oncol 1995;21:83–84.

44. Renard TH, Morton RL, Mathews R, Poulos E. Primary lymphoma of the rectum. Am Surg 1992;58:634–37.

45. Pais JR, Garcia-Segovia J, Rodriguez-Garcia JL, Alvarez-Baleriola I, Garcia-Gonzalez M. Solitary plasmacytoma of the rectum: report of a case treated by endoscopic polypectomy and radiotherapy. Eur J Surg Oncol 1994;20:592–94.

46. Price A, Quilty PM, Ludgate SM. Extramedullary plasmacytoma of the rectum: two cases treated by radiotherapy. Clin Radiol 1987;38:283–85.

47. Sagar S, Selby P, Sloane J, McElwain TJ. Colorectal lymphoma simulating inflammatory colitis and diagnosed by immunohistochemistry. Postgrad Med J 1986;62:51–53.

48. Werdin C, Limas C, Knodell RG. Primary malignant melanoma of the rectum: evidence for origination from rectal mucosal melanocytes. Cancer 1988;61:1364–70.

49. Nicholson AG, Cox PM, Marks CG, Cook MG. Primary malignant melanoma of the rectum. Histopathology 1993;22:261–64.

50. Alexander RM, Cone LA. Malignant melanoma of the rectal ampulla: report of a case and review of the literature. Dis Colon Rectum 1977;20:53–55.

51. Slingluff CL, Vollmer RT, Seigler HF. Anorectal melanoma: clinical characteristics and results of surgical management in twenty-four patients. Surgery 1990;107:1–9.

52. Goldman S, Glimelius B, Pahlman L. Anorectal malignant melanoma in Sweden: report of 49 patients. Dis Colon Rectum 1990;33:874–77.

53. Weinstock MA. Epidemiology and prognosis of anorectal melanoma. Gastroenterology 1993;104:174–78.

54. Pack GT, Oropeza R. A comparative study of melanoma and epidermoid carcinoma of the anal canal: a review of 20 melanomas and 29 epidermoid carcinomas. Dis Colon Rectum 1967;10:161–76.

55. Longo WE, Vernava AM, Wade TP, Coplin MA, Virgo KS, Johnson FE. Rare anal canal cancers in the US veteran: patterns of disease and results of treatment. Am Surg 1995;61:495–500.

56. Brady MS, Kavolius JP, Quan SHQ. Anorectal melanoma: a 64-year experience at Memorial Sloan-Kettering Cancer Center. Dis Colon Rectum 1995;38:146–51.

57. Thibault C, Sangar P, Nivatvongs S, Ilstrup DM, Wolff BG. Anorectal melanoma: an incurable disease? Dis Colon Rectum 1997;40:661–68.

58. Ben-Izhak O, Levy R, Weill S, et al. Anorectal malignant melanoma: a clinicopathologic study, including immunohistochemistry and DNA flow cytometry. Cancer 1997;79:18–25.

59. Wanebo H, Woodruff JM, Farr GH, Quan SH. Anorectal melanoma. Cancer 1981;47:1891–900.

60. Konstadoulakis MM, Ricaniadis N, Walsh D, Karakousis CP. Malignant melanoma of the anorectal region. J Surg Oncol 1995;58:118–20.

61. Cooper PH, Mills SE, Allen MS. Malignant melanoma of the anus: report of 12 patients and analysis of 255 additional cases. Dis Colon Rectum 1982;25:693–703.

62. Ross M, Pezzi C, Pezzi T, Meurer D, Hickey R, Balch C. Patterns of failure in anorectal melanoma: a guide to surgical therapy. Arch Surg 1990;125:313–16.

63. Freedman LS. Malignant melanoma of the anorectal region: two cases of prolonged survival. Br J Surg 1984;71:164–65.

64. Bolivar JC, Harris JW, Branch W, Sherman RT. Melanoma of the anorectal region. Surg Gynecol Obstet 1982;154:337–41.

65. Ruscainai L, Petraglia S, Alotto M, Calvieri S, Vezzoni G. Postsurgical adjuvant therapy for melanoma: evaluation of a 3-year randomized trial with recombinant interferon-alpha after 3 and 5 years of follow up. Cancer 1997;70:2354–60.

66. Grob JJ, Dreno B, Salmoniere P, et al. Randomized trial of interferon-alpha-2a as adjuvant therapy in resected primary melanoma thicker than 1.5 mm without clinically detectable node metastasis. Lancet 1998;351:1905–10.

67. Saclarides TJ, Szeluga D, Staren ED. Neuroendocrine cancers of the colon and rectum. Dis Colon Rectum 1994;37:635–42.

68. Schwartz AM, Orenstein JM. Small-cell undifferentiated carcinoma of the rectosigmoid colon. Arch Pathol Lab Med 1985;109:629–32.

69. Vortmeyer AO, Lubensky IA, Merino MJ, et al. Concordance of genetic alterations in poorly differentiated colorectal neuroendocrine carcinomas and associated adenocarcinomas. J. Natl Cancer Inst 1997;89:1448–53.

70. Cox WF, Pierce GB. The endodermal origin of the endocrine cells of an adenocarcinoma of the colon of the rat. Cancer 1982;50:1530–38.

71. Sidhu GS. The endodermal origin of digestive and respiratory tract APUD cells. Am J Pathol 1979;96:5–20.

72. Gaffy MJ, Mills SE, Lack EE. Neuroendocrine carcinoma of the colon and rectum. Am J Surg Pathol 1990;14:1010–23.

73. Wick MR, Wetherby RP, Weiland LH. Small cell neuroendocrine carcinoma of the colon and rectum: clinical, histologic, and ultrastructural study and immunohistochemical comparison with cloacogenic carcinoma. Hum Pathol 1987;18:9–21.

74. Khansur TK, Routh A, Mihas TA, Underwood JA, Smith GF, Mihas AA. Syndrome of inappropriate ADH secretion and diplopia: oat cell (small cell) rectal carcinoma metastatic to the central nervous system. Am J Gastroenterol 1995;90:1173–74.

75. Robidoux A, Monte M, Heppell J, Schurch W. Small-cell carcinoma of the rectum. Dis Colon Rectum 1984;28:594–96.

76. Shirouzu K, Morodomi T, Isomoto H, Yamauchi Y, Kakegawa T, Morimatsu M. Small-cell carcinoma of the rectum. Dis Colon Rectum 1985;28:434–39.

77. Cunningham JA, Garcia VF, Uispe G. Diffuse cavernous rectal hemangioma – sphincter-sparing approach to therapy. Report of a case. Dis Colon Rectum 1989;32:344–47.

78. Phillips B. Erectile tumor of the anus. Lond Med Gazette 1839;1:514–17.

79. Ghahremani GG, Kangarloo H, Volberg F, Meyers MA. Diffuse hemangioma of the colon in the Klippel–Trenaunay–Weber syndrome. Radiology 1976;118:673–78.

80. Azizkhan RG. Life-threatening hematochezia from a rectosigmoid vascular malformation in Klippel–Trenauray syndrome: long-term palliation using an argon laser. J Pediatr Surg 1991;26:1125–28.

81. Demircan O, Sonmez H, Zeren S, Cosar E, Bicacki K, Ozkan S. Diffuse cavernous hemangioma of the rectum and sigmoid colon. Dig Surg 1998;15:713–15.

82. Bland KI, Abney HT, MacGregor AMC, Hawkin IF. Hemangiomatosis of the colon and anorectum: a case report and a review of the literature. Am Surg 1974;40:626–35.

83. Coppa GF, Eng K, Localio SA. Surgical management of diffuse hemangioma of the colon, rectum and anus. Surg Gynecol Obstet 1984;159:17–22.

84. Djouhri H, Arrive L, Bouras T, Martin B, Monnier-Cholley L, Tubiana JM. MR imaging of diffuse cavernous hemangioma of the rectosigmoid colon. AJR Am J Roentgenol 1998;171:413–17.

85. Ner Z, Altaca G. Diffuse cavernous rectal hemangioma: clinical appearance, diagnostic modalities and sphincter-saving approach to therapy – report of 2 and a collective review of 79 cases. Acta Chir Belg 1993;93:173–76.

86. Djouhri H, Arrive L, Bouras T, Martin B, Monnier-Cholley L, Tubiana JM. Diffuse cavernous hemangioma of the rectosigmoid colon: imaging findings. J Comput Assist Tomogr 1998;22:851–55.

87. Lupetin AR. Diffuse cavernous hemangioma of the rectum: evaluation and MRI. Gastrointest Radiol 1990;15: 343–45.

88. Hasegawa H, Teramoto T, Watanabe M. Diffuse cavernous hemangioma of the rectum: MR imaging with endorectal surface coil and sphincter-saving surgery. J Gastroenterol 1996;31:875–79.

89. Tan RCF, Wang JY, Cheung YC, Wan WYL. Diffuse cavernous hemangioma of the rectum complicated by invasion of the pelvic structures. Dis Colon Rectum 1998;41:1062–66.

90. Katsinelos P, Eugenidis N, Paroutoglou G, Katsos J, Vasiliadis T. A case of diffuse cavernous hemangioma of the rectum with unusual clinical manifestations. Endoscopy 1995;27:405.

91. Grasso G, Greco P, Tricoli D, Carullo F. Cavernous hemangioma of the colon and rectum: a case report. Tumori 1982;68:173–76.

92. Popovici A, Mitulescu G, Hortopan M, Jianu C, Iliescu CA. Rectal hemangioma – a pseudo neoplastic form. A case report and review of the literature. Chirurgia (Bucur) 1998;93:261–65.

93. Jeffery PJ, Hawley PR, Parks AG. Colo-anal sleeve anastomosis in the treatment of diffuse cavernous hemangioma involving the rectum. Br J Surg 1976;63:678–82.

94. Chisholm AJ, Hillkowitz P. Lymphangioma of the rectum. Am J Surg 1932;17:281.

95. Kuramoto S, Sasaki S, Tsuda K, et al. Lymphangioma of the large intestine. Report of a case. Dis Colon Rectum 1998;31:900–905.

96. Takano K, Suzuki N, Saito H, et al. A case of hemangiopericytoma in the pelvic retroperitoneum and review of the literature on hemangiopericytoma in the retroperitoneal space in Japan. Nippon Geka Gakkai Zasshi 1985;86:959–65.

97. Schneider TA, Birkett DH, Vernava AM. Primary adenosquamous and squamous cell carcinoma of the colon and rectum. Int J Colorectal Dis 1992;7:144–47.

98. Lafreniere R, Ketcham AS. Primary squamous cell carcinoma of the rectum: report of a case and review of the literature. Dis Colon Rectum 1985;28:967–72.

99. DiSario JA, Randall WB, Kendrick ML, McWhorter WP. Colorectal cancers of rare histologic types compared with adenocarcinomas. Dis Colon Rectum 1994;37:1277–80.

100. Comer TP, Beahrs OH, Dockerty MB. Primary squamous cell carcinoma of the colon and rectum. Cancer 1971;28: 1111–17.

101. David VC, Loring M. The relation of chronic inflammation and especially lymphogranuloma to the development of squamous cell carcinoma of the rectum. Ann Surg 1939;109:837–43.

102. Lorenzsonn V, Trier JS. The fine structure of human rectal mucosa. Gastroenterology 1968;55:88–101.

103. Cabrera A, Pickren JW. Squamous metaplasia and squamous-cell carcinoma of the rectosigmoid. Dis Colon Rectum 1967;10:288–97.

104. Williams GT, Blackshaw AJ, Morson BC. Squamous carcinoma of the colorectum and its genesis. J Pathol 1979;129: 139–47.

105. Cerezo L, Alvarez M, Edwards O, Price G. Adenosquamous carcinoma of the colon. Dis Colon Rectum 1985;28:597–603.

106. Beradi RS, Chen HP, Lee SS. Squamous cell carcinoma of the colon and rectum. Surg Gynecol Obstet 1986;163:493–96.

107. Vezeridis MP, Herrera LO, Lopez GE, Ledesma EJ, Mittleman A. Squamous-cell carcinoma of the colon and rectum. Dis Colon Rectum 1983;26:188–91.

108. Lafreniere R, Ketcham AS. Squamous cell carcinoma of the rectum: a multimodality approach. J Surg Oncol 1986;32:106–109.

109. Nigro ND, Vaitkevicius VK, Considine B. Combined therapy for cancer of the anal canal: a preliminary report. Dis Colon Rectum 1974;17:354–56.

110. Nigro ND, Vaitkevicius VK, Buroker T, Bradley GT, Considine B. Combined therapy for cancer of the anal canal. Dis Colon Rectum 1981;24:73–75.

111. Pigott JP, Williams GB. Primary squamous cell carcinoma of the colorectum: case report and literature review of a rare clinical entity. J Surg Oncol 1987;35:117–19.

112. Cagir B, Nagy MW, Topham A, Rakinic J, Fry RD. Adenosquamous carcinoma of the colon, rectum, and anus. Dis Colon Rectum 1999;42:258–63.

113. Petrelli NJ, Valle AA, Weber TK, Rodriqurez-Bigas M. Adenosquamous carcinoma of the colon and rectum. Dis Colon Rectum 1996;39:1265–68.

114. Cerezo L, Alvarez M, Edwards O, Price G. Adenosquamous carcinoma of the colon. Dis Colon Rectum 1985;28:597–603.

115. Meijer S, Peretz T, Gaynor JJ, Tan C, Hajdu SI, Brennan MF. Primary colorectal sarcoma. Arch Surg 1990;125:1163–68.

116. Feldtman RW, Oram-Smith JC, Teears RJ, Kircher T. Leiomyosarcoma of the rectum: the military experience. Dis Colon Rectum 1981;24:402–403.

117. Khalifa AA, Bong WL, Rao VK, Williams MJ. Leiomyosarcoma of the rectum: report of a case and review of the literature. Dis Colon Rectum 1986;29:427–32.

118. Asbun J, Asbun HJ, Padilla A, Lang A, Bloch J. Leiomyosarcoma of the rectum. Am Surg 1992;58:311–14.

119. Haque S, Dean PJ. Stromal neoplasms of the rectum and anal canal. Hum Pathol 1992;23:762–67.

120. Walsh TH, Mann CV. Smooth muscle neoplasms of the rectal and anal canal. Br J Surg 1984;71:597–99.

121. Luna-Perez P, Rodriguez DF, Lujan L, et al. Colorectal sarcoma: analysis of failure patterns. J Surg Oncol 1998;69: 36–40.

122. Berridge DC. Leimyosarcoma of the rectum: report of two cases illustrating an unusual presentation and the need for repeated biopsy. Dis Colon Rectum 1987;30:721–22.

123. Randleman CD, Wolff BG, Dozois RR, Spencer RJ, Weiland LH, Ilstrup DM. Leiomyosarcoma of the rectum and anus. Int J Colorect Dis 1989;4:91–96.

124. Minsky BD, Cohen AM, Hajdu SI, Nori D. Sphincter preservation in rectal sarcoma. Dis Colon Rectum 1990;33: 319–22.

125. Lorenz HP, Wilson W, Leigh B, Schecter WP. Kaposi's sacoma of the rectum in patients with the acquired immunodeficiency syndrome. Am J Surg 1990;160:681–83.

126. Kaufmann T, Nisce LZ, Coleman M. Case report: Kaposi's sarcoma of the rectum – treatment with radiation therapy. Br J Radiol 1996;69:573–74.

127. Endean ED, Ross CW, Strodel WE. Kaposi's sarcoma appearing as a rectal ulcer. Surgery 1987;101:767–69.

16. Quality of Life and Palliative Care in Rectal Cancer Patients

A. Filiberti, A. Sbanotto and R.A. Audisio

Introduction

This chapter deals with quality of life (QoL) and palliative care in rectal cancer. The impact of rectal cancer and its treatment will be discussed as well as the medical management of the symptoms of advanced rectal cancer. We have combined these two core subjects because it is well known that QoL and palliative care are closely linked. Palliative care is not addressed to alter the underlying disease process; it is a symptomatic therapy administered with the goal of improving QoL in the advanced stages of disease, usually cancer. It does not aim to prolong life. Indeed, QoL assessment is becoming a relevant study endpoint in current rectal cancer clinical trials, particularly in those involving patients with advanced cancer.

Quality of Life: Defining and Measurement Issues

Disease-free and overall survival, tumor response, and toxicity have been the traditional endpoints for evaluating treatment effect in clinical trials of cancer therapy [1–3]. The 1990s have witnessed an increasing interest in including and assessing the impact of the disease and its treatment on patients' QoL. Consideration of QoL has become more common in medical research, particularly in oncology. Today, several very important clinical organizations have a policy to introduce QoL assessment as a standard procedure when evaluating the efficacy of a new trial [1–3]. It is important to stress that, even if QoL is used as if it is an absolute value, no gold standard is available for its assessment. Some authors have questioned the current use of QoL data

because they do not consider that a well-validated questionnaire is satisfactory for clinicians' goal of indicating what patients perceive as QoL [4–7]. QoL is an individual perception; a good QoL as defined by one person may differ dramatically from another. Subjectivity is a really thorny point when measuring QoL. As stated by Cella [6], the severe degree of one side effect (e.g. nausea) in two patients may lead to acute social impairment in one and to little change in another. QoL in these terms may be too highly subjective and seems to be a concept that is very hard to turn into a quantity. A patient's report of his or her QoL often differs from that of the closest relatives and of health professionals. Another critical set of issues pertains to social anthropology. Constructs such as QoL may vary dramatically according to culture or national context [4]. Creating cross-cultural questionnaires could be a solution to the questions concerning cultural variations [5].

In spite of these current critical opinions, a consensus has been reached on which QoL components should be measured. The term QoL refers to a multidimensional concept that encompasses at least four different domains such as physical, emotional, social and cognitive functioning [2,3,6,7]. In addition to evaluating the efficacy of a new cancer therapy, QoL data have been shown to be useful in several clinical areas such as alerting physicians and nurses to patients' common concerns, informing patients of common reactions to their cancer and therapy, aiding patients in medical decision making, developing training programs for health professionals, and designing psychosocial intervention in oncology [8]. QoL is also relevant in the economic appraisal of cancer therapy [9], and may be of prognostic importance for survival [10,11]. A study assessed the relationship between survival, tumor size and quality of life in 50 patients with liver metastases from a colorectal tumor. Results indicated that QoL provides a better survival esti-mate than measurement of tumor size [12]. Furthermore, QoL assessment favors the assump-tion of an ethical attitude directed towards patients. It allows patients to play an active role in medical decision making, and diminishes the risk that health professsionals will make assumptions on behalf of their patients on what would be in the patients' best medical and psychosocial interests [13].

The increasing recognition of the value of the QoL variables for supplementing biological end-points are owing to other reasons. First, the toxicity associated with the newer and very aggressive drugs has generated concerns about patient tolerance [2]. New therapeutic interventions may produce side effects and functional impairment. Moreover, long-term cancer patient survival has been lengthened by the amelioration of cancer therapies. As mentioned above, another reason for the increasing attention devoted to QoL is the prevalence of chronic diseases with the aging of society. The outcome in such diseases cannot be complete cure but QoL [1].

Multidimensional Quality of Life Questionnaires

Many instruments are available to measure QoL. This section summarizes some of the most com-monly used QoL questionnaires in colorectal trials. These are divided into generic instruments, which are designed to measure QoL in a wide range of chronic disease populations (e.g. the Rand 36-item survey 1.0 (SF-36) [14]), to specific cancer measures (e.g. Functional Living Index for Cancer (FLIC) [15], Cancer Rehabilitation Evaluation System (CARES) [16], Rotterdam Symptom Check List (RCSL) [17], Functional Assessment of Cancer Therapy (FACT) [18], and the European Organization for Research on Treatment of Cancer Quality of Life Question-naire C30 (EORTC QLQ-C30 [19])). This designation is rather arbitrary because these instruments could be applied to other diseases.

The SF-36 [14] is a self-administered question-naire that measures eight QoL factors, such as phys-ical functioning, limitations in role functioning due to physical problems, social functioning, physical pain, and overall mental health. Responses range from the dichotomous to a maximum of five choices. The SF-36 is reported to have quite satisfactory reliability and validity. It has been demonstrated to have sensitivity to distinguish patients with or without chronic conditions and has been applied to different diseases.

The FLIC [15] addresses physical symptoms and activity, mood, work and social interaction by using linear analog scales. It is a 22-item scale on which patients indicate the impact of cancer on day-to-day living issues representing the global construct of functional quality of life by using a seven-point Likert scale. It is easy to use, administer and score. Psychometric validation procedures indicate that the FLIC is more highly correlated with measures of physical functioning than emotional distress. Despite these results only a single global score is as yet available. It has been used in several clinical trials for different pathologies in oncology.

The CARES-Short Form (CARES-SF) [16] includes 59 of the total 139 items. It as a self-admin-istered rehabilitation and QoL instrument. The measure yields: a global score reflecting overall QoL; five summary scores reflecting physical, psycho-social, medical interaction, marital and sexual dimensions; and 13 subscales. Adequate test–retest reliability, internal consistency, and concurrent validity with other QoL measures are calculated. Summary scores have replicated global CARES scores, particularly in colorectal and lung cancer. The RSCL [17] includes 30 symptom items with eight scales to assess daily activities. It is useful for assessing physical symptoms, treatment toxicity and psychosocial morbidity. It has highly sensitivity, particularly in advanced cancer patients. It is easily administered, well validated and rapidly scored. The FACT scales [18] were developed by Cella et al. [14] to be used in Eastern Cooperative Oncology Group trials. The 28-item FACT-G is the core version, which is applicable to any oncology patient. At the end of each set of items assessing a QoL dimension, a single item asks patients to rate how much this dimension affects QoL. Reliability, validity and sens-itivity over time of this instrument has been demonstrated.

The EORTC QLQ-C30 [19] is a cross-cultural instrument, available in different European and North American languages and to suit individual cultures. In 1986, the EORTC Study Group on Quality of Life started a research program address-ing the development of instruments for the assess-ment of QoL in international oncology clinical trials. This working group developed the EORTC QLQ-C36, which has been further refined and is known as the QLQ-C30. This is a cancer-specific, structured, self-administered questionnaire. It is copyrighted and contains 30 items, 24 of which aggregate into nine multiple scales, representing various aspects, or dimensions, of QoL: one global scale, five functional scales (physical, role, emo-tional, cognitive and social), and three symptoms scales (fatigue, pain, and nausea and vomiting). The remaining six items are intended to be mono-item scales describing relevant cancer-orientated symptoms such as dyspnea, sleep disturbance, appetite loss, constipation, diarrhea, and the financial impact of the disease. The last part consists of two items addressing global health and QoL on a 7-point Likert scale. This is a multidimensional questionnaire designed for heterogeneous groups of cancer patients. Its psychometric properties have been tested in several studies: non-resectable lung cancer, head and neck cancer, a hetergeneous cancer population, multiple myeloma patients receiving palliative care, and a mixed population of Canadian cancer patients. All of these studies validated the psychometric properties of the QLQ-C30. Recently, these have been tested in a large cohort of Italian cancer long-term survivors. Six hundred and four patients (199 suffering from colorectal cancer and 405 from breast cancer) have been accrued to validate the Italian version of this QoL core questionnaire [20]. An additional EORTC colorectal module, different for colostomy and non-colostomy patients, is also available [21].

All these questionnaires are well validated. Psychometric properties such as validity and reliability have been calculated for each measurement tool. It is important not to forget that, in QoL research, validity can be rated only indirectly because no gold standard exists. Nevertheless, the psychological testing theory describes in detail the criteria for rating reliability and validity of QoL questionnaires [22]. Attention must be given to the choice of measurement instrument. As stated by Osoba, QoL is a multidimensional construct and should be rated through multidimensional questionnaires. Unidimensional instruments are insufficient to measure a very complex construct and should not be called QoL measures [3].

Psychosocial Aspects of Rectal Cancer: A Brief Historical Review

The psychosocial adjustment of ostomy patients has claimed the attention of both clinicians and researchers for many years. Rectal surgery was associated in the past with severe esthetic damage, and bowel and sexual dysfunction. Urological difficulties after rectal surgery have also been identified. Rectal cancer therefore drew the early attention of psycho-oncology's forerunners. In 1947 Dukes reported on a series of 100 patients from the St Mark's Hospital in London [23], where he identified a high level of reactive depression after surgery when patients became aware of the presence of a colostomy. The following year, McLamham and Gilmore [24] reported a series of 40 colostomy patients, more than half of whom had varying degrees of curtail-

ment of their activities, but these were not specified. Ewing [25] identified serious impairments in social life activities in a group of 20 patients. Sutherland [26], a pioneer of psycho-oncology, set up a study in which different features of the lives of patients with stomas were considered, including sexuality, work activity, and family and social adaptation. Of the 29 men and 28 women who were investigated, 14 males were wholly impotent while five had marked impairment of erection. Four of the women had ceased sexual activity, while in two it was severely curtailed after surgery. The women appeared to be resistant to discussion relating to sexual matters. Work activity was also clearly impaired in this sample population and social life was damaged by the anxiety evoked by the loss of sphincter control. Ostomy has been demonstrated historically to be associated also with several psychosocial difficulties specifically related to the fear of spillage and related problems.

Symptoms Associated with Rectal Surgery

Psychosocial studies have generated many data concerning the impact of rectal cancer and its treatment on patients' daily life. The psychological and psychiatric sequelae to either sphincter scarifying or sphincter saving surgical interventions are now well known. Almost all of these countless studies were carried out by means of unstructured instruments that had not been well validated psychometrically. Moreover, they did not assess a formal QoL in all its dimensions but investigated only isolated symptoms. In spite of these methodologic shortcomings, inferences can be drawn from the existing literature that evaluates the psychological impact of rectal cancer and its therapy [27].

To date, a large amount of literature is available that evaluates the impact of amputation surgery for rectal cancer on at least one of the components of overall QoL. Physical well-being such as bowel and urinary functions and sexuality, as well as social life and mood in patients who have undergone ostomy surgery have been extensively investigated [21,27–29].

Sexual and Urological Dysfunction

Studies have compared postoperative psychosocial adjustment in ostomy and non-ostomy patients. Sprangers et al. [30] identified 17 studies taking into account at least one of the overall QoL aspects. Sexuality received most attention in these studies; sexual function is frequently affected in male patients with a stoma. Males who have undergone abdominoperineal resection (APR) report an incidence of neurologic impotency ranging from 62% to 92%, while patients who have had sphincter preservating surgery reported a slightly lower degree of sexual dysfunction, ranging from a 33% to 75% [31]. Ejaculation dysfunction is significantly associated with APR and low anterior resection compared with high anterior resection. In our previous report, 70% of the patients who underwent APR revealed ejaculation difficulties versus 5% of patients who had a high anterior resection. Ejaculation disturbance ranged from 25% to 100% in patients with APR or high anterior resection [28].

In similar fashion, 50–60% female patients with a stoma were reported to have sexual difficulties, whereas sphincter preserving surgery was associated with a lesser degree of sexual problems [32,33]. Sexual problems in women are identified as loss of libido, anorgasmia, dyspareunia, and cessation of intercourse. APR is associated with more sexual problems than anterior resection, but the difference is not statistically significant [28,31].

Our psychosexual evaluation of males treated with a coloanal hand-sewn anastomosis suggests that sexual potency could be preserved by such conservative surgery: 23 patients were investigated [33] and only two of them reported impotency after surgery. Ejaculation disturbance was, conversely, reported by 90% of our patients. Good functional outcome has also been reported by other researchers, especially when a colonic pouch has been performed [34].

Sexuality and urologic function may also be affected by supraradical lymphadenectomy. When this is performed for rectal cancer, and when it includes the excision of the mesenteric and extramesenteric lymphatic drainage, long-term difficulties in the passage of urine seem to affect one-third of these patients and 20% require the long-term use of urinary catheters, while impotence is reported in 76% of patients under the age of 60 years [35].

Urologic problems after rectal surgery have been well investigated. The major urinary symptoms are incontinence, retention and dysuria. As with sexuality, urinary difficulties are more often associated with APR than with anterior resection but again the difference is not statistically significant [28]. Balslev and Harling [36] identified urologic symptoms such as dysuria and incontinence in 29 of 31 patients who underwent APR. According to Camilleri-Brennan and Steele, reactive urologic disorders in patients with a colostomy range from 12% to 93% [28]. Sexual and urologic symptoms usually occur secondary to damage of the pelvic autonomic nerves and the pelvic floor, sustained during dissection of the rectum [28,31].

Bowel Dysfunction

Bowel symptoms have been reported after colorectal surgery [37], and many studies have been carried out to assess sphincter function [28]. The most common symptoms are frequency of bowel motion, urgency and fecal leakage, and incontinence. Some authors also report a prevalence of diarrhea, constipation and flatus [32,37,38]. Williams and Johnston [37] suggest that the frequency of bowel motions is usually greater after APR than anterior resection. Other studies stress that colostomy surgery tends to cause more problems with flatus and bad odor, but the prevalence of diarrhea is similar in both groups [37–39].

Bowel function after a sphincter saving intervention depends on more than one issue. The level of the anastomosis may be relevant. A low colorectal or coloanal anastomosis has been reported to be associated with a higher frequency of defecation, and more fecal leakage and incontinence than a high colorectal anastomosis [28], although some authors disagree [38]. Defecatory problems may be also due to surgical trauma to the anal sphincter and its innervation.

Mood and Social Life

Psychiatric dysfunction such as depression, suicidal thoughts, feelings of stigmatization and low self-esteem were identified as being prevalent among rectal cancer patients [37,38,40]. Wirsching et al. [40] described colostomy being associated with a significant degree of depression, loneliness and hopelessness. They used the Heidelberg Colostomy Questionnaire, which covers the psychological and social aspects of ostomy surgery to compare a cohort of 214 colostomy patients with 110 patients who underwent sphincter saving surgery.

Patients with an ostomy also reported mood disturbances, most commonly depression and anxiety, in 14–50% of cases, while non-ostomy patients were demonstrated to have a lower degree of mood disturbance. [30]. It is interesting to note that stoma patients resumed their working activity in 20–72% of instances, compared with 79–93% of those without an ostomy [30]. Stronger feelings of stigma have been described in colostomy patients than in patients who have undergone anterior resection [39]. They participated less in social events than those who underwent restorative surgery. Similar results have been obtained by others [37].

Colostomy may seriously affect patients' social life. Many feel isolated and want to be so for fear of causing embarrassment to others or being the cause of foul-smelling odors. Concerns about appearance and body change (body image impairment) were also prominent [39]. Furthermore, it has been demonstrated that younger and female patients have more difficulties in coping with a stoma than do older or male patients [38]. Emotional relationships with partners are also impaired in 25–30% of stoma patients; this is less in patients who have under-gone anterior resection, as we have previously demonstrated [31].

Available data suggest that patients' social life may deteriorate after rectal surgery, but results are contradictory. In our previous survey, no difference has been found between APR and anterior resection. Although complications have been demonstrated, some studies suggest that overall QoL may improve after rectal surgery, irrespective of the type of operation performed [41,42].

Psychological functioning has been measured with unstandardized instruments (e.g. a clinical interview) without known validity and reliability. Clinical inferences concerning the psychological functioning of stoma patients are available for the planning of psychosocial rehabiliation projects to favor their adjustment skills.

The studies that compare symptoms experienced after different rectal cancer surgical operations are biased by the methodologic variability, such as in the stage of the disease, the surgical procedures performed and the length of time elapsed since surgery. Nevertheless, the clear message emerging from the literature is that patients with a permanent colostomy suffer more from psychosocial symptoms than those who have undergone restorative surgery.

Quality of Life Studies

In this section, we will discuss only clinical or research reports that contain a formal assessment of QoL. As noted above, the psychological and sexual debilitating consequences of colorectal surgery are well known. Furthermore, QoL researchers have generated information on several clinical matters concerning surgery, chemotherapy, radiotherapy, supportive therapy and palliative care, and have contributed to the identification of the rehabilitation needs of rectal cancer survivors. To review current literature on QoL in rectal cancer patients, a MEDLINE search was carried out for the years 1995–1998. The subject heading "Quality of life" was matched with "Rectal cancer", "Colorectal cancer" and "Colonic cancer". This search identified 97 arti-

cles, most concerning advanced colorectal cancer patients. Only a few contained a formal evaluation of QoL in all its components. In addition, Qol English language reviews were consulted [27–29]. A total of 17 articles in which QoL was a relevant endpoint have been identified.

Chemotherapy

The evaluation of some chemotherapy trials has been supplemented by QoL assessment. Patients with advanced colorectal cancer participated in two international comparative studies of raltitrexed (Tomudex) versus standard 5-fluorouracil (5-FU) plus leucovorin (LV). QoL was assessed by the EORTC QLQ-C30 and the RSCL. Early significant advantageous effects of raltitrexed versus 5-FU plus LV on QoL were observed at week 2, but necessary dose delays and different dose scheduling made it difficult to evaluate QoL [43]. Streit et al. [44] studied 88 patients suffering from advanced colorectal cancer and identified that a 5-day continuous infusion of 5-FU and folinic acid is an effective second line regimen that preserves QoL. Ross et al. [45] studied 200 patients with advanced colorectal cancer, who were randomized to protracted venous infusional (PVI) 5-FU with and without Mitomycin C and studied for tumor response, survival, toxicity and QoL. They concluded that PVI 5-FU plus Mitomycin C resulted in failure-free survival and a response advantage, tolerable toxicity and better QoL when compared with PVI 5-FU alone.

Another study reported QoL measurements in 210 advanced colorectal cancer patients receiving equitoxic regimens of weekly 5-FU plus LV or 5-FU alone in a multicenter, placebo-controlled, double-blind, randomized trial. No significant difference in QoL was detected between the groups, as measured by the FLIC questionnaire, or in any measurements of efficacy or toxicity. A change in the FLIC score was not associated with tumor response or improvement in pain, but a decline in the score was associated with survival [46].

Finally, a randomized trial compared bolus fluorouracil plus LV, continuous flourouracil infusion (FUcont), and FuCont plus cyclophosphamide and Mitomicyn C in 129 eligible patients with measurable advanced colorectal cancer. QoL was assessed by linear analog scales. Similar scores were obtained in the patients receiving bolus fluorouracil plus LV and those receiving Fucont. The authors suggested FUcont as the more suitable schedule in terms of response and survival, and in QoL [47].

Qol measures may also play a role in economic appraisal. QoL data have been useful in the cost-effectiveness analysis of an adjuvant chemotherapy trial in Dukes' B and C patients randomized to surgery plus adjuvant chemotherapy or surgery alone. QoL was measured by the EORTC questionnaire. The data showed that the adjuvant chemotherapy did not affect short-term QoL [48]. The long-term QoL assessment is not yet available.

The Medical Research Council Colorectal Working Party [49] carried out a randomized study to evaluate if interferon-alpha (IFN-α) improved the efficacy of Fura/LV. Two hundred and sixty chemotherapy-naive patients with advanced colorectal cancer were involved. QoL (RSCL questionnaire, Hospital Anxiety and Depression Scale (HADS)) was adversely affected by IFN-α; moreover, at a dose that impaired QoL, IFN-α did not improve the efficacy of FUra/LV. Similar results were obtained by Hill et al. [50], who investigated the effects of adding IFN-α2b to PVI 5-FU. A total of 160 patients with advanced colorectal cancer were randomized. QoL was measured by the EORTC QLQ-C30. There were no toxic deaths and few notable differences in QoL between the groups. IFN did not enhance the palliative benefits of PVI 5-FU.

Laufmann et al. [51] found no difference in QoL scores between patients receiving 5-FU and placebo and those receiving 5-FU and LV. All patients suffered from advanced colorectal cancer. QoL was measured with the RSCL and the HADS. This study suggests that patients with advanced colorectal disease should receive 5-FU at doses sufficient to produce toxicity.

Infusion of the hepatic artery with floxuridine for colorectal liver metastases was found to prolong life and its quality when compared with conventional palliative care and using the RSCL and the HADS [52].

The Nordic trial [53] compared 5-FU alone with a combination of sequential methotrexate, 5-FU and LV (MFL). Forty-four advanced colorectal cancer patients were randomized into two arms, 22 in each group. This study reported that either quality or quantity of life was better in the MFL group.

The Nordic Gastrointestinal Tumour Adjuvant Therapy Group [54] reported an improvement in the overall QoL scores in approximately one-third of patients with symptomatic colorectal cancer who were receiving chemotherapy.

Radiotherapy

The evaluation of the efficacy of radiotherapy has also been supplemented by QoL assessment. Both preoperative and postoperative adjuvant radiotherapy have been shown to reduce the local recurrence rate of rectal cancer. In the long term, both preoperative and postoperative radiotherapy may be associated with different physical side effects such as colovesical and colovaginal fistula, urinary tract infection, and an increased risk of venous thromboembolic arterial disease and intestinal obstruction [55]. However, the North Central Cancer Treatment Group carried out a randomized study to compare adjuvant chemotherapy in association with radiation therapy with adjuvant radiation therapy alone. Two hundred and four rectal cancer patients with poor prognosis were eligible. A Q-TWIST (quality adjusted time without symptoms or toxicity) analysis indicated that the combined therapy conferred significantly greater benefit concerning coping with the toxicity of treatment and the symptoms of overt disease than radiation therapy alone [56].

Padilla et al. [57] assessed QoL by means of the Health Quality of Life Index in a cohort of patients receiving pelvic radiotherapy for colorectal cancer. QoL scores remained at an acceptable level throughout the treatment.

Surgery

To date only a few English language reports are available that formally evaluate the impact on QoL after rectal surgery. However, QoL data contributed to the evaluation of the efficacy of a surgical trial. Forty-five patients suffering from rectal cancer were randomized to straight and colonic J-pouch anastomosis after rectal excision. QoL, measured by the Nottingham Health Profile questionnaire, improved in both groups after surgery. No significant differences were obtained. The trial reflected an advantage of the pouch group regarding bowel function. However, it did not reflect an improved QoL score according to the questionnaire used [58].

Whynes et al. [41], in 1994, evaluated QoL retrospectively in more than 400 patients who underwent rectal surgery. No difference was found between the QoL scores of the 77 colostomy patients and those of patients who underwent restorative surgery. The Health Measurement questionnaire was used. In 1997, Whynes and Neikon [42] carried out a prospective study to evaluate QoL in 49 rectal cancer patients who were undergoing different surgical procedures. Postoperative QoL scores were improved when compared with the preoperative scores for all colorectal surgical procedures. Patients were administered part of the Nottingham Health Profile and part of the RSCL questionnaire before surgery and 3 months after discharge. Such results are amazing because, commonly, patients with a stoma are perceived to have a low QoL due to the several iatrogenic effects associated with a colostomy.

Rehabilitation Needs

Rehabilitation needs were evaluated in 86 patients undergoing surgery for colorectal cancer. Two validated instruments, the QLQ-C30 and the Katz Index of independence in activities of daily living, were used 5–8 months after surgery [59]. When compared with preoperative scores, the patients with colon cancer had significantly less pain and less constipation at follow-up than did those with rectal cancer. The patients with rectal cancer, having undergone preoperative radiotherapy treatment, had significantly lower 95% confidence intervals for physical functioning and role functioning scales at follow-up when compared with their preoperative scores.

Palliative Care in Rectal Cancer Patients

Patients with cancer, especially those undergoing active therapy and those with advanced disease, may experience severe symptom distress, which may influence their social and physical functioning levels, curtail patient–caregiver interaction, and lead to emotional responses of anger, frustration, or depression [60]. Palliative care aims to improve the QoL of patients, drawing attention to the global aspects of patient distress. Most patients with advanced rectal cancer present with liver metastases; this complication accounts for about 50% of the deaths from colorectal cancer [61]. The clinical course of patients with metastatic rectal cancer depends on tumor behavior and responsiveness to therapy, with death usually occurring within 6 months from the diagnosis of inoperable metastases. In a survey of 6451 hospice patients, Christakis and Escarce [62] found that the median survival of those affected by colorectal disease was 31 days, with 15.8% dying within 7 days of admission. The site of the cancer, the patient's age and limitations in functioning do not alter greatly the presentation of symptoms [63–65]. We will therefore discuss mainly data deriving from cancer patients with advanced disease, usually with gastrointestinal malignancy.

Evaluation

Different studies have attempted to investigate the impact of symptoms on the QoL and distress of patients with advanced cancer, most of whom experience a wide range of physical and psychological symptoms (Table 16.1.) Usually, a reported high prevalence of symptoms relates to a poorer QoL.

Table 16.1. Prevalence of main symptoms in patients affected by cancer (modified from Portenoy et al. [73])[a]

Symptom	%
Lack of energy	75
Worrying	70
Feeling Sad	65
Pain	65
Sleepiness	60
Nervous feeling	60
Insomnia	50
Xerostomia	55
Anorexia	45
Nausea	45
Sweating	40
Taste alterations	35
Constipation	35
Cough	30
Weight loss	30
Edema	30
Dyspnea	25
Vomiting	20

[a] This survey included 243 inpatients and outpatients of a cancer center; 2/3 had metastatic disease, 1/3 earlier disease.

Portenoy et al., in a survey including patients with colon cancer, found that the vast majority presented with multiple concurrent symptoms (mean 11.5, range 0–25), and that those with a higher number of symptoms had more significant psychological distress and a worse QoL [66]. In another survey, Holmes et al. found a high correlation between the intensity of symptoms and a deterioration in the activities of daily life [67]. Most symptoms are characterized by rates of prevalence that are higher than 50% [60,64,68–73], although it should be noted that surveys are generally conducted in patients with advanced disease, utilizing different methods of data collection that make very difficult the comparison of results.

Symptom evaluation relies upon an interdisciplinary approach, which should consider as a gold standard the subjective nature of symptoms and the possible interactions among them. A comprehensive assessment of the patient, including data from past medical and cancer histories, the relevant psychosocial issues, the current symptomatology and medication, is especially important.

Several symptom evaluation tools have been described [66,74–78]. Each of these instruments is feasible for the assessment and follow-up of different patient populations. Some of them are com-

Table 16.2. Some important steps in the assessment of symptoms

Cancer history
Past medical history (including drug allergies, abuse and
    addiction)
Current symptoms (including their meaning for the patient)
Psychosocial and financial aspects (with special attention to the
    patient's knowledge of the disease and its extent)
Global distress due to symptoms
QoL evaluation
Current medications
Physical examination
Available imaging and laboratory data
Other diagnostic investigations needed
Consider colleagues' and patient's relatives' opinions

plete but lengthy and require special training before their implementation. Others are simple and suitable for repeated use. Whenever possible, the effects of the symptoms should be discussed within the health care team, identifying the most relevant areas of impact of the illness. If indicated, specific investigations may be required to obtain a full understanding of the pathophysiology of the symptoms. Gonzales et al., in a survey evaluating the impact of a comprehensive approach to cancer pain, found that a previously undiagnosed etiology for pain was present in 64% of the patients, and that 20% of these etiologies were treatable by primary therapy [79]. In the following paragraphs we will discuss briefly some of the most relevant symptoms affecting patients with advanced rectal cancer.

Pain

Pain is a common problem in metastatic cancer. About 75% of all patients with advanced cancer have pain; its incidence depends on the type and stage of the disease. At diagnosis and during the intermediate stages, about 30–45% of all patients experience moderate to severe pain [80]. Curless et al. report a prevalence of abdominal pain in recently diagnosed colorectal cancer of 48–54% [81]. Forty to fifty percent of all cancer patients who are experiencing pain report it as moderate to severe, while another 25% describe it as very severe [82]. Most of these patients present with multiple pains [60]. In three different surveys, covering all stages of colorectal cancer, a range of 32–63% for pain prevalence was identified [83–85]. Cancer pain may be mainly due to:

- Progression of the disease and the related complications
- Diagnostic and therapeutic procedures
- Side effects of treatments

- Musculoskeletal pain, often related to immobility [86]

The assessment of pain is fundamental for its correct management; evaluation should include:

- A detailed history, including the use of analgesics and other drugs, the pain's intensity and its characteristics
- A physical examination
- A brief psychosocial assessment
- Appropriate diagnostic workup; whenever possible, a diagnosis of the prevalent pain syndrome should be made [87]

Pain evaluation is carried out according to the patient's perception of the symptom. Two main classes of evaluation tools are available: intensity scales, such as visual analog scales or numerical and verbal scales [88]; and pain questionnaires, such as the Brief Pain Inventory [89], or the Memorial Pain Assessment Card [90]. It is important to reassess the patient regularly, evaluating the effectiveness of treatment, and the appearance of new pain.

Common Pain Syndromes in Advanced Rectal Cancer

Common pain syndromes may arise from the spreading of the rectal cancer towards the lumbosacral plexus.

Table 16.3. Common pain syndromes in advanced rectal cancer

Cancer history
Lumbosacral plexopathy
Malignant perineal pain
Ureteric obstruction
Chronic intestinal obstruction
Peritoneal carcinomatosis
Phantom anus pain syndrome

In most patients the nerve tissue is involved by direct extension of the neoplasm, less frequently by metastases. Pain is the first symptom reported by patients with lumbosacral plexopathy; in about 20% it may be the only disturbance experienced. It has an aching, pressure-like quality, often associated with paresthesia and episodes of stabbing pain, leg weakness, sensory loss, asymmetric reflexes, distal leg edema, and positive straight legs tests. According to the portion of the plexus involved, pain may be perceived in the back, lower abdomen, iliac crest, or anterolateral thigh. A low plexopathy occurs in about 50% of patients, with buttock and perineal distributions. The posterolateral aspect of the thigh and leg may be affected, often with an L4–S1 distribution. Leg edema, bladder dysfunction and positive straight leg raising tests are frequently found. In about 25% of these patients, pain may present as a panplexopathy, with an L1–S3 involvement. Another clinical picture is radiation-induced plexopathy. It can be difficult to distinguish this from the previous malignant clinical picture; pain is not usually prominent, while progressive weakness and leg edema are more evident. Electromyography can show myokymic discharges, and a computed tomographic scan and a needle biopsy may be necessary to establish a differential diagnosis.

Neoplasms of the colon or rectum are often responsible for perineal pain [91]. This may constitute a signal of alarm in those patients who have been previously treated with antineoplastic therapies, being the sole sign of recurrent disease, even months before instrumental detection [91,92]. It has been proposed that microscopic perineural invasion could cause this clinical picture [93]. The pain is usually of constant quality, often aggravated by sitting or standing, and may be associated with bladder or rectal tenesmus [91].

Intrapelvic tumor spread may result in ureteric compression or obstruction, causing a typical dull chronic discomfort in the flank, sometimes irradiating to the inguinal region. Painless hydronephrosis may develop, and there may be subsequent episodes of urinary tract infection, with added loin pain and dysuria. Another pain syndrome related to rectal cancer is caused by peritoneal carcinomatosis [94], which may cause peritoneal adhesions and inflammation. Ascites is a common occurrence. Pain can be due either to bowel obstruction, when it has a colicky quality, or to abdominal wall involvement. Referred low back pain is not infrequent. Chronic intestinal obstruction is often closely related to peritoneal carcinomatosis; symptoms may depend on a combination of mechanical partial obstruction and ileus. Autonomic neuropathy and drug side effects may also play a role [94]. Colicky pain is very frequent.

Among patients who have undergone APR, about 20% may complain of phantom anus pain [95]. This may appear just days or weeks postoperatively, or later, after months or even years. In the former group it usually has an aching or burning quality. In the latter, the intensity is usually greater and the pain has an aching quality. iI about 25% of patients it is related to cancer recurrence. Sitting on hard surfaces is the most common precipitating factor, with tiredness as a contributing factor [5].

Principles of Pain Management
Drugs constitute the mainstay of cancer pain management [96]. The World Health Organization

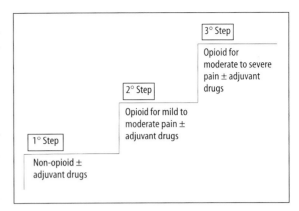

Fig. 16.1. The World Health Organization analgesic ladder (modified from Portenoy et al. [97]).

has proposed a simple and effective method for the control of cancer pain [97], which is based on a sequential (ladder) approach (Fig. 16.1). This has been shown to be useful in about 90% of patients with cancer and in about 75% of cancer patients during the terminal phase of their illness [98]. It can be summarized as:

- By the mouth
- By the clock
- By the ladder
- For the individual
- With attention to detal

Patients with mild to moderate pain should receive non-steroidal anti-inflammatory drugs (NSAIDs), according to the above-mentioned principles. Patients with moderate to severe pain, or those failing to obtain satisfactory relief from the first step, should receive an opioid for mild pain (e.g. codeine), generally combined with an NSAID. If pain control is not satisfactory with this second step, then opioids for more severe pain are indicated (e.g. morphine), again combined with an NSAID. Adjuvant drugs may be added at any step, to treat side effects (e.g. constipation), other concurrent symptoms (e.g. anorexia) or as adjuvant analgesics (e.g. steroids, anticonvulsants). Table 16.4 reports the most common analgesics used.

Syringe drivers and other portable devices have been used extensively in recent years to perform continuous subcutaneous infusions. This is a simple way of administration, characterized by the high bioavailability of drugs, a reduction in side effects, and a more stable 24-hour analgesic profile [99,100]. Similar results can be obtained with intravenous infusions, but there may be practical problems due

Table 16.4. Common analgesics used for cancer pain.

Drug	Schedule of administration	Notes
NSAIDs		
Aspirin	500–1000 mg p.o. 6-hourly	Gastrointestinal disturbances are common; contraindicated in bleeding dyscrasias
Paracetamol	500–1000 mg p.o. 4–6-hourly	Weak anti-inflammatory action; no adverse effects on gastric mucosa and platelets
Ibuprofen	200–1000 mg p.o. 6-hourly	Less gastrolesive than other NSAIDs; Contraindicated in bleeding dyscrasias
Naproxen	200–250 mg p.o. b.i.d.	Gastrointestinal disturbances are less common than with aspirin; contraindicated in bleeding dyscrasias
Opioids for moderate pain		
Codeine	60 mg p.o. 4–6-hourly	Constipation is common; has both analgesic and antitussive action; drowsiness
Oxycodone	5 mg p.o. 4–6-hourly (starting dose)	Drowsiness; constipation; nausea and vomiting; no antitussive activity
Tramadol	50–100 mg p.o. 6–8-hourly (parenteral (i.v./i.m./s.c.) also available)	Drowsiness; constipation; nausea and vomiting; has a codeine-equivalent antitussive action
Opioids for severe pain		
Morphine	5–10 mg p.o. 4-hourly (starting dose in opioid-naive patients); no maximum limiting dose (also available for i.v./i.m./s.c./rectal/nebulized routes)	The most important analgesic for cancer pain; drowsiness (especially at the beginning of therapy); constipation; nausea and vomiting; has antitussive action
Methadone	3–5 mg p.o. 8–12-hourly (in opioid-naive patients) (also available for i.m./i.v. administration)	Drowsiness; constipation. nausea and vomiting; because of its dual phase kinetics, it can accumulate, especially in elderly patients; contraindicated in confused patients; can be an alternative in patients with morphine unresponsiveness
Hydromorphone	1 mg p.o. 4-hourly (in opioid-naive patients) (can also be administered by i.v./i.m./s.c./rectal routes)	As for other opioids: drowsiness; constipation; nausea and vomiting; can be an alternative in patients with morphine unresponsiveness

to the venous access required and limitations on patients' mobility [101]. Subcutaneous infusions of opioids are usually considered to be equianalgesic with intravenous infusions [102]. The indications for continuous opioid infusions are several, namely dysphagia, gastrointestinal tract obstruction, opioid-related side effects due to bolus administration (e.g. nausea and drowsiness), and chronic nausea [99–101]. The correct application of the World Health Organization analgesic ladder achieves good or satisfactory pain control in about 80–90% of patients [97,103,104]. Nerve blocks and neurosurgical techniques may supplement or reduce the use of systemic analgesic drugs. Among the neurolysive techniques used for cancer pain management, the celiac plexus block is probably the most common one used for abdominal pain [96]. This is indicated for pain due to cancer infiltration of upper abdominal viscera, including the pancreas, liver, gall bladder and proximal small bowel [105]. It should be used for those patients who have failed to

obtain satisfactory analgesia by drugs or have suffered intolerable side effects. Various techniques are available, which give similar results [106–109]. Ischia et al., in a randomized trial, compared three different techniques for performing celiac blocks and found no significant differences in the analgesic results [110]. Three studies compared the efficacy of pharmacological treatment with celiac plexus block, showing similar results with both treatments [111–113]. Two of the studies showed a lower consumption of opioids in the celiac plexus block group [111,113]. This technique can be extremely efficacious in relieving true visceral pain, while somatic pain (e.g. pain due to retroperitoneal spread) is less sensitive. Most authors report good immediate analgesia in about 80–90% of patients, but pain relief is usually short lasting, on average for 2–4 weeks. After this period, most treated patients need some form of pharmacological treatment, usually opioids [112,113]. Orthostatic hypotension is the most common side effect of this technique, occurring in about 50–70% of patients [112]. Less frequent side effects include transient diarrhea and pain at the injection site. The most serious side effects are those associated with accidental injection of the neurolytic solution into the subarachnoidal lumbar space or towards the spinal roots [106,114–116].

In selected patients who present with perineal pain, a caudal neurolytic block may be used. Owing to the high degree of bladder and rectal compromise this should be reserved for patients with a colostomy and no bladder function. Hyperbaric phenol in glycerine is usually used to block the rootlets of the lower sacral and coccygeal nerves. Correct positioning of the patient is especially important.

These invasive procedures should be considered only as part of a continuing care program and reserved for a few selected patients.

A relatively common and severe pain syndrome that affects patients with abdominal malignancy is that caused by gastrointestinal obstruction [117]. This occurs in up to 28% of patients with colorectal cancer [118]. The symptoms include continuous and colicky abdominal pain (in about 90% and 75% of patients respectively), and nausea and vomiting (in most patients). Nasogastric suction and intravenous fluids can be useful in preparing patients for surgery, but they are generally contraindicated in those who are terminally ill. Nasogastric suction is uncomfortable and creates a physical barrier between the patient and the family. It can be indicated in the presence of high-level obstruction when pharmacologic measures have failed. A percutaneous venting gastrostomy is indicated in patients with a high-level obstruction and possible longer survival [119,120]. In patients who are in poor general condition or not fit for surgery (e.g. with liver failure, ascites, palpable abdominal masses), different non-operative options are available, among which is a pharmacological approach based on the concurrent use of analgesics, antiemetics and antisecretive drugs [117,121]. The results appear promising with regard to the QoL of these patients [122,123].

Cachexia–Anorexia

Cancer cachexia is a condition characterized by anorexia, progressive wasting and weight loss [124,125], which is more frequent in patients affected by lung, pancreatic and gastric cancer [125]. Current evidence suggests that it is more common in patients with solid tumors compared with hematological malignancies, with breast cancer being the main exception to this rule. However, breast cancer

patients may suffer from cachexia during the advanced stages of the disease [126]. The exact incidence of this syndrome varies widely. Different surveys show that between 50% and 65% of patients affected by stomach, esophagus, pancreas, colonic and rectal cancer have significant weight loss and evidence of malnutrition at the time of operation [127–129]. Curless et al., in a survey of consecutive unselected patients with a histological diagnosis of colorectal carcinoma considered for two age groups (younger or older than 70 years), found a prevalence of 35% and 54% respectively of anorexia, and of 47% and 48% of subjective weight loss [81]. In that study, malaise was reported by 38% of the younger patients and 49% of the older ones. The Eastern Cooperative Oncology Group study by de Wys et al. substantially failed to show a close relationship between the extent of cancer and weight loss [130]. In patients undergoing antineoplastic treatments, chemotherapy plays an important role in weight loss, with a variety of mechanisms involved [131]. Weight loss can be present in about 50% of patients undergoing chemotherapy; this possibly underestimates the size of the problem [130]. Radiotherapy may also cause weight loss, depending on the site treated and the dose administered [132]. Major gastrointestinal surgery usually causes weight loss and a fall in the serum albumin level. Part of the weight loss may be due to neoplasm removal and fluid losses [128,129,132]. Patients admitted to palliative care services or to hospices present a higher incidence of weight loss, ranging from 55% to 80% [69].

A lack of appetite, or anorexia, affects from 30% to 80% of patients with cancer [64,68,69,72,73,126, 133]. It can be influenced by many other symptoms, such as xerostomia, dysphagia, taste alterations, dyspepsia, nausea and constipation [64,68, 70–72,126,134]. Depressed mood also can be significant [135].

The cachexia syndrome has been related to different mechanisms, including tumor necrosis factor and other cytokines (interleukin IL-1, IL-6, IFN-γ), abnormal eicosanoid production, hormones, monocyte/macrophage activation, impairment of lymphocyte function (with inadequate IL-2 production) and leukemia inhibitory factor [136–139]. Despite all these suggested mechanisms, it has been difficult to correlate them clearly with cancer cachexia and weight loss. Todorov et al. isolated, in mice, a circulatory catabolic factor, identified as a proteoglycan of relative molecular mass 24 KDa, which produces cachexia in vivo by inducing muscle catabolism [140]. This substance was also present in the urine of cachectic patients suffering from various neoplasms and a weight loss of more than 1.5 kg per month. It was not detectable in normal subjects or in patients whose weight loss was due to trauma, or was less than 1.3 kg per month.

Limiting the wasting process and improving QoL are the main goals of cachexia–anorexia syndrome management. The assessment of cachectic patients should be simple. A weight loss >10% is usually considered as an index of severe depletion. Ascites, edema or tumor mass can influence such data. Appetite assessment is usually conducted by means of a visual analog scale or a questionnaire [141,142], the latter being more appropriate in patients with advanced cancer because a decrease in appetite affects QoL.

Dietary counseling, and parenteral and enteral nutrition may be suggested as adjuvant treatment in the management of anorexia and cachexia. The nutritional counseling is aimed at improving QoL by giving the patient greater enjoyment from eating. The reader who is interested in a comprehensive review of these issues is referred to the monograph by Bruera and Higginson [143]. The pharmacological treatment of cachexia–anorexia is limited to a few groups of drugs. Corticosteroids, especially prednisolone, methylprednisolone and dexamethasone, have been studied. In one investigation of 116 patients affected by advanced gastrointestinal malignancies and treated with dexamethasone, a significant increase in strength and appetite was noted. In this placebo-controlled trial, the stimulant effect of two different daily dosages of dexamethasone appeared after about 2 weeks of treatment, but subsided after 4 weeks. Side effects were minimal, with one case of gastrointestinal hemorrhage [144]. In a double-blind cross-over trial, Willcox et al. reported a significant improvement in appetite and well-being in patients receiving chemotherapy [145]. In another randomized, double-blinded crossover study, Bruera et al. showed that methylprednisolone twice a day significantly reduced pain and analgesic consumption. In addition, performance status, appetite and food intake improved significantly, although the effect on appetite was no longer present 3 weeks after the beginning of the study [144]. Two other multicenter studies have evaluated the use of intravenous methylprednisolone, with similar results. In the first study, preterminal cancer patients achieved a significant increase in QoL indexes by the administration of methylprednisolone 125 mg daily intravenously, for 8 weeks [146]. In the second study, female patients with terminal cancer received the same daily dosage of methylprednisolone. Their QoL improved significantly for the duration of the study [147]. The exact mechanism of action of corticosteroids in

patients with advanced and terminal disease is not known. Despite this fact, corticosteroids are currently used for a wide range of symptoms [148–150]. Their side effects may be relevant, especially with long-term use. Weakness, delirium, proximal myopathy, osteoporosis and immunodepression have been reported in patients with cancer.

Synthetic progestational agents, mainly medroxyprogesterone acetate (MPA) and, more recently, megestrol acetate (MA), have been shown to improve appetite and possible non-fluid weight gain in advanced cancer, particularly in patients affected by breast cancer [151,152]. MA has been the special object of several controlled studies, which have shown it to have a significantly positive effect on appetite [153–156]. Two of these studies also reported a favorable effect on weight gain in a patient subgroup [154,157]. A multicenter randomized, double-blind trial was carried out to study the effect of oral MPA 500 mg twice daily in patients suffering from advanced non-hormone-sensitive cancer, including digestive cancers [157]. This study failed to show a significant increase in QoL as evaluated by the EORTC QLQ-C30, but it confirmed the mild side effects profile, mainly slight peripheral edema, and the beneficial effect on appetite and weight. The mechanism of action of MA is not clear, but it possibly acts as a steroid, thereby stimulating appetite. Weight gain is mainly due to an increase in body fat stores and only in part to hydration of the fat-free mass [158]. Most studies have reported few side effects for MA.

Other agents used in the treatment of cachexia-anorexia include hydrazine sulfate [159,160], cyproheptadine [161], cannabinoids [162] and pentoxifylline [134]. None of these agents has been shown to be active in cachexia–anorexia. Recently eicosapentaenoic acid has been proposed as a possible useful agent because of its ability to inhibit tumor-produced lipid-mobilizing factor and to reduce protein degradation [163]. Clinical controlled studies are necessary to determine the role of eicosapentaenoic acid in advanced cancer patients.

In summary, the management of cachexia-anorexia should always take account of the possibility of increasing oral intake with frequent, small, tempting high-protein meals, and reducing concurrent symptoms that are potentially interfering with the appetite. The support of a dietitian is desirable. A pharmacological approach is currently based on MA. The correct starting dose is 160 mg/day, titrating upwards according to the patient's response. When life expectancy is short and/or other problems suggest the use of steroids (e.g. for pain or neurologic complications), dexamethasone 4 mg/day can be recommended as a starting medication.

Ascites

Ascites usually represents a poor prognostic sign in patients with cancer [164] and is associated with a median survival of about 8–10 weeks from diagnosis [165]. It is extremely important to balance the best control of this complication with minimal hospitalization and distress. Patients with malignant ascites usually have extensive intra-abdominal disease in the form of hepatic metastases and/or peritoneal seeding. They may complain of abdominal swelling, respiratory discomfort, difficulty with ambulation, and other symptoms of esophageal reflux and squashed stomach syndrome. Pain and other symptoms may coexist. Extensive hepatic metastases may distort the normal hepatic structure, leading to a rise in portal venous pressure. This combines with poor nutritional status and liver damage to reduce albumin synthesis and thereby colloid osmotic pressure. In patients with widespread peritoneal disease, the fluid loss to the peritoneal cavity is due to a combination of lymphatic obstruction and increased peritoneal fluid production [166], as studies conducted with intraperitoneal radiolabelled colloid have shown [167]. Diffusable factors produced by the tumor and alterations in microvasular permeability have also been proposed [165].

The management of ascites is often disappointing. No gold standard exists and current treatments vary from simple oral medication to peritoneovenous shunts. Treatment should begin with paracentesis, which has diagnostic and possible therapeutic value because sometimes the fluid does not reaccumulate. The protein content and bacterial and cytologic evaluation can be checked at this time; a detailed biochemical analysis is rarely required. The measurement of the ratios of lactate dehydrogenase, protein and carcinoembryonic antigen or other tumor markers in serum and ascitic fluid may be helpful when the diagnosis of ascites secondary to cancer is doubtful [164,168, 169]. Other non-neoplastic causes of ascites, such as congestive heart failure, cirrhosis, nephrosis and, less frequently, complications of radiotherapy and chemotherapy, should be ruled out. Paracentesis is considered as a satisfactory way to control tense ascites, especially in patients in whom the fluid reaccumulates at a relatively slow rate. This approach is much more debatable when the general condition of the patient is poor and protein depletion induced by the procedure causes further debilitation. Under these conditions, the major criterion is to perform the paracentesis only if a substantial symptomatic advantage is to be gained (e.g. relief from secondary dyspnea or abdominal discomfort and pain).

Among the medications used, diuretic treatment is usually indicated, even if it is not possible to predict which patients will respond and which will not. Commonly, good or partial responses are seen in about 40–50% of these patients [170,171]. Spironolactone (100–400 mg/day p.o.) and/or furosemide (40 mg q.a.m. p.o.), increased gradually, are the most widely used drugs. Water and salt restriction, when used in the treatment of cirrhotic ascites, causes unnecessary discomfort and is not indicated, especially in dying patients. Intracavitary radiocolloids, mainly ^{32}P, are now rarely used. Response rates vary between 30% and 50%, but most studies are incomplete and do not include QoL evaluation. Moreover, the onset of the therapeutic effect is slow, usually taking 2–3 months to reach the maximum [172]. The intracavitary injection of irritating agents such as bleomycin, and *Corynebacterium parvum* to induce obliteration of the space between the visceral and parietal peritoneum has been used, with 40–60% of partial or complete results [173,174]. The intraperitoneal instillation of chemotherapeutic agents may have a role, especially in ascites caused by gastrointestinal and ovarian carcinomatosis; it can be combined with systemic antineoplastic agents. Commonly used drugs include cisplatin, 5-FU, bleomycin and doxorubicin. These agents produce partial or complete results in 45–60% of patients [175–178]. Their administration through a catheter is usually warranted, which may be complicated by malfunction and sepsis, requiring strict selection and follow-up of suitable patients [179,180]. In patients who are in good general condition and have rapidly recurring ascites and a longer life expectancy, the implantation of a peritoneovenous shunt may be considered. This technique involves implanting a shunt with a one-way valve, allowing the collection of ascitic fluid from the abdominal cavity into the intravascular space, usually the superior vena cava or the right atrium. Shunts were first introduced for the management of refractory ascites in patients with either cirrhosis or malignancy [181]. Currently, two main types of shunt are in use: the LeVeen and the Denver shunt, both of which are equally efficient [182,183]. Some relative contraindications to their use must be mentioned. A serum bilirubin level higher than 3 mg/dl in the presence of hepatic metastases increases the risk of disseminated intravascular coagulation in the postoperative period. Patients suffering from congestive heart failure may not be able to tolerate the increased preload resulting from a peritoneovenous shunt [184]. If the ascitic fluid is infected, a shunt clearly cannot be inserted. Problems can arise also if the ascitic fluid has a high protein or cell content (e.g. blood cells); this can produce clots that will block the shunt. From a general point of view, patients with a short life expectancy (e.g. less than 1–2 months) are not candidates for this procedure. Long-term rates of ascites control by means of a shunt average about 70%, comparing favorably with intracavitary radiocolloids and chemotherapy. The most frequent complication, arising in about 10–40% of patients, is shunt occlusion, usually due to tube kinking, malpositioning or clot formation [184–186]. However, because of complications and the need for admission, this technique should be reserved for a few selected patients.

Nausea and Vomiting

This section will deal mainly with chronic nausea. By this term we refer to a nausea existing for longer than 2–4 weeks in the absence of more defined causes such as radiotherapy, chemotherapy or post-surgical syndromes.

Nausea and vomiting affects 20–70% of patients with advanced or terminal cancer [60,71,187,188]. The prevalence of nausea and vomiting during the last 6 weeks of illness is reported to be around 40% [187]. Dunlop studied the perception of gastrointestinal symptoms in a group of 50 patients with advanced cancer, in whom nausea was ranked as the eighth most frequent and distressing symptom, especially in female patients [126]. Owing to the involvement of several pathways and neurotransmitters, a range of antiemetics with different mechanisms and sites of action may be necessary. While nausea and vomiting due to chemotherapy and radiotherapy are generally related to a simple model of nausea, patients with advanced cancer often present a more complex clinical picture, where several factors may be involved. These will be briefly discussed.

A possible cause of chronic nausea is autonomic failure, originally described in patients affected by diabetes, chronic renal disease or neurologic disorders [189,190]. Some of the common clinical characteristics of diabetic autonomic neuropathy, such as nausea, anorexia, early satiety and cardiovascular dysfunction, are also present in advanced cancer patients, especially those with a poorer performance status [191]. A possible multifactorial etiology may be involved for autonomic failure in advanced cancer. Malnutrition itself may play a relevant role [190]. Other causes are radiation damage, chemotherapeutic agents (e.g. vinca alkaloids) direct tumor involvement and human immunodeficiency virus infection [192,193].

Another common cause of chronic nausea is the use of opioids. Usually, opioid-related nausea is of short duration and sensitive to most antiemetics.

Some patients, especially those receiving high doses of opioids, may develop severe nausea, accompanied by abdominal distension and severe constipation. Nausea may correlate with changes in body position, such as in vestibular disturbances. Opioid-induced constipation, delayed gastric emptying and direct stimulation of the chemoreceptor trigger zone (CTZ), can be involved.

In the presence of renal insufficiency in particular [194], metabolite accumulation may explain chronic nausea that develops in patients receiving long-term opioids. The evaluation of nausea and vomiting should take into account other symptoms such as pain, dyspnea and psychologic factors.

Some possible common causes of chronic nausea to be checked are:

- Opioid therapy
- Iatrogenic damage (e.g. chemotherapy or radiotherapy)
- Constipation
- Bowel obstruction
- Metabolic imbalance
- Drugs other than opioids and antineoplastic agents (e.g. digitalis)
- Gastritis or peptic ulcer
- Autonomic failure
- Raised intracranial pressure

Whenever possible, underlying causes should be corrected. Metabolic changes, such as hypercalcemia, drug-related side effects (e.g. opioids) or simple constipation are common causes of chronic nausea, and general measures like regular follow-up of the patient and good bowel care are most important. The pharmacologic treatment of chronic nausea relies upon a "step by step" approach. The initial treatment is made with prokinetic drugs, namely metoclopramide, domperidone and cisapride. Various trials have studied the efficacy of prokinetics in gastroparesis [195]. In addition to its peripheral antiemetic properties, metoclopramide presents a central antiemetic action due to antagonism of D2 receptors in the CTZ. Domperidone has mainly a peripheral activity because it does not cross the blood–brain barrier; it causes a reduction in central extrapyramidal side effects. The action of cisapride is characterized by a reduction in gastroduodenal reflux and by an increase in intestinal peristalsis. Because they stimulate peristalsis, prokinetic agents are usually contraindicated in the presence of gastrointestinal obstruction as they may increase pain and vomiting. Neuroleptics, such as the phenothiazines and butyrophenones, are another group of antiemetic agents. They can produce sedation, which limits their use. Haloperidol is the most widely used of these agents, especially for chronic nausea related to opioids, where its main central mechanism of action on the CTZ is particularly useful. Occasionally, adjuvant drugs may be necessary. By the term, adjuvant drug, we refer to a miscellaneous group of pharmacologic agents, such as corticosteroids, anticonvulsants, antidepressants, neuroleptics and others. Corticosteroids are among the most widely used, owing to their non-specific antiemetic effect. In addition, they may exert a direct anti-inflammatory effect, which can be extremely useful in conditions characterized by edema (e.g. in brain metastases or during radiotherapy or chemotherapy). Octreotide, a synthetic analog of somatostatin, may have a role in gastrointestinal obstruction and subobstructive conditions, where it reduces the amount of gastrointestinal secretion and increases fluid reabsorption [121].

Pereira and Bruera have proposed a therapeutic ladder for the management of chronic nausea [195]. The first step involves the use of oral or subcutaneous metoclopramide (10 mg), administered every 4 hours because of its short half-life. The second step involves the addition of oral or parenteral dexamethasone because of the synergistic effect of steroids and metoclopramide [196]. If the second step fails after 2–3 days of treatment, step 3 relies upon the administration of higher doses [60–120 mg daily) of metoclopramide by subcutaneous continuous infusion, plus dexamethasone [197]. Step 4 involves the use of other antiemetics such as haloperidol and cisapride, to be used when metoclopramide is contraindicated or if the previous steps have failed to control the nausea. The new 5-HT$_3$ antagonists, such as ondansetron and granisetron, may be indicated when the standard antiemetics have failed [198].

Dyspnea

Dyspnea can be defined as an unpleasant awareness of a difficulty in breathing. It is important to keep in mind such a definition because the subjectivity of the symptom is especially important in breathlessness. It can affect about 50% of terminally ill cancer patients, about 70% with lung cancer [199,200]. Its incidence increases during the last weeks of life [201]. Different causes may be involved, relating to cancer and to cancer therapies, but even pre-existing conditions, such as chronic obstructive pulmonary disease may be relevant. It is important to establish whether or not the causes of this symptom are reversible [202]. In the first instance, specific measures such as radiotherapy, antibiotics, or parancen-

tesis may be used. Frequently, the causes are not reversible, as in advanced or terminal disease. It is then important to modify the patient's general situation (e.g. by correct positioning in the bed and/or the use of oxygen) and start respiratory sedatives, aiming to reducing the perception of breathlessness. Morphine is the main respiratory sedative used. It has respiratory and analgesic properties, which are especially useful in those patients with concomitant pain (e.g. due to a pathological fracture of ribs), and it can be administered by different routes [203,204]. Starting doses are usually 20–40 mg daily by mouth. In more acute situations, intravenous or subcutaneous routes are best. If the patient is already on morphine for pain, it may be sufficient to increase the current dose by 50%. If the symptom is characterized by acute attacks, the use of nebulized morphine may be tried, when 20 mg of morphine sulfate in 10 ml of saline solution are administered by a nebulizer in air or oxygen. The rate of absorption of the drug is negligible and the action is mainly local [205,206]. Oxygen administered by nasal prongs or a mask is not useful in many cancer patients; a trial of therapy is the best way to determine any benefit [207]. When it is helpful, it can be given for 5–10 minutes before exertion. Respiratory panic attacks benefit from regular oral morphine. Additional measures are regular lorazepam or diazepam.

Conclusions

The psychologic and psychiatric literature identified outlined the prominent adverse reactions to ostomy surgery for rectal cancer. Surgery has been moving towards more conservative procedures to avoid patients having to live with a stoma. As we have illustrated above, conservative surgery for rectal cancer may be associated with less sexual and relationship difficulties.

QoL data revealed their importance when evaluating the efficacy of a new trial, so it is mandatory to make a correct assessment of this multidimensional construct, particularly in the realm of clinical trials. The science of QoL has evolved during the 1990s, and a great deal of effort has been devoted to developing QoL questionnares that have a satisfactory degree of reliability and validity. There are still many challenges that need to be faced and resolved, such as how to distinguish the effect of the disease on QoL from the effects of the treatment. However, how correct is it to measure an individual construct by means of a general and structured instrument? Finally, how should weighting be assigned to QoL when evaluating the efficacy or cost-effectiveness of a trial [3]? Biases may be introduced because of different dosage schedules or different timings of treatment administration, which make it difficult to compare QoL between two or more treatments, as we have noted above [31]. More prospective studies are needed for rectal cancer to assess the QoL changes over time (i.e. before and after surgery) in a large sample of patients. Studies that have so far assessed QoL have shown an improvement after surgery, irrespective of the type of operation performed.

Special procedures should be introduced to ensure compliance and quality control of QoL data. The timing of the administration of QoL questionnaires should be the same for all arms of a study. The Southwest Oncology Study Group suggested the administration of questionnaires for at least a minimum of three times, such as at baseline, during the therapy and at the end of the treatment [2]. Adequate study design should include the following methodological issues. It is mandatory to provide: a clear rationale for the study; satisfactory administration procedures; a well-trained data manger; and a protocol document [208].

An updated solution concerning the best instrument for the collection of QoL data has been introduced by the EORTC Quality of Life Study Group and the Eastern Cooperative Onology Group. This relates to the utilization of a modular approach, which requires the combined use of a core questionnaire with the addition of a site-specific module to address symptoms that are either not included or are included in only general terms by the core questionnaire. A complementary colorectal module has been developed by these study groups. A validated and reliable scoring scale was developed and popularised by Jorge and Wexner [209] in 1993. This scale is applicable to patients with fecal incontinence as well as to those who have undergone rectal surgery. Several other instruments with the same aim have been proposed.

QoL assessment has contributed to the evaluation of the efficacy of several clinical trials spanning different therapy domains as well as to cost-effectiveness analysis. Furthermore, QoL data would be very useful in the medical decision-making process in rectal cancer [210]. Patients' survival rate is not the sole factor influencing treatment choice. The number of patients who are willing to trade off the probability of survival (quantity of life) to improve their chance of maintaining a higher QoL will undoubtedly increase in the future. QoL issues have thus become a part of the physician's armamentarium. Moreover, several ethical committees and distinguished scientific institutions demand that all new study proposals must contain information about the intention to assess QoL measurements in new clinical trials.

Finally, the approach towards patients who are in the advanced stages of disease should be global and multidisciplinary. The control of symptoms is not sufficient in itself because they are only part (if an important part) of the management and care of patients and their families. Symptom evaluation should be part of everyday clinical activity and of clinical trials, especially Phase III trials, in which new cancer treatments are compared with standard therapies and the possible benefits should at least be symptomatic.

References

1. Quality of life in clinical trials [editorial]. Lancet 1994;346: 1–2.
2. Moinpour CM. Measuring quality of life: an emerging science. Semin Oncol 1994;21:48–60.
3. Osoba D. Lessons learned from measuring health-related quality of life in oncology. J Clin Oncol 1994;12:608–16.
4. Kleinman A, Eisenberg L, Good B. Culture, illness and care: clinical lessons from anthropologic and cross-cultural research. Ann Intern Med 1978;88:251–58.
5. Bullinger M, Power M, Aaronson NK. Creating and evaluating cross-cultural instruments. In: Spilker B, editor. Quality of life and pharmacoeconomics in clinical trials. Philadelphia, PA: Lippincott-Raven, 1996:659–68.
6. Cella D. Quality of life: concepts and definition. J Pain Symptom Manage 1994;9:186–92.
7. Testa M, Simonson D. Assessments of quality of life outcomes. N Engl J Med 1996;334:835–39.
8. Meyerowitz BE. Quality of life in breast cancer patients: the contribution of data to the care of patients. Eur J Cancer 1993;29A Suppl 1:S59–S62.
9. Uyl-de Groot CA, Rutten FF, Bonsel GJ. Measurement and valuation of quality of life in economic appraisal of cancer treatment. Eur J Cancer 1994;30A:111–17.
10. Ganz PA, Lee JJ, Siau J. Quality of life assessment. An independent prognostic variable for survival in lung cancer. Cancer 1991;67:3131–35.
11. Coates A, Gebski V, Signorini D, et al. Prognostic value of quality-of-life scores during chemotherapy for advanced breast cancer. Australian New Zealand Breast Cancer Trials Group. J Clin Oncol 1992;10:1833–38.
12. Earlam S, Glover C. Frody C, et al. Relation between tumor size, quality of life, and survival in patients with colorectal metastases. J Clin Oncol 1996;14:171–75.
13. Singer PA, Tasch ES, Stacking C, et al. Sex and survival: trade-offs between quality of life and quantity of life. J Clin Oncol 1991;9:328–34.
14. Ware J, Sherbourne CD. The MOS 36-item short form for health survey. Med Care 1992;30:473–83.
15. Shipper H, Clinch J, McMurray J, Levitt M. Measuring the quality of life of cancer patients. The Functional Living Index – Cancer. Development and validation. J Clin Oncol 1984;2:472–83.
16. Ganz PA, Schag CA, Lee JJ, Sim MS. The CARES: a generic measure of health-related quality of life for patients with cancer. Qual Life Res 1992;1:19–29.
17. deHaes JC, Raatgever JW, van der Burg ME, et al. Evaluation of the quality of life of patients with advanced ovarian cancer treated with combination chemotherapy. Qual Life Res 1987;1:19–29.

18. Cella D, Tulsky DS, Gray G, et al. The Functional Assessment of Cancer Therapy (FACT) scale: development and validation of the general measure. J Clin Oncol 1993;11:570–79.

19. Aaronson NK, Ahmedzai S, Bergman B, et al. The European Organization for Research and Treatment of Cancer QLQ-C30: a quality-of-life instrument for use in international clinical trials in oncology. J Natl Cancer Inst 1993;85:365–76.

20. Apolone G, Filiberti A, Cifani R, Ruggiata R, Mosconi P. The evaluation of the EORTC QLQ-C30 questionnaire: a comparison with the SF-36 Health Survey in a cohort of Italian lung survival cancer patients. Ann Oncol 1997;9:549–57.

21. Sprangers M, Taal BG, Aaronson N, et al. Quality of life in colorectal cancer. Dis Colon Rectum 1995;38:361–69.

22. Ware J. Standards for validating health measures: definition and content. J Chronic Dis 1987;40:473–80.

23. Dukes CE. Management of a permanent colostomy: study of 100 patients at home. Lancet 1947;ii:12–14.

24. McLamham S, Gilmore WE. Colostomies: a follow up study of functional results. South Med J 1947;408–12.

25. Ewing MR. Colostomy: the patient's point of view. Postgrad Med J 1950;26:584–89.

26. Sutherland AM, Orbach CE, Dyk RB, Bard M. Adaptation to the dry colostomy: preliminary report and summary of findings. Cancer 1952;5:857–72.

27. Sprangers M, de Velde A, Aaronson NK. Quality of life following surgery for colorectal cancer: a literature review. Psychooncology 1993;2:247–59.

28. Camilleri-Brennan J, Steele RJ. Quality of life after treatment for rectal cancer. Br J Surg 1998;85:1036–43.

29. Audisio RA, Filiberti A, Geraghty J, et al. Personalized surgery for rectal tumours: the patient's opinion counts. Support Care Cancer 1996;5:17–21.

30. Sprangers MA, Taal BG, Aaronson NK, Te VA. Quality of life in colorectal cancer. Stoma vs. nonstoma patients. Dis Colon Rectum 1995;38:361–69.

31. LaMonica G, Audisio RA, Tamburini M, Filiberti A, Ventafridda V. Incidence of sexual dysfunction in male patients treated surgically for rectal malignancy. Dis Colon Rectum 1985;28:937–40.

32. Devlin HB, Plant JA, Griffin M. Aftermath of surgery for anorectal cancer. BMJ 1971;3:413–18.

33. Filiberti A, Audisio RA, Gangeri L, et al. Prevalence of sexual dysfunction in male cancer patients treated with rectal excision and coloanal anastomosis. Eur J Surg Oncol 1994;20:43–46.

34. Ortiz H, DeMiguel M, Armendariz P, et al. Coloanal anastomosis: are functional results better with a pouch? Dis Colon Rectum 1995;38:375–77.

35. Hojo K. Extended wide lymphadenectomy and preservation of pelvic autonomic nerves in rectal cancer surgery. G Chir 1989;10:149–53.

36. Balslev I, Harling H. Sexual dysfunction following operation for carcinoma of the rectum. Dis Colon Rectum 1983;26:785–88.

37. Williams NS, Johnston D. The quality of life after rectal excision for low rectal cancer. Br J Surg 1983;70:460–62.

38. Frigell A, Ottander M. Stenbeck H. Quality of life of patients treated with abdominoperineal resection or anterior resection for rectal carcinoma. Ann Chir Gynaecol 1990;79:26–30.

39. McDonald LD, Anderson HR. The health of rectal cancer patients in the community. Eur J Surg Oncol 1985;11:235–41.

40. Wirsching M, Druner HU, Hermann G. Result of psychosocial adjustment to long-term colostomy. Br J Surg 1975;70:60–62.

41. Whynes DK, Neilson AR, Robinson MH, Hardcastle JD. Colorectal cancer screening and quality of life. Qual Life Res 1994;3:191–98.

42. Whynes DK, Neilson AR. Symptoms before and after surgery for colorectal cancer. Qual Life Res 1997;6:61–66.

43. Anderson H, Palmer MK. Measuring quality of life: impact of chemotherapy for advanced colorectal cancer. Experience from two recent large Phase III trials. Br J Cancer 1998;77 Suppl 2:9–14.

44. Streit M, Jaende U, Stremetzne G, et al. Five-day continuous infusion of 5-fluorouracil and pulsed folinic acid in patients with metastatic colorectal carcinoma: an effective regimen. Ann Oncol 1997;8:163–65.

45. Ross P, Norman A, Cunningham D, et al. A prospective randomized trial of protracted venous infusion 5-fluorouracil with or without mitomycin C in advanced colorectal cancer. Ann Oncol 1997;8:995–1001.

46. Sullivan BA, McKinnis R, Laufman LR. Quality of life in patients with metastatic colorectal cancer receiving chemotherapy: a randomized, double-blind trial comparing 5-FU versus 5-FU with leucovorin. Pharmacotherapy 1995;15:600–607.

47. Caudry M, Bonnel C, Floquet A, et al. A randomized study of bolus fluorouracil plus folinic acid versus 21-day fluorouracil infusion alone or in association with cyclophosphamide and mytomicin C in advanced colorectal carcinoma. J Clin Oncol 1995;18:118–25.

48. Norum J, Vonen B, Olsen JA, Revhaug A. Adjuvant chemotherapy (5-fluorouracil and levamisole) in Dukes' B and C colorectal carcinoma. A cost effectiveness analysis. Ann Oncol 1997;8:65–70.

49. Seymour MT, Slevin ML, Kerr DJ, et al. Randomized trial assessing the addition of interferon alpha-2a to fluorouracil and leucovorin in advanced colorectal cancer. Colorectal Cancer Working Party of the United Kingdom Medical Research Council. J Clin Oncol 1996;14:2280–88.

50. Hill M, Norman A, Cunningham D, et al. Impact of protracted venous infusion fluorouracil with or without interferon alfa-2b on tumor response, survival, and quality of life in advanced colorectal cancer. J Clin Oncol 1995;13:2317–23.

51. Laufman LR, Bukowski RM, Collier MA, et al. A randomized, double-blind trial of fluorouracil plus placebo versus fluorouracil plus oral leucovorin in patients with metastatic colorectal cancer. J Clin Oncol 1993;11:1888–93.

52. Allen-Mersh TG, Earlam S, Fordy C, Abrams K, Houghton J. Quality of life and survival with continuous hepatic-artery floxuridine infusion for colorectal liver metastases. Lancet 1994;334:1255–60.

53. Glimelius B, Hoffman K, Olafsdottir M, Pahlman L, Sjoden PO, Wennberg A. Quality of life during cytostatic therapy for advanced symptomatic colorectal carcinoma: a randomized comparison of two regimens. Eur J Cancer Clin Oncol 1989;25:829–35.

54. Glimelius B, Hoffman K, Graf W, Pahlman L, Sjoden PO. Quality of life during chemotherapy in patients with symptomatic advanced colorectal cancer. The Nordic Gastrointestinal Tumor Adjuvant Therapy Group. Cancer 1994;73:556–62.

55. Mak AC, Rich TA, Schultheiss TE, Kavanagh B, Ota DM, Romsdahl MM. Late complications of postoperative radiation therapy for cancer of the rectum and rectosigmoid. Int J Radiat Oncol Biol Phys 1994;28:597–603.

56. Gelber RD, Goldhirsch A, Cole BF, Wieand HS, Schroeder G, Krook JE. A quality-adjusted time without symptoms or toxicity (Q-TWIST) analysis of adjuvant radiation therapy and chemotherapy for resectable rectal cancer. J Natl Cancer Inst 1996;88:1039–45.

57. Padilla GV, Grant MM, Lipsett J, Anderson PR, Rhiner M, Bogen C. Health quality of life and colorectal cancer. Cancer 1992;70:1450–56.

58. Hallbrook O, Hass U, Wanstrom A, Sjodahl R. Quality of life measurement after rectal excision for cancer. Comparison

between straight and colonic J-pouch anastomosis. Scand J Gastroenterol 1997;32:490–93.

59. Ulander K, Jeppsson B, Grahn G. Quality of life and independence in activities of daily living preoperatively and at follow-up in patients with colorectal cancer. Support Care Cancer 1997;5:402–409.

60. Coyle N, Adelhardt J, Foley KM, Portenoy RK. Character of terminal illness in the advanced cancer patient: pain and other symptoms during the last four weeks of life. J Pain Symptom Manage 1990;5:83–93.

61. Pickren J, Tsukada Y, Lane W. Liver metastasis: analysis of autopsy data. In: Weiss L, Gilbert HA, editors. Liver metastases. Boston, MA: GK Hall, 1982:2–18.

62. Christakis N, Escarce JJ. Survival of Medicare patients after enrollment in hospice programs. N Engl J Med 1996;335:172–78.

63. Given CW, Given B, Stommel M. The impact of age, treatment, and symptoms on the physical and mental health of cancer patients. A longitudinal perspective. Cancer 1994;74:2128–38.

64. Reuben DB, Mor V, Hiris J. Clinical symptoms and length of survival in patients with terminal cancer. Arch Intern Med 1998;148:1586–91.

65. Mor V, Masterson Allen S, Houts PS, Siegel K. The changing needs of patients with cancer at home. Cancer 1992;69:829–38.

66. Portenoy RK, Thaler HT, Kornblith AB, et al. The Memorial Symptom Assessment Scale: an instrument for the evaluation of symptom prevalence, characteristics and distress. Eur J Cancer 1994;30A:1326–36.

67. Holmes S, Dickerson J. The quality of life: design and evaluation of a self-assessment instrument for use with cancer patients. Int J Nurs Stud 1987;24:15–24.

68. Brescia F, Adler D, Gray G, Ryan M, Cimino J, Mamtani R. Hospitalized advanced cancer patients: a profile. J Pain Symptom Manage 1990;5:221–27.

69. Curtis EB, Krech R, Walsh TD. Common symptoms in patients with advanced cancer. J Palliat Care 1991;7:25–29.

70. Ventafridda V, DeConno F, Ripamonti C, Gamba A, Tamburini M. Quality-of-life assessment during a palliative care programme. Ann Oncol 1990;1:415–20.

71. Fainsinger R, Miller MJ, Bruera E, Hanson J, MacEachern T. Symptom control during the last week of life on a palliative care unit. J Palliat Care 1991;7:5–11.

72. Grosvenor M, Bulcavage L, Chlebowsky RT. Symptoms potentially influencing weight loss in a cancer population. Correlation with primary site, nutritional status, and chemotherapy administration. Cancer 1989;63:330–34.

73. Portenoy RK, Thaler HT, Kornblith AB, et al. Symptom prevalence, characteristics and distress in a cancer population. Qual Life Res 1994;3:183–89.

74. Bruera E, Kuehn N, Miller MJ, Selmser P, MacMillan K. The Edmonton Symptom Assessment System (ESAS): a simple method for the assessment of palliative care patients. J Palliat Care 1991;7:6–9.

75. Melzack R. The McGill Pain Questionnaire: major properties and scoring methods. Pain 1975;1:277–99.

76. Price DD, McGrath P, Rafti A, et al. The validation of a visual analog scale or a ratio pain scale. Pain 1983;17:45–46.

77. Mahler D, Weinberg D, Wells C, et al. The measurement of dyspnoea. Chest 1984;85:751–58.

78. Folstein MF, Folstein SE, McHugh PR. "Mini-mental State". A practical method for grading the cognitive state of patients for the clinician. J Psychiatr Res 1975;12:189–98.

79. Gonzales GR, Elliott KJ, Portenoy RK, Foley KM. The impact of a comprehensive evaluation in the management of cancer pain. Pain 1991;47:141–44.

80. Daut RL, Cleeland CS. The prevalence and severity of pain in cancer. Cancer 1982;50:1913–18.

81. Curless R, French J, Williams GV, James OF. Comparison of gastrointestinal symptoms in colorectal carcinoma patients and community controls with respect to age. Gut 1994;35:1267–70.

82. Bonica JJ. Cancer pain. In: Bonica JJ, editor. The management of pain. Philadelphia, PA: Lea and Febiger, 1990:400–60.

83. Basset ML, Goulston KJ. Colorectal cancer – a study of 230 patients. Med J Aust 1979;1:589–92.

84. Pheils MT, Barnett JE, Newland RC, Macpherson JG. Colorectal carcinoma: a prospective clinicopathological study. Med J Aust 1976;1:17–21.

85. Najem AZ, Hennessey M, Malfitan RC, Cheung NK, Hobson RW. Colon and rectal carcinoma: clinical experience. Am Surg 1977;43:583–88.

86. Tiniakos DG, Lee JA, Burt AD. Innervation of the liver: morphology and function. Liver 1996;16:151–60.

87. Foley KM. Cancer pain syndromes. J Pain Symptom Manage 1987;2:S13–S17.

88. Jensen MP, Karoly P, Braver S. The measurement of clinical pain intensity: a comparison of six methods. Pain 1986 Oct;27(1):117–26.

89. Daut RL, Cleeland CS, Flanery RC. Development of the Wisconsin Brief Pain Questionnaire to assess pain in cancer and other diseases. Pain 1983 Oct;17(2):197–210.

90. Fishman B, Pasternak S, Wallenstein SL, Houde RW, Holland JC, Foley KM. The Memorial Pain Assessment Card. A valid instrument for the evaluation of cancer pain. Cancer 1987;60:1151–58.

91. Stillman MJ. Diagnosis and management, with particular attention to perineal pain of cancer. In: Foley KM, Bonica JJ, Ventafridda V, editors. Proceedings of the Second International Congress on Cancer Pain;1988 July 14–17; Rye (NY). New York: Raven Press, 1990;359–77.

92. Radbruch L, Zech D, Grond S, Meuser T, Lehmann KA. Perineal pain and rectal cancer – prevalence in local recurrence. Med Klin 1991;86:180–85,228.

93. Seefeld PH, Bargen JA. The spread of carcinoma of the rectum: invasion of lymphatics, veins and nerves. Ann Surg 1943;118:76–90.

94. Ventafridda V, Ripamonti C, Caraceni A, Spoldi E, Messina L, DeConno F. The management of inoperable gastrointestinal obstruction in terminal cancer patients. Tumori 1990;76:389–93.

95. Boas RA, Schug SA, Acland RH. Perineal pain after rectal amputation: a 5-year follow up. Pain 1993;52:67–70.

96. Ventafridda V, Caraceni A, Sbanotto A. Cancer pain management. Pain Rev 1996;3:153–79.

97. World Health Organization. Cancer pain relief. Geneva: WHO, 1986.

98. Grond S, Zech D, Schug SA, Lynch J, Lehmann KA. Validation of World Health Organization guidelines for cancer pain relief during the last days and hours of life. J Pain Symptom Manage 1991;6:411–22.

99. Ventafridda V, Spoldi E, Caraceni A, Tamburini M. The importance of subcutaneous morphine administration for cancer pain control. Pain Clinic 1986;1:47–55.

100. Bruera E, Brenneis C, Michaus M, et al. Use of the subcutaneous route for the administration of narcotics in patients with cancer pain. Cancer 1988;62:407–11.

101. Portenoy RK, Moulin DE, Rogers A, Inturrisi CE, Foley KM. IV infusion of opioids for cancer pain: clinical review and guidelines for use. Cancer Treat Rep 1986;70:575–81.

102. Moulin DE, Kreeft JH, Murray-Parsons N, Bouquillon AI. Comparison of continuous subcutaneous and intravenous hydromorphone infusions for management of cancer pain. Lancet 1991;337:465–68.

103. Walker VA, Hoskin PJ, Hanks GW, White ID. Evaluation of WHO analgesic guidelines for cancer pain in a hospital-

based palliative care unit. J Pain Symptom Manage 1988;3: 145–49.

104. Zech DF, Grond S, Lynch J, Hertel D, Lehmann KA. Validation of World Health Organization guidelines for cancer pain relief: a 10-year prospective study. Pain 1995;63:65–76.

105. Black A, Dwyer B. Coeliac plexus block. Anaesth Intensive Care 1973;1:315–18.

106. Thompson GE, Moore DC, Bridenbaugh LD, Artin RY. Abdominal pain and alcohol celiac plexus nerve block. Anesth Analg 1977;56:1–5.

107. Singler RC. An improved technique for alcohol neurolysis of the celiac plexus. Anesthesiology 1982;56:137–41.

108. Ischia S, Luzzani A, Ischia A, Faggion S. A new approach to the neurolytic block of the coeliac plexus: the transaortic technique. Pain 1983;16:333–41.

109. Montero MA, Vidal LF, Aguilar SJ, Donoso BL. Percutaneous anterior approach to the coeliac plexus using ultrasound. Br J Anaesth 1989;62:637–40.

110. Ischia S, Ischia A, Polati E, Finco G. Three posterior percutaneous celiac plexus block techniques. A prospective, randomized study in 61 patients with pancreatic cancer pain. Anesthesiology 1992;76:534–40.

111. Ventafridda GV, Caraceni AT, Sbanotto AM, Barletta L, DeConno F. Pain treatment in cancer of the pancreas. Eur J Surg Oncol 1990;16:1–6.

112. Mercadante S. Celiac plexus block versus analgesics in pancreatic cancer pain. Pain 1993;52:187–92.

113. Polati E, Finco G, Gottin L, Bassi C, Pederzoli P, Ischia S. Prospective randomized double-blind trial of neurolytic coeliac plexus block in patients with pancreatic cancer. Br J Surg 1998;85:199–201.

114. Davies DD. Incidence of major complications of neurolytic coeliac plexus block. J R Soc Med 1993;86:264–66.

115. van Dongen RT, Crul BJ. Paraplegia following coeliac plexus block. Anaesthesia 1991;46:862–63.

116. Jabbal SS, Hunton J. Reversible paraplegia following coeliac plexus block. Anaesthesia 1992;47:857–58.

117. Ripamonti C. Management of bowel obstruction in advanced cancer. Curr Opin Oncol 1994;6:361–57.

118. Ripamonti C, DeConno F, Ventafridda V, Rossi B, Baines MJ. Management of bowel obstruction in advanced and terminal cancer patients. Ann Oncol 1993;4:15–21.

119. Malone JMJ, Koonce T, Larson DM. Freedman RS, Carrasco CH, Saul PB. Palliation of small bowel obstruction by percutaneous gastrostomy in patients with progressive ovarian carcinoma. Obstet Gynecol 1986;68:431–33.

120. Campagnutta E, Cannizzaro R, Galo A, et al. Palliative treatment of upper intestinal obstruction by gynecological malignancy: the usefulness of percutaneous endoscopic gastrostomy. Gynecol Oncol 1996;62:103–105.

121. Mercadante S. The role of octreotide in palliative care. J Pain Symptom Manage 1994;9:406–11.

122. Steadman K, Franks A. A woman with malignant bowel obstruction who did not want to die with tubes. Lancet 1996;347:944.

123. Mangili G, Franchi M, Mariani A, et al. Octreotide in the management of bowel obstruction in terminal ovarian cancer. Gynecol Oncol 1996;6:345–48.

124. Fearon KC, Carter DC. Cancer cachexia. Ann Surg 1988;208:1–5.

125. Kern KA, Norton JA. Cancer cachexia. JPEN J Parenter Enteral Nutr 1988;12:286–98.

126. Dunlop GM. A study of the relative frequency and importnce of gastrointestinal symptoms and weakness in patients with advanced cancer. Palliat Med 1989;63:37–43.

127. Thompson BR, Julian TB, Stremple JF. Perioperative total parenteral nutrition in patients with gastrointestinal cancer. J Surg Res 1981;30:497–500.

128. Muller JM, Brenner U, Dienst C, Pichlmeier H. Preoperative parenteral feeding in patients with gastrointestinal carcinoma. Lancet 1982;i:68–71.

129. Holter AR, Fischer JE. The effect of perioperative hyperalimentation on complications in patients with carcinoma and weight loss. J Surg Res 1977;23:31–43.

130. DeWys WD, Begg C, Lavin PT, et al. Prognostic effect of weight loss prior to chemotherapy in cancer patients. Eastern Cooperative Oncology Group. Am J Med 1980;69:491–97.

131. Mitchell EP, Schein PS. Gastrointestinal toxicity of chemotherapeutic agents. Semin Oncol 1982;9:52–64.

132. Sloan GM, Maher M, Brennan MF. Nutritional effects of surgery, radiation therapy, and adjuvant chemotherapy for soft tissue sarcomas. Am J Clin Nutr 1981;34:1094–102.

133. McCarthy M. Hospice patients: a pilot study in 12 services. Palliat Med 1990;4:93–104.

134. Goldberg RM, Loprinzi CL, Mailliard JA, et al. Pentoxifylline for treatment of cancer anorexia and cachexia? A randomized, double-blind, placebo-controlled trial. J Clin Oncol 1995;13:2856–59.

135. Plumb MM, Holland J. Comparative studies of psychological function in patients with advanced cancer. II: Interviewer-rated current and past psychological symptoms. Psychosom Med 1981;43:243–54.

136. Beutler B, Cerami A. Cachectin and tumour necrosis factor as two sides of the same biological coin. Nature 1986;320:584–88.

137. Strassmann G, Fong M, Kenney JS, Jacob CO. Evidence for the involvement of interleukin-6 in experimental cancer cachexia. J Clinc Invest 1992;89:1681–84.

138. Matthys D, Dijkmann R, Proost P, et al. Severe cachexia in mice inoculated with interferon-gamma-producing tumour cells. Int J Cancer 1991;49:77–82.

139. Heber D, Tchekmedyian NS. Pathophysiology of cancer: hormonal and metabolic abnormalities. Oncology 1992;49: 28–31.

140. Todorov P, Cariuk P, McDevitt T, Coles B, Fearon KC, Tisdale M. Characterization of a cancer cachetic factor. Nature 1996;379:739–42.

141. Portenoy RK. Therapeutic use of opioids: prescribing and control issues. NIDA Res Monogr 1993;131:35–50.

142. Loprinzi CL, Michalak JC, Schaid DJ, et al. Phase III evaluation of four doses of megestrol acetate as therapy for patients with cancer anorexia and/or cachexia. J Clin Oncol 1993;11:762–67.

143. Bruera E, Higginson I. Cachexia-anorexia in cancer patients. Oxford: Oxford University Press, 1996.

144. Moertel CG, Schutt AJ, Reitemeier RJ, Hahn RG. Corticosteroid therapy of preterminal gastrointestinal cancer. Cancer 1974;33:1607–609.

145. Willcox JC, Corr J, Shaw J, Richardson M, Calman KC, Drennan M. Prednisone as an appetite stimulant in patients with cancer. Br Med J (Clin Res) 1984;288:27.

146. Della CG, Pellegrini A, Piazai M. Effect of methylprednisolone sodium succinate on quality of life in preterminal cancer patients: a placebo-controlled, multicenter study. The Methylprednisolone Preterminal Cancer Study Group. Eur J Cancer Clin Oncol 1989;25:1823–29.

147. Popiela T, Lucchi R, Giongo F. Methylprednisolone as a palliative therapy for female terminal cancer patients. The Methylprednisolone Female Preterminal Cancer Study Group. Eur J Cancer Clin Oncol 1989;25:1823–29.

148. Ettinger AB, Portenoy RK. The use of corticosteroids in the treatment of symptoms associated with cancer. J Pain Symptom Manage 1988;3:99–103.

149. Farr WC. The use of corticosteroids for symptom management in terminally ill patients. Am J Hosp Care 1990;7:41–46.

150. Needham PR, Dale A, Lennard RF. Steroids in advanced cancer: survey of current practice. BMJ 1992;305:999.

151. Tchekmedyian NS, Hickman M, Heber D. Treatment of anorexia and weight loss with megestrol acetate in patients with cancer or acquired immunodeficiency syndrome. Semin Oncol 1991;18:35–42.

152. Downer S, Joel S, Allbright A, et al. A double-blind placebo controlled trial of medoxyprogesterone acetate (MPA) in cancer cachexia. Br J Cancer 1993;67:1102–105.

153. Bruera E, MacMillan K, Kuehn N, Hanson J, MacDonald RN. A controlled trial of megestrol acetate on appetite, caloric intake, nutritional status, and other symptoms in patients with advanced cancer. Cancer 1990;66:1279–82.

154. Loprinzi CL, Ellison NM, Schaid DJ, et al. Controlled trial of megestrol acetate for the treatment of cancer anorexia and cachexia. J Natl Cancer Inst 1990;82:1127–32.

155. Tchekmedyian NS, Hickman M, Siau J, et al. Megestrol acetate in cancer cachexia and anorexia and weight loss. Cancer 1992;69:1268–74.

156. Feliu J, Gonzalez-Baron M, Berrocal A, et al. Usefulness of megestrol acetate in cancer cachexia and anor-exia. A placebo-controlled study. Am J Clin Oncol 1992;15:436–40.

157. Simons JP, Aaronson NK, Vansteenkiste JF, et al. Effects of medroxyprogesterone acetate on appetite, weight, and quality of life in advanced-stage, non-hormone-sensitive cancer: a placebo-controlled multicenter study. J Clin Oncol 1996;14:1077–84.

158. Loprinzi CL, Schaid DJ, Dose AM, Burnham NL, Jensen MD. Body-composition changes in patients who gain weight while receiving megestrol acetate. J Clin Oncol 1993;11:152–54.

159. Loprinzi CL, Goldberg RM, Su JQ, et al. Placebo-controlled trial of hydrazine sulfate in patients with newly diagnosed non-small-cell lung cancer. J Clin Oncol 1994;12:1126–29.

160. Loprinzi CL, Kuross SA, O'Fallon JR, et al. Randomized placebo-controlled evaluation of hydrazine sulfate in patients with advanced colorectal cancer. J Clin Oncol 1994;12:1121–25.

161. Kardinal CG, Loprinzi CL, Schaid DJ, et al. A controlled trial of cyproheptadine in cancer patients with anorexai and/or cachexia. Cancer 1990;65:2657–62.

162. Nelson K, Walsh D, Deeter P, Sheehan F. A Phase II study of delta-9-tetrahydrocannabinol for appetite stimulation in cancer-associated anorexia. J Palliat Care 1994;10:14–18.

163. Beck SA, Smith KL, Tisdale MJ. Anticachectic and anti-tumour effect of eicosapentaenoic acid and its effect on protein turnover. Cancer Res 1991;51:6089–93.

164. Appelqvist P, Silvo J, Salmela L, Kostiainen S. On the treatment and prognosis of malignant ascites: is the survival time determined when the abdominal paracentesis is needed? J Surg Oncol 1982;20:238–42.

165. Garrison RN, Kaelin LD, Galloway RH, Heuser LS. Malignant ascites. Clinical and experimental observations. Ann Surg 1986;203:644–51.

166. Lacy JH, Wieman TJ, Shively EH. Management of malignant ascites. Surg Gynecol Obstet 1984;159:397–412.

167. Coates G, Bush RS, Aspin N. A study of ascites using lymphoscintigraphy with ^{99m}Tc-sulfur colloid. Radiology 1973;107:577–83.

168. Green LS, Levine R, Gross MJ, Gordon S. Distinguishing between malignant and cirrhotic ascites by computerised stepwise discriminant function analysis of its biochemistry. Am J Gastroenterol 1978;70:448–54.

169. Loewenstein MS, Rittgers RA, Kupchik HZ, Zamcheck N. Carcinoembryonic antigen gradients between plasma and malignant ascites: use in detecting peritoneal and liver metastases. J Natl Cancer Inst 1981;66:803–806.

170. Sharma S, Walsh D. Management of symptomatic malignant ascites with diuretics: two case reports and a review of the literature. J Pain Symptom Manage 1995;10:237–42.

171. Razis DV, Athanasiou D, Dadiotis L. Diuretics in malignant effusions and edemas of generalized cancer. J Med 1976;7:449–61.

172. Jackson GL, Blosser NM. Intracavitary chronic phospate ^{32}P colloidal suspension therapy. Cancer 1981;48:2596–98.

173. Olson K, Cunningham TJ, Sponzo R, Donavan M, Horton J. Intracavitary bleomycin in the management of malignant effusions. Cancer 1976;38:1903–908.

174. Ostrowski MJ, Priestman TJ, Houston RF, Martin WM. A randomized trial of intracavitary bleomycin and *Corynebacterium parvum* in the control of malignant pleural effusions. Radiother Oncol 1989;14:19–26.

175. Hagiwara A, Takahashi T, Sawai K, et al. Clinical trials with intraperitoneal cisplatin microspheres for malignant ascites – a pilot study. Anticancer Drug Res 1993;8:463–70.

176. Lind SE, Cashavelly B, Fuller AF. Resolution of malignant ascites after intraperitoneal chemotherapy in women with carcinoma of the ovary. Surg Gynecol Obstet 1988;166:519–22.

177. Lucas WE, Markman M, Howell SB. Intraperitoneal chemotherapy for advanced ovarian cancer. Am J Obstet Gynecol 1985;152:474–78.

178. Bitran JD. Intraperitoneal bleomycin. Pharmacokinetics and results of a Phase II trial. Cancer 1985;56:2420–23.

179. Kaplan RA, Markman M, Lucas WE. Infectious peritonitis in patients receiving intraperitoneal chemotherapy. Am J Med 1985;78:49–53.

180. Piccart MJ, Speyer JL, Markman M, et al. Intraperitoneal chemotherapy: technical experience at five institutions. Semin Oncol 1985;12:90–96.

181. Leveen HH, Christoudias G, Ip M, Luft R, Falk G, Grosberg S. Peritoneovenous shunting for ascites. Ann Surg 1974;180:580–91.

182. Gough IR, Balderson GA. Malignant ascites. A comparison of peritoneovenous shunting and nonoperative management. Cancer 1993;71:2377–82.

183. Cheung DK, Raaf JH. Selection of patients with malignant ascites for a peritoneovenous shunt. Cancer 1982;50:1204–209.

184. Lund RH, Moritz MW. Complications of Denver peritoneovenous shunting. Arch Surg 1982;117:924–28.

185. Lokich J, Reinhold R, Silverman M, Tullis J. Complications of peritoneovenous shunts for malignant ascites. Cancer Treat Rep 1980;64:305–309.

186. Campioni N, Pasquali LR, Vitucci C, et al. Peritoneovenous shunt and neoplastic ascites: a 5-year experience report. J Surg Oncol 1986;33:31–35.

187. Reuben DB, Mor V. Nausea and vomiting in terminal cancer patients. Arch Intern Med 1986;146:2021–23.

188. Ventafridda V, Ripamonti C, DeConno F, Tamburini M, Cassileth BR. Symptom prevalence and control during cancer patients' last days of life. J Palliat Care 1990;6:7–11.

189. Hosking DJ, Bennet T, Hampton JR. Diabetic autonomic neuropathy. Diabetes 1978;27:1043–55.

190. Henrich WL. Autonomic insufficiency. Arch Intern Med 1982;142:339–44.

191. Bruera E, Chadwick S, Fox R, Hanson J, MacDonald N. Study of cardiovascular autonomic insufficiency in advanced cancer patients. Cancer Treat Rep 1986;70:1383–87.

192. Mamdani MB, Walsh RL, Rubino FA, Brannegan RT, Hwang MH. Autonomic dysfunction and Eaton Lambert syndrome. J Auton Nerv Syst 1985;12:315–20.

193. Villa A, Foresti V, Confalonieri F. Autonomic neuropathy and HIV infection. Lancet 1987;ii:915.

194. Hagen NA, Foley KM, Cerbone DJ, Portenoy RK, Inturrisi CE. Chronic nausea and morphine-6-glucuronide. J Pain Symptom Manage 1991;6:125–28.

195. Pereira CA, Bruera E. Chronic nausea. In: Bruera E, Higginson I, editors. Cachexia–anorexia in cancer patients. Oxford: Oxford University Press, 1996:23–37.

196. Bruera ED, Roca E, Cedaro L, Chacon R, Estevez R. Improved control of chemotherapy-induced emesis by the addition of dexamethasone to metoclopramide in patients resistant to metoclopramide. Cancer Treat Rep 1983;67:381–83.

197. Bruera E, Brenneis C, Michaud M, MacDonald N. Continuous sc infusion of metoclopramide for treatment of narcotic bowel syndrome [letter]. Cancer Treat Rep 1987;71:1121–22.

198. Cole RM, Robinson F, Harvey L, Trethowan K, Murdoch V. Successful control of intractable nausea and vomiting requiring combined ondansetron and haloperidol in a patient with advanced cancer. J Pain Symptom Manage 194;9:48–50.

199. Cowcher K, Hanks GW. Long-term management of respiratory symptoms in advanced cancer. J Pain Symptom Manage 1990;5:320–30.

200. Reuben DB, Mor V. Dyspnea in terminally ill cancer patients. Chest 1986;9:234–36.

201. Higginson I, McCarthy M. Measuring symptoms in terminal cancer: are pain and dyspnoea controlled? J R Soc Med 1989;82:264–67.

202. Ripamonti C, Fulfaro F, Bruera E. Dyspnoea in patients with advanced cancer: incidence, causes and treatments. Cancer Treat Rev 1998;24:69–80.

203. Bruera E, MacMillan K, Pither J, MacDonald RN. Effects of morphine on the dyspnea of terminal cancer patients. J Pain Symptom Manage 1990;5:341–44.

204. Boyd KJ, Kelly M. Oral morphine as symptomatic treatment of dyspnoea in patients with advanced cancer. Palliat Med 1997;11:277–81.

205. Zeppetella G. Nebulized morphine in the palliation of dyspnoea. Palliat Med 1997;11:267–75.

206. Farncombe M, Chater S. Clinical application of nebulized opioids for treatment of dyspnoea in patients with malignant disease. Support Care Cancer 1994;2:184–87.

207. Bruera E, deStoutz N, Velasco-Leiva A, Schoeller T, Hanson J. Effects of oxygen on dyspnoea in hypoxaemic terminal cancer patients. Lancet 1993;342:13–14.

208. Cella DF. Methods and problems in measuring quality of life. Support Care Cancer 1995;3:11–22.

209. Jorge JM, Wexner SD. Etiology and management of fecal incontinence. Dis Colon Rectum 1993;36:77–97.

210. Stiggelbout AM, deHaes JC, Kiebert GM, Kievit J, Leer JW. Tradeoffs between quality and quantity of life: development of the QQ Questionnaire for Cancer Patient Attitudes. Med Decis Making 1996;16:184–92.

17. Costs of Rectal Cancer Patient Management

K.S. Virgo, W.E. Longo and F.E. Johnson

Introduction

It was estimated that $37 billion would be expended in direct medical costs for cancer care in 2000 [1]. In addition, the costs of lost productivity and mortality were estimated at $11 billion and $59 billion, respectively [1]. These figures do not include the psychosocial costs associated with living with cancer. Such patients may suffer prolonged and often intense pain, as well as live with the constant threat of disability, recurrence and death. Despite the resources devoted to cancer care, there is little patient-level information available regarding the costs of care. Such information can provide valuable input on patterns and intensity of care as they change over time. These data are also crucial in comparisons of alternative therapies in terms of patient outcomes. Cancers such as of the breast, lung and ovary are generally the focus of the few cost analyses that exist [2–4]. Much less common are analyses of the costs of rectal cancer patient management.

A substantial number of patients are diagnosed with rectal cancer each year. Approximately 36 400 new cases were predicted in the USA for 2000 [5]. The majority are treated with curative intent and enter follow-up programs. Although rectal cancer can occur early in life, it affects disproportionately those aged 65 years and over. The incidence rate for this age group is 73.6 per 100 000 population compared with 5.7 per 100 000 for those under 65 years of age [6]. The number of patients dying of rectal cancer each year in the USA is 8600 [5]. The 5-year relative survival rate is 59.5% [6]. If rectal cancer is detected while it is still localized, the 5-year relative survival rate is 85.7%. These rates fall dramatically if the tumor is more widespread at diagnosis, to 56.9% if regional lymph nodes are involved and 6.4% if distant metastases are present [6].

The options available to rectal cancer patients for treatment of the initial primary lesion are essen-tially surgical and can impose a great financial burden, particularly if the patient lacks sufficient insurance coverage. Alternatively, palliative therapy is also costly. The primary treatment modality for most patients is radical surgical resection. Adjuvant radiation and chemotherapy are often used to improve the results attained with this surgical approach. Tumors in the upper third of the rectum are generally treated with a low anterior resection. Sphincter saving surgical therapies are preferred for cancers in the middle third of the rectum and selected lower third lesions. Many cancers in the lower third of the rectum still require abdomino-perineal resection with a colostomy [7]. Although a substantial portion of the direct medical costs to the patient of treatment for rectal cancer may be covered by insurance (private, Medicare, Medicaid), many of the hidden costs are often not covered and can be substantial, such as the costs of prescription and non-prescription medicines, transportation, child care, homemaker services, orphan drugs and lost wages [8]. In one study of a single community in Washington State, 33% of colorectal cancer patients in fee-for-service health care plans stated that their portion of the total costs of cancer care had at least a moderate effect on their family's finances; 10% of these said that the effect was serious [9].

This chapter will analyze the costs of rectal cancer patient management by phase of disease progression as defined by Baker et al. [10]: (1) initial care phase (3 months after diagnosis); (2) continuing care phase (period between initial care and last 6 months of life); and (3) terminal care phase (last 6 months of life). This methodology is based on both clinical considerations and analyses of Medicare charge data [11–13]. The initial care phase corresponds with the period spanning the initial course of therapy. (Over time the definition of the length of the initial care phase has been expanded by others to 6 months after diagnosis [14–17].) The continuing care phase is equivalent to the period of follow-up after treatment. The terminal care phase is a period of particularly high costs resulting from an increased need for inpatient care, nursing home care, and hospice care just preceding death. Although the majority of articles reviewed did not mention explicitly the phases of disease progression as defined by Baker et al. [10], they could all be readily categorized by using this scheme. Screening costs and costs related to diagnosis of the initial primary will not be analyzed here.

Methods

Literature Review

A Medline search of the literature spanning 15 years (1984–1998) was performed to identify citations covering the measurement of the costs of rectal cancer patient management. Keywords used in the search included: rectal neoplasms, costs, charges, fees, economics, resection, treatment, and therapy. Articles were eliminated: if they examined costs for patients with non-invasive tumors only; if they examined the costs of procedures approved only for use in clinical trials; if they lacked average (per patient) cost or charge data; or if only nationwide or statewide totals were provided and insufficient data were available to calculate costs or charges on a per-patient level. Also eliminated were many studies that were described as dealing with cost-effectiveness or cost–benefit analyses, but which were merely statements that patient care can be expensive and lacked objective data or formal analyses to substantiate such statements.

Cost Analyses

All data were identified as either costs or charges. In those instances where it was unclear whether costs or charges were the basis of the analysis, charges were assumed because complete cost data are generally difficult to obtain [18,19]. Costs are generally defined as resources expended by the manufacturer to produce a given unit of output. These resources typically include such items as personnel, supplies, capital equipment and overhead. Charges are defined as the price paid by the purchaser of the output to the producer of the output. Charges are generally derived from a facility's cost of producing the unit of output plus some percentage profit. In the case of health services; purchasers are patients or third-party payers such as insurance companies.

An exception to the assumption of charges in the presence of ambiguity was made for studies con-ducted in countries with national health insurance schemes. One might presume that a national health insurance system would not bill itself for more than the cost of a given service and, therefore, it could be assumed that the data reported in such studies referred to costs. However, private hospitals operate within many of these countries. Therefore, unless the article specifically stated that the data were derived from the national health insurance system, the data were interpreted as charges.

The year associated with the cost or charge data was then identified for each article. For those articles that did not provide this information, the year preceding publication of the article was assumed if the publication date was in the first 6 months of the year. The current year was assumed if the publication date was in the last 6 months of the year. For example, if the publication date was March 1997, 1996 data were assumed; if the publication date was November 1997, 1997 data were assumed. The importance of identifying the year associated with the data was twofold. First, for articles authored by individuals from outside the USA, such data are needed to permit selection of an appropriate exchange rate for conversion of the cost or charge data to a common currency (US dollars). This is necessary to facilitate the use of all studies that meet the inclusion criteria in the analyses. For the eight articles presenting cost or charge data in other than US dollars [16,20–26], the average exchange rate for the year of the data was used for conversion ((Ruesch International, New York: unpublished data, 1998) and [27]). The applicable US dollar exchange rates for the British pound were 0.64 for 1996, 0.57 for 1991, 0.68 for 1986, and 0.66 for 1983. The applicable US dollar exchange rates for the remaining currencies were 1.18 for the 1989 Canadian dollar, 1.12 for the 1979 Australian dollar, 1.76 for the 1988 German mark, and 1270.67 for the 1987 Italian lire.

The second reason for identifying the year associated with the data was to permit the establishment of a baseline from which cost or charge estimates could be inflated to a common year. All costs or charges were inflated to 1999 US dollars by using the medical care component of the Consumer Price Index [28]. Since 1960, this component has never been negative. The medical care component increased by 11.0% in 1980, 10.7% in 1981, 11.6% in 1982, 8.8% in 1983, 6.2% in 1984, 6.3% in 1985, 7.5% in 1986, 6.6% in 1987, 6.5% in 1988, 7.7% in 1989, 9.0% in 1990, 8.7% in 1991, 7.4% in 1992, 5.9% in 1993, 4.8% in 1994, 4.5% in 1995, 3.5% in 1996, 2.8% in 1997, 3.2% in 1998, and 3.5% in 1999.

Discounting to factor in the time value of money was not conducted owing to its lack of relevance to this analysis. The time value of money is the principle that $1 today is worth more than $1 in the future because current dollars can be invested and, by earning interest, yield more dollars. Discounting is generally used in a cost–benefit or a cost-effectiveness analysis to determine the present value of a stream of funds to be received in the future or costs to be incurred in the future. As the focus of this study is not to conduct a fully-fledged cost–benefit or cost-effectiveness analysis of two methods of patient management, owing to the unavailability of survival benefit or quality of life benefit for any of the surveillance strategies, discounting is not relevant [29].

Costs were compared separately from charges across studies within each phase. This was necessary owing to the differences in the definition of each mentioned earlier. For studies measuring costs, it was generally assumed, unless otherwise stated, that all direct medical costs were included and all indirect costs were excluded. Direct medical costs are defined as expenses to a facility or health care system (rather than to the patient) related solely to the conduct of a specific activity. Direct costs represent resources expended to provide such services as inpatient, outpatient, nursing home and hospice services. Components of direct costs include the costs of medical personnel, supplies and equipment. Indirect costs are defined as costs that cannot be identified with a single activity, service or product. Such costs are shared by all services based on some unit of service indicator (e.g. heating, lighting, air conditioning, security).

For studies measuring charges, it was generally assumed, unless otherwise stated, that total medical charges were included and all indirect and psychosocial costs were excluded. Total medical charges are defined for the purposes of this study as expenditures borne by the patient or third-party payer for inpatient, outpatient, nursing home and hospice services. Components of total medical charges include hospital charges, physician fees (inpatient and outpatient), nursing home charges, hospice charges and prescription drug charges. Indirect costs refer to the costs associated with time lost from work and reduced productivity while on the job due to morbidity and mortality. Psychosocial costs refer to deteriorations in quality of life such as economic dependence and social isolation [29].

Results

Twenty-five articles were identified that analyzed rectal cancer patient management costs or charges during one or more of the three phases of disease progression (Tables 17.1–17.3) [10,14–26,30–40]. Only four articles contained cost or charge data for

all three phases [10,14,15,17]. All remaining articles provided data for only a single phase or portion of a phase of disease progression. Many articles presented facility-specific cost or charge data. Few were nationwide in scope [10,17,30,33,34,38]. Two specifically analyzed costs of rectal cancer patient management in health maintenance organizations (HMOs) [14,15].

Initial Care Phase

Of the 25 articles containing rectal cancer patient management cost or charge data, 16 computed costs or charges for all or part of the initial care phase (Table 17.1). Only five articles analyzed costs or charges for the full three months [10,14–17]. All except Baker et al. [10] defined the initial care phase as at least the 6 months after diagnosis rather than 3 months. The remaining 11 calculated costs or charges for primary treatment only [18–24,30–33]. For seven of the 11, total costs or charges included any cost or charge associated with the hospital admission for receipt of primary treatment. For four of the 11, total costs or charges included only the cost of or charge for the procedure [18,19,21,31]. The main goal of the initial care phase is the delivery of primary treatment. In a best–case scenario, curative treatment with sphincter preservation is possible due to early detection.

Charges

Three Months After Diagnosis Even after separating the articles into cost and charge studies, comparative analyses are difficult owing to the varying operational definitions of the initial care phase and differences in the types of charges included. For example, only two studies analyzed charge data and defined the initial care phase as at least 3 months after diagnosis [10,17]. The results of these two studies initially seem counterintuitive because total charges for the study defining the initial care phase as exactly 3 months ($33 254) are 23.5% greater than those for the study with this phase defined as 7 months ($26 936). Some of the difference lies in the fact that the database for the study with a 7-month initial care phase did not contain charges for services rendered while Medicare beneficiaries were enrolled in HMOs. According to Riley et al., approximately 8% of patients in their database were enrolled in HMOs at some time during the study [17]. However, much of the difference is likely to be due to practice pattern variation between the time periods of the two studies (1974–1981 and 1973–1989), particularly the influence of the 1982–1989 era in Riley et al.'s study. The impact of

Table 17.1. Costs by phase of rectal cancer disease progression: initial care phase

Reference	Phase operational definition	Cost vs charges	Colorectal vs rectal	n	Costs/charges included	Cost/charges as reported in original study	Costs/charges in 1999 $
Riley et al. 1995 [17]	Month prior to diagnosis + 6 month after diagnosis	Medicare charges in 1990 $	Colorectal	27 788	Total medical charges, excluding prescribed medicines, nursing home services below the skilled level, and services rendered while enrolled in an HMO	$17 505 if survival >1 year	26 936
Fireman et al. 1997 [14]	6 months after diagnosis	Cost to Kaiser Permanente (HMO) in 1992 $	Rectal	790	Direct medical costs, including overhead and excluding costs when not enrolled in the HMO	$26 369	34 756
Taplin et al. 1993 [15]	6 months after diagnosis	Cost to Group Health Cooperative (HMO) in 1992 $	Rectal	141	Direct medical costs, including overhead and excluding costs when not enrolled in the HMO	$17 428	22 971
Whynes et al. 1993 [16]	6 months after diagnosis	Cost to the National Health Service in 1991 UK £	Colorectal	360	Direct medical costs; unclear if overhead included	£2319 control £2370 study	5 789 5 915
Baker et al. 1989 [10]	3 months after diagnosis	Medicare charges in 1984 $	Colorectal	19 673	Total medical charges, excluding prescribed medicines and nursing home care below the skilled level	$14 190	33 254
Mushinski 1998 [30]	Inpatient admission for receipt of primary treatment	MetLife charges in 1995 $	Rectal	482	Total medical care charges, excluding prescribed medicines and nursing home services	$20 944	23 802
Elixhauser et al. 1998 [33]	Inpatient admission for receipt of primary treatment	Nationwide hospital charges in 1995 $	Rectal	31 149	Hospital charges only	$24 020	27 298
McCarthy 1990 [23]	Inpatient admission for receipt of primary treatment	Cost to the Ontario Health Insurance Plan in 1989 Canadian $	Rectal	1	Direct medical costs; unclear if overhead included	Can $5339	7570
Mellow 1989 [32]	Inpatient admission for receipt of primary treatment	Presbyterian Hospital, Okla koma charges in 1988? $	Rectal	51	Total medical care charges, excluding surgical assistants' fees, consultants' fees, prescription medicines, nursing home care services	$23 156 surgery $5 333 endoscopic laser, inpatient	41 828 9 633
Tuck et al. 1989 [24]	Inpatient admission for receipt of primary treatment	Cost to Queen's Medical Centre, Nottingham, UK in 1986 UK £	Colorectal	85	Direct medical costs, including overhead	£1552 control £1477 study	4 651 4 426
Payne et al. 1987 [20]	Inpatient admission for receipt of primary treatment	Cost to Concord Hospital, NSW, Australia, in 1979 Australian $	Colorectal	97	Direct medical costs, including overhead	Aust $6310 After excluding 3 outliers Aust $5238	20 965 17 400
de la Hunt et al. 1986 [22]	Inpatient admission for receipt of primary treatment	Cost to Royal South Hants Hospital, UK, in 1983 UK £	Colorectal	4	Direct medical costs, including overhead	£1364	5 146

Table 17.1. Costs by phase of rectal cancer disease progression: initial care phase   (*continued*)

Reference	Phase operational definition	Cost vs charges	Colorectal vs rectal	n	Costs/charges included	Cost/charges as reported in original study	Costs/charges in 1999 $
Cajozzo et al. 1990 [21]	Anastomosis procedure only	Cost to the University of Palermo, Italy, in 1987? Italian lire	Colorectal	48	Materials cost only. No significant difference in all other costs	200 000 lire staples 48 000 lire sutures	302 73
Peller et al. 1989 [31]	Protective loop colostomy only	Moun Sinai Medical Center, NY, charges in 1988? $	Colorectal	61	Hospital charges only	$12 000	21 676
Eckhauser et al. 1989 [18]	Pre-resectional laser recanalization and resection vs diversion or diversion/resection	Cleveland Metropolitan General Hospital charges? in 1988? $	Colorectal	22	Total medical charges, excluding prescription medicines	$16 606 laser/resection $24 176 diversion/resection	29 996 43 670
MacDonald 1989 [19]	Short-term bolus fluorouracil vs continuous infusion as outpatient	Lucille Parker Markey Cancer Center charges? in 1989? $	Colorectal	1	Total medical charges	$684 bolus $3446 continous infusion	1 148 5 780

HMO, health maintenance organization.

Table 17.2. Costs by phase of rectal cancer disease progression: continuing care phase

Reference	Phase operational definition	Cost vs charges	Colorectal vs rectal	n	Costs/charges included	Cost/charges as reported in original study	Costs/charges in 1999 $
Virgo and Johnson 1997 [38]	5 years of follow-up, based on recommendations of experts in the field	Medicare charges in 1992 $	Colorectal	5 recommendations	Total medical charges for follow-up visits and tests only	$3661–$15717 Medicare-allowed charges $5931–$25477 actual charges	4825–20729 7817–33580
Audisio et al. 1996 [35]	5 years of follow-up	European Institute of Oncology charges in 1990 $	Rectal	146	Total medical charges for follow-up visits and tests only	$5400	8309
Bruinvels et al. 1995 [36]	5 years of follow-up, based on simulation data	Cost to Leiden University Hospital in 1994 $	Colorectal	N/A	Direct medical costs	$3270 no F/U $3288 minimum F/U $4637 intensive F/U 1 $4635 intensive F/U 2	3884 3905 5507 5505
Virgo et al. 1995 [34]	5 years of follow-up based on review of published surveillance strategies	Medicare charges in 1992 $	Colorectal	11 strategies	Total medical charges for follow-up visits and tests only	$561–$16492 Medicare-allowed charges $910–$26717 actual charges	739–21737 1191–35214
Müller et al. 1994 [25]	5 years of follow-up	Cost to Chirurgische Universitätsklinik, Cologne, Germany, in 1998 DM	Colorectal	366	Direct medical costs for follow-up visits and tests only	3184,35 DM	3263
Baker et al. 1989 [10]	Period as defined	Medicare charges in 1984 $	Colorectal	19673	Total medical charges, excluding prescribed medicines and nursing home care below the skilled level	$572 per month $34320 for 5 years[a]	1341 80426
Norum and Olsen 1997 [26]	4 years of follow-up, based on guideline recommendations	Cost to the Norwegian health care system reported in 1996 UK £	Colorectal	1 guideline	Direct medical costs plus travel costs	£1232, excludes workup of positive test results £1943, includes workup of positive test results and subsequent treatment surgical	2129 3356
Rocklin et al. 1990 [37]	4 years of follow-up	West Virginia University Hospital charges in 1988 $	Colorectal	65	Total medical charges for follow-up visits and tests only	$9768	17645
Fireman et al. 1997 [14]	Phase as defined less 3 months already included in the initial phase	Cost to Kaiser Permanente (HMO) in 1992 $	Rectal	1219	Direct medical costs, excluding costs when not enrolled in the HMO	$3187 per 6 months $31870 for 5 years[a]	4201 42006
Taplin et al. 1993 [15]	Phase as defined less 3 months already included in the initial phase	Cost to Group Health Cooperative (HMO) in 1992 $	Rectal	340	Direct medical costs, excluding costs when not enrolled in the HMO	$5999 per year $29995 for 5 years[a]	7907 39535
Riley et al. 1995 [17]	Phase as defined less 3 months already included in the initial phase and less 1 year at end and included in the pre-final phase	Medicare charges in 1990 $	Colorectal	42296 continuing care cases 24334 pre-final cases	Total medical charges, excluding prescribed medicines, nursing home services below the skilled level, and services rendered while enrolled in an HMO	$3625 per year $18125 for 5 years[a] $9056 for pre-final phase $23556 for 4 years + pre-final phase	5578 27889 13935 36248

[a] Extrapolated from data reported in the original study.
F/U, follow-up; N/A, not applicable; HMO, health maintenance organization.

Table 17.3. Costs by phase of rectal cancer disease progression: terminal care phase

Reference	Phase operational definition	Cost vs charges	Colorectal vs rectal	n	Costs/charges included	Cost/charges as reported in original study	Costs/charges in 1999 $
Fireman et al. 1997 [14]	Phase as defined.	Cost to Kaiser Permanente (HMO) in 1992 $	Rectal	142	Direct medical costs, including overhead and excluding costs when not enrolled in the HMO	18 310	24 133
Riley et al. 1995 [17]	Phase as defined	Medicare charges in 1990 $	Colorectal	21 829	Total medical charges, excluding prescribed medicines, nursing home services below the skilled level, and services rendered while enrolled in an HMO	12 028	18 507
Taplin et al. 1993 [15]	Phase as defined	Cost to Group Health Cooperative (HMO) in 1992 $	Rectal	76	Direct medical costs, including overhead and excluding costs when not enrolled in the HMO	15 051	19 838
Baker et al. 1989 [10]	Phase as defined	Medicare charges in 1984 $	Colorectal	19 673	Total medical charges, excluding prescribed medicines and nursing home care below the skilled level	15 776	36 969
Spector and Mor 1984 [39]	Phase as defined	Charges for both Medicare and non-Medicare patients in 1981? $	Colorectal and small intestine	2 104	Total medical charges, excluding prescribed medicines	9 803	29 622
Long et al. 1984 [40]	Phase as defined	Charges to non-Medicare patients with comprehensive benefit coverage underBlueCross Blue Shield plans in Michigan, Indiana, and Atlanta, Georgia, in 1980 $	Colorectal	206	Total medical charges	16 337	54 650

HMO, health maintenance organization.

the prospective payment system over that time forced health care providers to be more cost-conscious in scrutinizing the utilization of both inpatient and outpatient services. Given the large sample sizes and the nationwide scope of the databases that served as the basis for each study, both of these studies can be assumed to provide reliable estimates of primary treatment charges according to practice patterns of the relevant era.

Inpatient Admission for Receipt of Primary Treatment   Three studies analyzed charges and provided data for only the primary treatment inpatient admission portion of the initial care phase. Of the three, one would assume from the included charges that the study including hospital charges only (no physician fees) would produce the lowest charge estimate [33], the study including hospital charges and some physician fees (while excluding surgical assistants' fees, consultants' fees, prescription medicine charges, and nursing home care service charges) would produce a higher charge estimate [32], and the study excluding only prescription medicines and nursing home services would produce the highest estimate [30]. However, this was not the case. The study producing the lowest charge estimate was the most inclusive study [30]. One possible reason for this unusual result is that the $23 802 total inpatient charge estimate for receipt of primary treatment by rectal cancer patients may not be comparable with the estimates produced by the other studies owing to the selectivity of the dataset. Only patients insured by the Metropolitan Life Insurance Company (MetLife and Metra Health policyholders) are included in the database. Thus, the distribution of demographic and socioeconomic characteristics of the Metropolitan Life patient population may not reflect that of the US population in general. Therefore, results derived from this study may not be generalizable to the USA as a whole. Although not stated in the article, it is also possible that the Metropolitan Life charges appear low because only covered charges and not total submitted charges were analyzed.

For the study estimating total charges of $41 828 for surgically treated rectal cancer patients and $9633 for endoscopic-laser-treated patients (five of whom were curatively treated), the sample size is small and the charges are facility specific [32]. Thus, the data are most likely not generalizable beyond the Presbyterian Hospital in Oklahoma. The estimate of $27 298 for hospital charges only is generalizable nationwide because it is drawn from the Healthcare Cost and Utilization Project Nationwide Inpatient Sample database, which is a 20% stratified probability sample of hospital discharges from all US non-federal, short-term, general and other specialty hospitals [33]. Once again, understanding the limitations of these articles is the key to making use of the results.

Procedure Only   For the three articles that computed procedure charges only rather than the charge for the full admission or initial care phase, no two analyzed charges associated with the same procedure [18,19,31]. Peller et al. estimated the additional hospital charges associated with protective loop colostomy for patients undergoing elective anterior resection at $21 676 [31]. Eckhauser et al. compared the charges for pre-resectional laser recanalization and resection ($29 996) with the charges for diversion or diversion and resection ($43 670) for patients with obstructing carcinomas of the colon and rectum [18]. Macdonald compared the charges for short-term bolus fluorouracil ($1148) with the charges for outpatient continuous low-dose infusion of fluorouracil ($5780) for patients with advanced colorectal cancer [19]. Unfortunately, the charge data presented in each article are facility specific and the sample sizes are small, thus limiting generalizability.

Costs

Six Months After Diagnosis   Three studies analyzed cost data and defined the initial care phase as the 6-month period after diagnosis [14–16].

Filling an important niche in the literature, two articles analyzed costs to HMOs [14,15]. These articles provide comparable data in that both used similar inclusion criteria in their computations of total costs. It is interesting that the total costs to Kaiser Permanente for rectal cancer patients in San Francisco Bay area were 51% higher than total costs to Group Health Cooperative for rectal cancer patients in the Puget Sound area. The reason for this disparity is unclear. The majority of the difference may be due to variation in service coverage between Kaiser Permanente and Group Health Cooperative. The remainder is most likely due to variation in overhead costs and unit costs between these two HMOs.

The remaining article analyzed costs to the UK National Health Service (NHS) for the 6-month period after diagnosis [16]. This article compared the costs of treatment for patients whose cancers were detected through screening (cases) with the costs of treatment for those whose cancers were detected based on symptoms (controls). Surprisingly, the costs of treatment were not significantly less for patients whose cancers were screen detected. The costs of treatment varied by only 2.2% between cases and controls.

The substantially lower cost estimates for rectal cancer patients treated in the UK health care system [16] (compared with the cost estimates for patients treated in US model HMOs [14,15]) are most likely due to three factors. First, physicians in the UK health care system are salaried. Although not stated in the article by Whynes et al. [16], physician salaries are probably pro-rated across bed days of care, rather than across procedures, resulting in a fairly low cost per patient. Physician incomes in the NHS are often derived from two sources: directly from the NHS and from private consultative work. Often, the NHS salary is dwarfed by the income derived from private patients. It is safe to assume that patient costs overall are markedly higher if care is delivered in the non-NHS system, which has grown dramatically in recent years. Second, the treatment of overhead in the UK health care system is not covered by Whynes et al. It is likely that what is categorized as overhead in the UK is quite different from overhead as defined in the US model HMO. It is also likely that very little, if any, overhead is actually pro-rated across procedures. Third, somewhat greater capitation within the UK health care system than in the typical HMO may be an additional contributing factor to the differential in cost estimates. However, in the initial care phase, the effect of this factor is probably minor.

Inpatient Admission for Receipt of Primary Treatment   For the four studies that analyzed cost data and defined the initial care phase as the inpatient admission for receipt of primary treatment, all addressed costs to hospitals operating within national health systems [20,22–24]. Three clearly included overhead costs [20,22,24]. For the remaining article, whether overhead was included or not was unclear[23]. Cost estimates for the inpatient care of rectal cancer patients during the initial care phase ranged from $4426 for patients with screen-detected tumors in the UK health care system to $20 965 for patients treated in the Australian health care system [20,24]. This large cost differential was primarily due to major differences in the fee schedules of the two countries, particularly for medical and nursing staff.

Cost estimates for patients treated in the two British hospitals varied by 16.3% (range $4426–$5146) [22,24]. Variation in overhead costs in the two facilities may account for some of the difference. However, the majority of the difference is most likely due to the particularly small sample size ($n = 4$) of the de la Hunt et al. study and the restrictive nature of the patient population upon which the cost estimate was based [22]. The population comprised only those patients who underwent resection and primary anastomosis without postoperative complications. Studied separately to determine the cost of complications were ten patients who suffered complications after undergoing major abdominal surgery.

Procedure Only   For the one study that computed only anastomosis procedure costs rather than the cost for the full admission or initial care phase, the materials costs for staples was $302 compared with $73 for sutures [21]. The authors' reasoning for comparing materials costs only was that there was no significant difference in anastomosis construction time, postoperative stay, or complications; hence, there were no other costs to consider.

Continuing Care Phase

Of the 25 articles containing rectal cancer patient management cost or charge data, 11 computed costs or charges for all or part of the continuing care phase defined as the period between the 3-month initial care phase and the terminal care phase (Table 17.2) [10,14,15,17,25,26,34–38]. For three articles, the start date for the continuing care phase was 3 months later owing to the use of a 6-month definition of the initial care phase [14,15,17]. For one article, the end date for the continuing care phase was 1 year earlier owing to the definition of the year prior to the terminal care phase as its own category (pre-final phase) [17]. Only three studies analyzed costs of continuing care for rectal cancer patients separately from costs for colon cancer patients [14,15,35]. Most studies provided cost or charge data for 4 or more years of follow-up. For those studies where costs or charges were provided on a per-month, per-6-month, or per-year basis, it was assumed that a 5-year follow-up cost estimate could be derived by multiplying these estimates by 60, 10 and 5, respectively [10,14,15,17].

There are many goals of surveillance after potentially curative cancer therapy, including the provision of patient education regarding the negative effects of such modifiable risk factors as physical inactivity, high-fat low-fiber diets, and diets lacking in fruits and vegetables. However, the main goals of surveillance after treatment of the initial primary are often stated to be the detection of recurrence and second primaries. Whether post-treatment surveillance is worthwhile, however, is unclear. It is not enough to be able to detect recurrences and second primaries prior to the development of symptoms if effective treatment for detected disease is unavailable. Proof of lengthened survival or significant quality of life benefits are needed to substantiate the need for intensive follow-up.

Unlike in the initial care phase, where costs were expected to vary within a narrow range, as were charges, in the continuing care phase much greater variation should be anticipated for two reasons. First, there are no widely accepted guidelines for the follow-up of rectal cancer patients after treatment, although many guidelines have been published [37,41–58]. Secondly, little is known about how outcomes vary when a chosen surveillance strategy is altered.

Charges

Alternative Definition of the Continuing Care Phase
Other than the Baker et al. study itself [10], none of the other five studies that analyzed charges defined the continuing care phase in a similar manner [17,34,35,37,38]. One of the five specified that the continuing care phase began in month 7. This same study also used a different end date for the continuing care phase and will be discussed separately [17]. The remaining four specified that follow-up began at the conclusion of adjuvant therapy, which is generally at 6–12 months. Thus, the continuing care phase would have begun 7–13 months after diagnosis in these studies. In the Baker et al. study, the initial care phase was defined as 3 months after diagnosis and the continuing care phase would have begun 4 months after diagnosis.

A second characteristic distinguishing these four studies from the Baker et al. study is their definition of total charges as fees for follow-up visits and tests for asymptomatic patients only [34,35,37,38]. In Baker et al.'s study, charges for the workup and treatment of disease detected during follow-up for both symptomatic and asymptomatic patients were also included. Among the four studies with similar definitions of both the continuing care phase and total charges, the range of Medicare-allowed charges in 1998 dollars was $739, based on an American Society of Colon and Rectal Surgeons recommended follow-up strategy consisting of barium enema only [51], to a high of $21 737 based upon the intense strategy of Makela et al. [59] (both these studies were included in the Virgo et al. review [34]). The range of charges for non-Medicare patients was $1199–$35 214. The charge ranges originally identified by Virgo et al. in their review of the literature (inflated to 1999 US dollars) have held up well over time [34]. More recent studies have derived estimates well within these ranges [35,38].

Such wide variation in charges for the follow-up of asymptomatic patients reflects great differences in suggested surveillance strategies. Both the selection of tests for inclusion in follow-up and the frequencies with which selected tests are ordered vary widely. Guidelines and recommendations published after the Virgo et al. review were examined in comparison with those in the review article to identify any specific trends in follow-up, such as perhaps gravitation towards less frequent follow-up [35,38,41–50,54]. Although there has been much published debate, little has changed over the last approximately 5 years. Office visits in conjunction with serum carcinoembryonic antigen (CEA) level, chest radiography, colonoscopy and sigmoidoscopy, are still the most frequently used diagnostic tests in the follow-up of rectal cancer patients. The only trend identified was somewhat less reliance on blood tests, other than serum CEA levels.

Let us return now to our discussion of the one study that collected workup and treatment charge data [10]. To obtain a rough estimate of additional charges for workup and treatment of disease detected during follow-up, one might propose a comparison of charge estimates from this study with estimates from the four surveillance-charge-only studies. However, these studies are much more recent than Baker et al.'s report. Follow-up practice patterns in the Baker et al. study are more likely to reflect those recommended by Steele in the only text available at that time that was devoted exclusively to follow-up of the cancer patient [56]. An office visit and complete blood count were recommended at 1 month after treatment, quarterly in years 1 and 2, and yearly thereafter. CEA level assessment was suggested quarterly in years 1 and 2, every 6 months in year 3, and annually thereafter. Fecal occult blood tests were recommended quarterly, beginning at 6 months and throughout years 1 and 2, every 6 months in year 3, and annually thereafter. Sigmoidoscopy was recommended every 6 months in years 1 and 2, and annually thereafter. Barium enema and chest radiography were recommended every 6 months in years 1 and 2, and every other year thereafter.

However, even if the charges associated with the above strategy were calculated for purposes of comparison with the Baker et al. study, an additional problem is posed by the method used by these authors to calculate continuing care charges. On the positive side, because all patients who survived for less than 9 months were excluded from the continuing care charge calculations, it was assumed that all remaining patients had at least some follow-up. Unfortunately, because the average length of time that patients spent in the continuing care phase was not mentioned, it is unclear whether the charge estimate of $572 per month (as originally quoted in the article in 1984 $) can safely be extrapolated to the standard 5-year follow-up period for purposes of comparison. Keeping in mind that follow-up is generally more intensive in the first 2 years after treatment [60], if the majority of patients were in the continuing care phase for less than 2 years, extrapolating estimates derived from such a patient population would result in an overestimate of 5-year follow-up charges. The amount of the overestimate would be determined by the size of the decrease in follow-up frequency and the types of surveillance tests still utilized after year 2 post-treatment. At the same time, an underestimate of workup and treatment costs could result from the unavailability of data for the complete continuing care phase. Thus, the 5-year charge estimate printed in Table 17.2 is provided primarily for information purposes.

As mentioned earlier, Riley et al. not only used a different start date for the continuing care phase but also modified the end date, defined as 1 year earlier due to the categorization of the year prior to the terminal care phase as a pre-final phase. Patients who survived 11 months or less were considered to have had no follow-up and were excluded from charge calculations for this phase. The data presented in this study included charges for surveillance as well as for the workup and treatment of disease detected during surveillance.

It is unclear in the Riley et al. study whether per-year charge estimates for the continuing care phase can safely be extrapolated to a 5-year estimate for the following reason. As in Baker et al.'s study [10], the average length of time spent by patients in follow-up was not given, nor were any data provided on the utilization of surveillance tests. By extrapolating, an overestimate of 5-year continuing care charges could result if the original data represent 2 or less years of follow-up, as explained earlier. Even if one assumes that charges for the continuing care and pre-final phases of Riley et al.'s study [17] should be summed to ensure consistency in the definition of the continuing care phase across studies, it is still necessary to determine how many years patients spent in the continuing care phase prior to adding charges from the pre-final phase because charges are phase specific. Thus, it is difficult to draw any solid conclusions regarding the comparability of this study with the majority of the studies reviewed earlier. In Table 17.2, however, we have provided two estimates of 5-year continuing care charges. If patients are assumed to live for a full 5 years prior to entering the pre-final phase, that estimate is $27 889. More realistically, if patients are assumed to survive for 4 years prior to the start of the pre-final phase, the estimate is $36 248.

Although a comparison of the Riley et al. results with the results of the four studies reviewed earlier is not possible, comparison with the Baker et al. study can be performed after converting monthly ($1341) to annual ($16 092) estimates [10]. Extrapolating from monthly estimates to an annual estimate is relatively safe because patients who survived for 9 months or less were excluded from continuing care charge calculations in the Baker et al. study and it is likely that most of the remaining patients spent at least 1 year in follow-up. On an annual basis, a difference of $10 514 in continuing care charges was identified between the two studies. Some of the variation in estimates may be due to a limitation of the dataset used by Riley et al. Charges for services rendered to Medicare beneficiaries while enrolled in HMOs were not captured. Another major factor is the budget-tightening impact of the prospective payment system. Thorough reviews of health services utilization became more common over the period between these two studies, as discussed earlier. Although the estimated charges for both studies have been inflated to 1998 levels, the practice patterns being compared are still those of 1974–1981 and 1984–1990. Also present is nationwide variation in surveillance, workup and treatment approaches, as would be expected.

Costs

Continuing Care Phase as Defined by Baker et al. Three studies analyzed costs and are assumed to have defined continuing care in a manner approximating that used by Baker et al. [25,26,36]. As was the case for selected charge studies, for these cost studies the exact start date of follow-up was somewhat vague owing to the lack of a definition for the period of adjuvant therapy. Assuming adjuvant therapy is generally completed after 3 months, then the initial care phase would reach completion after 3 months and follow-up would begin as defined by Baker et al. [10].

Only one of the three reports analyzed costs associated with follow-up visits and tests only [25]. Office visits, multichannel blood tests, liver function tests, serum CEA levels, serum CA19-9 levels, and fecal occult blood tests were conducted quarterly in year 1, every 6 months in year 2, and annually thereafter. Abdominal ultrasound, chest radiography and colonoscopy were performed every 6 months for the first 2 years after treatment and annually thereafter. The estimated cost for 5 years of follow-up was $3263.

The remaining two reports calculated the cost of post-treatment surveillance, workup and treatment of disease detected during follow-up. One study examined the cost-effectiveness of surveillance guidelines issued by the Norwegian Gastrointestinal Cancer Group (NGICG) [26]. The guideline recommends an office visit and serum CEA level monitoring quarterly for the first 2 years and annually for the next 2 years. Although not a commonly used test in the USA, the NGICG recommends ultrasound examination of the liver every 6 months for 4 years. Chest radiography is suggested every 6 months for 2 years and annually for the next 2 years. For patients who have undergone low anterior resection or total mesorectal excision, rectoscopy is recommended quarterly in the first 2 years and every 6 months in the next 2 years. The estimated cost of the basic follow-up program exclusive of workup and treatment of positive test results was $2129. The cost inclusive of workup and treatment was $3356. This cost estimate is very similar to that of Müller et al. [25].

According to the result of the cost-effectiveness analysis, a survival gain of 0.12 years was required in all patients. The required quality-of-life score ranged from 0.46 to 0.81, depending on the survival gain. Sensitivity analysis showed that the estimated cost per quality adjusted life year (QALY) saved ranged from $19 695 to $33 480, depending on the percentage of patients who were assumed to be eligible for salvage surgery and to survive for the number of years expected in the general Norwegian population. (QALYs are a measure of well-being comprising mental, physical and social functioning). Using $30 000 per QALY as the cut-off point between cost-effectiveness and cost-ineffectiveness, the guideline was considered to be generally cost-effective. This cut-off point has been used for analyses of other conditions (e.g. transplantation, cancer screening).

The second study to include surveillance, workup and treatment costs in the analysis was based solely on an analysis of simulation models [36]. Assumptions drawn from the literature regarding decision probabilities associated with every step in the surveillance, workup and treatment decision-making process were fed into the models in conjunction with the follow-up protocols and their associated costs. Probabilities of survival, recurrence and development of a second primary obtained from the literature were also components of the model. Three surveillance strategies were examined. The minimal follow-up strategy consisted of office visits annually for 5 years. Intensive follow-up strategy I consisted of office visits and serum CEA levels quarterly in years 1 and 2, every 6 months in years 3 and 4, and annually thereafter. Colonoscopy was used in years 2 and 4 and every 2 years thereafter. Intensive follow-up strategy II consisted of office visits, alkaline phosphatase levels, serum CEA levels and fecal occult blood tests quarterly in years 1 and 2 and every 6 months in years 3–5. Colonoscopy, chest radiography and liver ultrasound were carried out every 6 months in years 1–5. Actual costs were used for

office visits and follow-up tests. Estimated costs were assigned to the evaluation of a positive test result ($660), surgical exploration ($1100), resection of recurrence ($1600), living 1 year without recurrence ($100), and living 1 year with recurrence ($400).

Once again, estimates of costs were very similar to those found in the previous two studies [25,26]. There was very little difference between the cost of no follow-up ($3884) and the cost of minimal follow-up ($3905). The costs of the intensive strategies were also similar to one another ($5507 and $5505 for intensive follow-up strategies I and II, respectively). Cost-effectiveness was highest for patients 60 years of age and younger. The maximum benefit of intensive follow-up was 6 months. For a patient with a Dukes' C tumor, the maximum benefit was approximately 3 months.

Alternative Definition of the Continuing Care Phase

Only two studies analyzed cost data using a definition of the continuing care phase that differed from that of Baker et al. [10]. In both of these reports, the start date for the continuing care phase was defined as 3 months later due to the use of a 6-month definition of the initial care phase [14,15]. In the Fireman et al. study, patients who survived less than 1 year were considered to have had no follow-up and were excluded from cost calculations for this phase [14]. It is unknown how such patients were handled in the Taplin et al. study [15]. It is assumed that a similar methodology was used because much of the remainder of their methods mirror one another. The cost data presented in both studies included charges for surveillance as well as for the workup and treatment of disease detected during surveillance. The sources of data in both studies were HMO databases. As patients can elect to disenroll at any time from an HMO, the costs of care while patients were disenrolled were excluded from both analyses. Whether a set follow-up protocol for patients with rectal cancer was used in either Kaiser Permanente or the Group Health Cooperative was not specified.

The major differences between these two analyses appear to be the geographic regions examined (San Francisco Bay area versus Puget Sound area) and the respective sample sizes (1219 versus 340). For purposes of comparison, if the cost estimate of Fireman et al. for 6 months of continuing care is extrapolated to 1 year ($8402), a difference of only $495 exists between the estimates of the two studies. In the Taplin et al. study, which spanned the period 1990–1991, the 340 patients for whom continuing care data were available spent on average less than 2 years in the continuing care phase. Extrapolating to 5 years of follow-up results in an estimate of $39 535 which, because of reasons explained earlier, most likely overestimates costs of follow-up in years 3–5 post-treatment. At the same time, the unavailability of data for the complete continuing care phase most likely results in some underestimation of workup and treatment costs.

Fireman et al. provided no data on time spent in continuing care, although it is known that the study in general collected data on patients from July 1987 to June 1991. Thus it is probably a safe assumption that the average number of years spent by patients in the continuing care phase was longer. The resulting 5-year estimate of continuing care costs was $42 006, only 6% higher than that derived from extrapolating Taplin et al.'s results.

Terminal Care Phase

Of the 25 articles containing rectal cancer patient management cost or charge data, six computed costs or charges for the terminal care phase defined as the last six months prior to death (Table 17.3) [10,14,15,17,39,40]. Only two reports analyzed the costs of terminal care for rectal cancer patients separately from costs for colon cancer patients [14,15]. The goals of the terminal care phase are twofold. For some patients, any and all attempts at treatment are preferred to "doing nothing" while awaiting death. For these patients, salvage therapy to control further spread of disease is the primary goal. For patients with no available salvage treatment options remaining and those who have elected to forego further salvage treatment, the palliation of symptoms such as pain, bleeding or obstruction is the primary goal.

The cost of pain management is an area that has been identified by the Agency for Health Policy and Research as requiring sizeable additional research efforts [61]. In the past, the costs of pain management were rarely analyzed because of the difficulty of assigning a price to relief of suffering and because, historically, inexpensive oral medications and intramuscular injections were the primary methods of pain relief. With the advent of newer and more expensive approaches to pain management, such as parenteral infusion devices, nerve blocks, neuroablative surgery, implantable pumps, venous access devices, and epidural catheters, the costs of cancer pain management have risen substantially. For example, although at high doses the costs of oral analgesics can exceed $1000 per month, the monthly cost of patient-controlled analgesia using an ambulatory pump is $4000 [62]. Failure to treat pain can also result in major costs. In a recent study of 5000 patients at a single medical center, the cost of hospital admissions for unrelieved pain surpassed $5 million for 1990 [63]. In that same year, $3 million was saved by

providing parenteral morphine infusions in the home rather than in the inpatient setting.

Expenditures rise dramatically for the families of cancer patients as death approaches. It was at one time suggested that medical expenditures for patients in the terminal cancer phase exceed constant dollar health care expenditures for these patients for the previous 35 years combined [40]. In recent years, a trend towards the use of less costly alternatives such as home care and hospice care has been in evidence. For patients with gastrointestinal cancer, the use of hospice care has been shown to result in a 28% reduction in expenditures in comparison with inpatient care for the last 3 months of life and a 43% reduction for the last month alone [64].

Charges

Four studies analyzed charges associated with the terminal care phase [10,17,39,40]. Two of the four focused exclusively on charges for Medicare patients [10,17]. One incorporated charges for both Medicare and non-Medicare patients alike [39]. The remaining study specifically excluded patients over 65 years of age as well as disabled persons under 65 years of age who were covered by Medicare [40]. For the three studies that provided data by type of charge (inpatient, outpatient, physician, home health/skilled nursing facility/hospice), inpatient care comprised 68–84% of the total charges and physician fees were responsible for 11–19% of the total charges [17,39,40]. Long-term care services represented only 3–8% of total charges.

The charge estimates for the two studies restricted to Medicare patients ($18 507 and $36 969) differ by approximately 100%. Both include similar categories of charges, have similar patient inclusion criteria, and are based on similar sample sizes, but differ substantially in the time periods analyzed (1984–1990 [17] and 1974–1981 [10]). Changing practice patterns due to cost constraints imposed by the prospective payment system are primarily responsible for this sharp downward trend in charge estimates. The need to identify less costly alternatives for the delivery of terminal cancer care is driven in part by this major change in the health care delivery system. Both figures should be considered as solid estimates of the charges associated with terminal cancer care practice patterns at the time the data were analyzed.

As the remaining studies are discussed, this same trend will be evidenced for those using data from the 1980s and earlier compared with reports of more recent data. An example is the study estimating terminal care charges for both Medicare and non-Medicare patients [39]. Based on a dataset of all patients who died in Rhode Island during 1980 and

1981, again a comparatively high estimate of charges ($29 622) was the result. The impact of including charges for the terminal care of patients with malignancies of the small intestine is unknown because separate data were not provided.

The study that specifically excluded patients over 65 years of age as well as disabled persons under 65 years of age covered by Medicare produced the highest charge estimate for the terminal care phase [40]. This study was further restricted to only those patients with comprehensive benefit coverage under Blue Cross Blue Shield plans in three states. As the sample size was small and the restrictions many, the generalizability of these results is questionable. The results do provide a reasonable starting point for understanding the costs of terminal cancer care for younger patients.

Costs

Two studies analyzed costs associated with the terminal care phase using HMO data [14,15]. Both analyzed costs for rectal cancer patients separately from those for colon cancer patients. In both instances, the sample sizes were very small (142 versus 76). Similar estimates of terminal care costs were derived for the San Francisco Bay area ($24 133) as for the Puget Sound area ($19 838). The major difference here may be due to variation in overhead and unit costs for services between the two HMOs.

Inpatient costs as a percentage of total costs ranged from 64% for Puget Sound to 80% for San Francisco Bay. Outpatient costs were 32% of total costs for Puget Sound and were unavailable for the other study.

Conclusion

As demonstrated above, the costs of rectal cancer patient management tend to be highest in the initial and terminal care phases. Although each of these phases lasts for only 6 months, resource utilization is high and the technology used is expensive. This is not to say that the continuing care phase is inexpensive. The relative cost of the continuing care phase is dependent upon the length of time spent in this phase and whether disease is detected during follow-up that requires workup and treatment.

The major difficulty in understanding the literature in this field is directly related to the varying definitions of the phases of care and the different inclusion and exclusion criteria. A major problem is the lack of information for many studies regarding the cost analysis methodology. Great detail is generally provided for the clinical aspects of these studies, but little or no detail is provided on whether cost or charge data were utilized, what year's currency the results were presented in, whether discounting was used and the reasoning, and so on. Economists have often called for standardization in the details provided in costing studies [65,66]. In reviews of the literature aimed at identifying whether any studies would meet various proposed criteria, few pass the test [67].

As a result of this lack of standardization, cost and charge estimates vary widely. It is hoped that the application of Baker et al.'s methodology (phases of cancer care) has helped in this review to organize the literature in a more understandable fashion. Limitations of the various studies have been highlighted as have major contributions of selected studies. Future research in this field should focus on areas such as comparison of the costs of alternative treatment approaches for the initial primary, clinical trials comparing minimal follow-up with intensive follow-up, and comparisons of the costs of alternative systems of care for the terminal care phase.

References

1. American Cancer Society. Cancer facts and figures – 2000. Atlanta: American Cancer Society, 2000.
2. Baker MS, Kessler LG, Urban N, et al. Estimating the treatment costs of breast and lung cancer. Med Care 1991;29:40–49.
3. Brown ML, Fintor L. Cost-effectiveness of breast cancer screening: preliminary results of a systematic review of the literature. Breast Cancer Res Treat 1993;8:113–18.
4. Etzioni R, Urban N, Baker M. Estimating the costs attributable to a disease with application to ovarian cancer. J Clin Epidemiol 1996;49:95–103.
5. Greenlee RT, Murray T, Bolden S, Wingo PA. Cancer statistics, 2000. CA Cancer J Clin 2000;50:7–33.
6. Ries LAG, Kosary CL, Hankey BF, Miller BA, Clegg LX, Edwards BK, editors. SEER cancer statistics review, 1973–1996. (NIH Publication no. 99-2789.) Bethesda, MD: National Cancer Institute, 1999, Table VI–5, PG. 168.
7. Cohen AM, Minsky BD, Schilsky RL. Cancer of the rectum. In: DeVita VT Jr, Hellman S, Rosenberg SA, editors. Cancer: principles and practice of oncology; vol. 1. 5th ed. Philadelphia, PA: Lippincott-Raven, 1997:1197–234.
8. Berkman BJ, Sampson SE. Psychosocial effects of cancer economics on patients and their families. Cancer 1993;72:2846–49.
9. Francis AM, Polissar L, Lorenz AB. Care of patients with colorectal cancer. Med Care 1984;22:418–29.
10. Baker MS, Kessler LG, Smucker RC. Site-specific treatment costs for cancer: an analysis of the Medicare continuous history sample file. In: Scheffler RM, Andrews NC, editors. Cancer care and cost: DRGs and beyond. Ann Arbor, MI: Health Administration Press, 1989:127–38.
11. Health Care Financing Administration. Medicare Part B Extract and Summary System (BESS) file, 1997 [computer file].

12. Health Care Financing Administration. Medicare Hospital Outpatient Bill (HOP) file, 1992 [computer file].

13. Health Care Financing Administration. Part B Medicare Annual Data (BMAD) file, 1992 [computer file].

14. Fireman BH, Quesenberry CP, Somkin CP, et al. Cost of care for cancer in a health maintenance organization. Health Care Financing Rev 1997;18:51–76.

15. Taplin SH, Barlow B, Mandelson M, Timlin D. Direct costs of cancer treatment. National Cancer Institute final report, December 31, 1993 [on file].

16. Whynes DK, Walker AR, Chamberlain JO, Hardcastle JD. Screening and the costs of treating colorectal cancer. Br J Cancer 1993;68:965–68.

17. Riley GF, Potosky AL, Lubitz JD, Kessler LG. Medicare payments from diagnosis to death for elderly cancer patients by stage at diagnosis. Med Care 1995;33:828–41.

18. Eckhauser ML, Imbembo AL, Mansour EG. The role of pre-resectional laser recanalization for obstructing carcinomas of the colon and rectum. Surg 1989;106:710–17.

19. Macdonald JS. Continuous low-dose infusion of fluoro-uracil: is the benefit worth the cost [editorial]? J Clin Oncol 1989;7:412–14.

20. Payne JE, Murdoch CW, Dent OF, Chapuis PH. The cost of resection for colorectal cancer. Aust N Z J Surg 1987;57:627–33.

21. Cajozzo M, Compagno G, DiTora P, Spallitta SI, Bazan P. Advantages and disadvantages of mechanical vs. manual anastomosis in colorectal surgery: a prospective study. Acta Chir Scand 1990;156:167–69.

22. de la Hunt MN, Chan AYC, Karran SJ. Postoperative complications: how much do they cost? Ann R Coll Surg Engl 1986;68:199–202.

23. McCarthy E. Tracking the cost of health care: the bill came to $5339. Can Med Assoc J 1990;142:1271–73.

24. Tuck J, Walker A, Whynes DK, Pye G, Hardcastle JD, Chamberlain J. Screening and the costs of treating colo-rectal cancer: some preliminary results. Public Health 1989;103:413–19.

25. Müller JM, Tübergen D, Zieren U. Nachsorge beim kolo-rektalen Karzinom—Eine daten- und patientenorientierte Bewertung Zentralbl Chir 1994;119:65–74.

26. Norum J, Olsen JA. A cost-effectiveness approach to the Norwegian follow-up programme in colorectal cancer. Ann Oncol 1997;8:1081–87.

27. Board of Governors of the Federal Reserve System, Federal Reserve Bulletin, 1979, 1983, 1986–1989, 1991, 1996.

28. US Bureau of Labor Statistics. Consumer Price Index, detailed report, 1982–1997.

29. Hodgson TA, Meiners MR. Cost-of-illness methodology: a guide to current practices and procedures. Milbank Memorial Fund Q Health Soc 1982;60:429–62.

30. Mushinski M. Variation in in-hospital charges for colorectal cancer treatment. Cancer Manage 1998;3:28–34.

31. Peller CA, Froymovich O, Tartter PI. The true cost of pro-tective loop colostomy. Am J Gastroenterol 1989;84:1034–37.

32. Mellow MH. Endoscopic laser therapy as an alternative to palliative surgery for adenocarcinoma of the rectum – comparison of costs and complications. Gastrointest Endosc 1989;35:283–87.

33. Elixhauser A, Steiner CA, Whittington CA, McCarthy E. Clinical classifications for health policy research: hospital inpatient statistics 1995. Healthcare Cost and Utilization Project, HCUP-3 Research Note. (AHCPR publication no. 98-0049.) Rockville, MD: Agency for Health Care Policy and Research: 1998.

34. Virgo KS, Vernava AM, Longo WE, McKirgan LW, Johnson FE. Cost of patient follow-up after potentially curative colorectal cancer treatment. JAMA 1995;273:1837–41.

35. Audisio RA, Setti-Carraro P, Segala M, Capko D, Andreoni B, Tiberio G. Follow-up in colorectal cancer patients: a cost–benefit analysis. Ann Surg Oncol 1996;3:349–57.

36. Bruinvels DJ, Eijkemans MJC, Roberts MS, Kievit J, Habbema JDF, van de Velde CJH. First-order Monte Carlo simulation of a Markov decision model: follow-up of pa-tients with colorectal cancer. In: Bruinvels DJ. Follow-up of patients with colorectal cancer [dissertation]. Leiden: Rijksuniversiteit, 1995:73–89.

37. Rocklin MS, Slomski CA, Watne AL. Postoperative sur-veillance of patients with carcinoma of the colon and rectum. Am Surg 1990;56:22–27.

38. Virgo KS, Johnson FE. Costs of surveillance after potentially curative treatment for cancer. In: Johnson FE, Virgo KS, editors. Cancer patient follow-up. St Louis, MO: Mosby, 1997:23–47.

39. Spector WD, Mor V. Utilization and charges for terminal cancer patients in Rhode Island. Inquiry 1984;21:328–37.

40. Long SH, Gibbs JO, Crozier JP, et al. Medical expenditures of terminal cancer patients during the last year of life. Inquiry 1984;21:315–27.

41. Macintosh EL, Rodriguez-Bigas MA, Petrelli NJ. Colorectal carcinoma. In: Johnson FE, Virgo KS, editors. Cancer patient follow-up. St Louis, MO: Mosby, 1997:118–31.

42. Swallow CJ, Guillem JG. Counterpoint. In: Johnson FE, Virgo KS, editors. Cancer patient follow-up. St Louis, MO: Mosby, 1997:131–35.

43. Moriya Y. Counterpoint. In: Johnson FE, Virgo KS, editors. Cancer patient follow-up. St Louis, MO: Mosby, 1997:135–38.

44. Thomas MG, Hershman MJ. Counterpoint. In: Johnson FE, Virgo KS, editors. Cancer patient follow-up. St Louis, MO: Mosby, 1997:138–45.

45. Sinanan MN. Counterpoint. In: Johnson FE, Virgo KS, editors. Cancer patient follow-up. St Louis, MO: Mosby, 1997:145–47.

46. Cohen AM. Rectal cancer. In: Fischer DS, editor. Follow-up of cancer: a handbook for physicians. 4th ed. (Under the auspices of the Connecticut State Medical Society, Connecticut Division of the American Cancer Society, Connecticut State Department of Health Services, Yale Cancer Center.) Philadelphia, PA: Lippincott-Raven, 1996:52–53.

47. Engstrom PF, Benson AB, Cohen A, et al. NCCN colorectal cancer practice guidelines. Oncology 1996;10:140–75.

48. Venook A, Goodnight J, Kumar S, et al. Practice guidelines for colorectal cancer. Cancer J 1996;2 (Suppl):S23–S36.

49. Parikh SR, Attiyeh FF. Rationale for follow-up strategies. In: Cohen AM, Winawer SJ, Friedman MA, et al., editors. Cancer of the colon, rectum, and anus. New York: McGraw-Hill, 1995:713–24.

50. Averbach AM, Sugarbaker PH. Use of tumor markers and radiologic tests in follow-up. In: Cohen AM, Winawer SJ, Friedman MA, et al., editors. Cancer of the colon, rectum, and anus. New York: McGraw-Hill, 1995:725–51.

51. The Standards Task Force of the American Society of Colon and Rectal Surgeons. Practice parameters for the detection of colorectal neoplasms. Dis Colon Rectum 1992;35:389–94.

52. Sugarbaker PH, Gianola FJ, Dwyer A, Newman NR. A simplified plan for follow-up of patients with colon and rectal cancer supported by prospective studies of laboratory and radiologic test results. Surgery 1987;102:79–87.

53. Biggs CG, Ballantyne GH. Sensitivity versus cost effective-ness in postoperative follow-up for colorectal cancer. Curr Opin Gen Surg 1994;2:94–102.

54. Hurd T, Gutman H. Cancer of the colon, rectum, and anus. In: Berger DH, Feig BW, Fuhrman GM, editors. The MD Anderson surgical oncology handbook. Boston, MA: Little, Brown, 1995:160–93.

55. Buie WD, Rothenberger DA. Surveillance after curative resection of colorectal cancer. Gastrointest Endosc Clin North Am 1993;3:691–713.

56. Steele G. Colorectal cancer. In: Eiseman B, Robinson WA, Steele G Jr, editors. Follow-up of the cancer patient. New York: Thieme-Stratton, 1982:104–109.

57. Fleischer DE, Goldberg SB, Browning TH, et al. Detection and surveillance of colorectal cancer. JAMA 1989;261: 580–85.

58. Ovaska J, Jarvinen H, Kujari H, Perttila I, Mecklin JP. Follow-up of patients operated on for colorectal carcinoma. Am J Surg 1990;159:593–96.

59. Makela J, Laitinen S, Kairaluoma I. Early results of follow-up after radical resection for colorectal cancer: preliminary results of a prospective randomized trial. Surg Oncol 1992;1:157–61.

60. Virgo KS, Wade TP, Longo WE, et al. Surveillance after curative colon cancer resection: practice patterns of surgical subspecialists. Ann Surg Oncol 1995;2:472–82.

61. Ferrell BR, Griffith H. Cost issues related to pain management: report from the cancer pain panel of the Agency for Health Care Policy and Research. J Pain Symptom Manage 1994;9:221–34.

62. Swanson G, Smith J, Bulich R, et al. Patient-controlled analgesia for chronic cancer pain in the ambulatory setting: a report of 117 patients. J Clin Oncol 1989;7: 1903–908.

63. Ferrell B. Cost issues surrounding the treatment of cancer related pain. J Pharm Care Pain Symptom Control 1993;1:9–23.

64. Brooks CH, Smyth-Staruch K. Hospice home care cost savings to third-party insurers. Med Care 1984;22: 691–703.

65. Drummond MF, Richardson WS, O'Brien BJ, et al. Users' guides to the medical literature. XIII: How to use an article on economic analysis of clinical practice. A. Are the results of the study valid? JAMA 1997;277:1552–57.

66. O'Brien BJ, Heyland D, Richardson WS, et al. Users' guides to the medical literature. XIII: How to use an article on economic analysis of clinical practice. B. What are the results and will they help me in caring for my patients? JAMA 1997;277:1802–806.

67. Balas EA, Kretschmer RAC, Gnann W, et al. Interpreting cost analyses of clinical interventions. JAMA 1998;279:54–57.

Index